Disability and Society

Disability and Society

A Reader

Edited by

Renu Addlakha
Stuart Blume
Patrick Devlieger
Osamu Nagase
Myriam Winance

Orient BlackSwan

ORIENT BLACKSWAN PRIVATE LIMITED

Registered Office
3-6-752 Himayatnagar, Hyderabad 500 029 (A.P.), INDIA
e-mail: centraloffice@orientblackswan.com

Other Offices
Bangalore, Bhopal, Bhubaneshwar, Chennai, Ernakulam, Guwahati, Hyderabad, Jaipur, Kolkata, Lucknow, Mumbai, New Delhi, Patna

First published 2009
Reprinted 2009

ISBN: 978 81 250 3686 9

Typeset in Adobe Garamond 10.5/13 by
InoSoft Systems, Noida

Printed in India at
Glorious Printers
Delhi

Published by
Orient Blackswan Private Limited
1/24 Asaf Ali Road, New Delhi 110 002
e-mail: delhi@orientblackswan.com

Contents

Acknowledgements

J-F. Ravaud and H-J. Stiker. 'Inclusion/exclusion: An analysis of historical and cultural meanings', in G. Albrecht, K. Seelman and M. Bury (eds), *Handbook of Disability Studies.* London: Sage Publications Inc. (2001) pp. 490–512. © Sage Publications Inc. Reprinted by permission of Sage Publications Inc.

Patrick J. Devlieger. 'From handicap to disability: Language use and cultural meaning in the United States', *Disability and Rehabilitation* (1999) 21: 346–54. Reprinted by permission of Taylor & Francis (http://www.tandf.co.uk/journals).

M. Miles. 'Community, individual or information development? Dilemmas of concept and culture in South Asian disability planning', *Disability and Society* (1996) 11: 485–500. Reprinted by permission of Taylor & Francis.

M.H. Rioux. 'Disability: The place of judgement in a world of fact', *Journal of Intellectual Disability Research* (1997) 41 (2): 102–11. © Blackwell. Reprinted by permission of Wiley-Blackwell.

M. Bury 'Chronic illness as biographical disruption', *Sociology of Health and Illness* (1982) 4 (2): 167–82. © Blackwell Publishing. Reprinted by permission of Wiley-Blackwell.

R.F. Murphy. *The Body Silent.* New York: W.W. Norton, 1990 edition, pages 85–104. We have been unable to contact the copyright holders of this work, believed to be the estate of the late R.F. Murphy. Any correspondence in respect of the use of this work should be addressed to the volume editors.

G. Taleporos and M.T. McCabe. 'Body image and physical disability—personal perspectives', *Social Science and Medicine* (2002), 54, 971–80. Copyright 2002. Reprinted by permission by of Elsevier.

Ronald F. Barrett. 'Self mortification and the stigma of leprosy in Northern India', *Medical Anthropology Quarterly* (2005). Reprinted by permission of University of California Press.

Renu Addlakha. 'Living with chronic schitzophrenia: An ethnographic account of family burden and coping strategies', *Indian Journal of Psychiatry*, (1999) 41: 91–95. © Indian Psychiatric Society. Reprinted by permission from the Indian Psychiatric Society.

F. Davis. 'Deviance disavowal: The management of strained interaction by the visibly handicapped', *Social Problems* (1961) 9 (2): 120–32. Reprinted by permission of the University of California Press.

J.T. Hinnant. 'Adaptation to deafness in a Balinese community', in John T. Hinnant, I. Berlin and B. Keats (eds), *Genetics and Hearing Loss*, Delmar Learning, pp. 111–23. © 2000 Delmar Learning, a part of Cengage Learning Inc. Reproduced by permission of www.cengage.com/permissions.

Meenu Bhambani. 'Societal responses to women with disabilities in India', in Asha Hans and Annie Patri (eds), *Women, Disability and Identity*. New Delhi: Sage Publication. © Asha Hans and Annie Patri (2003). All rights reserved. Reproduced with the permission of the copyright holders and the publisher, Sage Publications India Pvt. Ltd., New Delhi, India.

C. Thomas. 'The baby and the bath water: Disabled women and motherhood in a social context', *Sociology of Health and Illness* (1997) 19 (3): 622–43. © Blackwell Publishing. Reprinted by permission of Wiley-Blackwell.

S. Kurzman. 'There's no language for this', in K. Ott, D. Serlin and S. Mihm (eds), *Artificial Parts, Practical Lives* (2002), pp. 227–48. Reprinted by permission of the author and of New York University Press.

M. Kohrman. 'Motorcycles for the disabled', *Culture Medicine and Psychiatry* (1999) 23: 133–55. Reprinted by permission of Springer Science and Business Media BV.

S. Miles. 'Engaging with the disability rights movement: The experience of community-based rehabilitation in Southern Africa', *Disability and Society* (1996) 11: 501–17. Reprinted by permission of Taylor & Francis.

R. Scotch. 'Disability as the basis for a social movement', *Journal of Social Issues* (1988) 44 (1): 159–72. © Blackwell Publishing. Reprinted by permission of Wiley-Blackwell.

T. Shakespeare. 'Disabled people's self organisation: A new social movement?', *Disability, Handicap and Society*, (1993) 8: 249–64. Reprinted by permission of Taylor & Francis.

R. Hyashi and M. Okuhira. 'The disability rights movement in Japan: Past, present and future', *Disability and Society* (2001) 9: 855–69. Reprinted by permission of Taylor & Francis.

A. Ghai. 'Disabled women: An excluded agenda of Indian feminism', *Hypatia* (2002) 17 (3): 49–66. © Anita Ghai. Reprinted by permission of the author and Indiana University Press.

Preface

Wachara Riewpaiboon and *Stuart Blume*

DISABILITY AND REHABILITATION IN EUROPE AND NORTH AMERICA

The origins of disability and rehabilitation programmes in the northern countries of Europe and in North America are deeply entwined with processes of industrialisation and with the emergence of welfare states and entitlements. In *The Disabled State*, Deborah Stone explains how the emergence of a category called 'disabled' was intimately connected with determining which people should be granted support and relief without having to work. She explains how medicine came to be accepted as providing scientific and objective ways of measuring physical or mental impairments, which were then used to assess the ability to work. Medicine would provide the concepts and instruments needed to administer new programmes of relief and support (Stone, 1984). Both the First World War (1914–18) and the Second World War (1939–45) led to huge increases in the numbers of impaired people. But soldiers, returning mutilated from combat, had a significance for disability and rehabilitation that went beyond sheer numbers. These were young men and women in the prime of their lives who had sacrificed a leg, an arm or more in the service of their country. They were mutilated and impaired—but they were also heroes. Their moral claim on society's best efforts was clear and widely accepted. Out of a collective commitment to try to compensate these wounded heroes, to enable them to resume some vestige of the life they might have had, emerged what we now call rehabilitation medicine (Gritzer and Arluke, 1985). This same commitment also led to new and innovative approaches to the making and fitting of artificial limbs (Guyatt, 2001).

The history of the terms and practices applied to people with disabilities is rooted in a constantly-shifting tension between commitment to equality (the equal rights of all citizens) on the one hand, and a sometimes uncomfortable awareness of difference on the other (Stiker, 1982).

> Euro-American assumptions about disability are not only based in a particular political philosophy, but are elaborated through a set of laws, administrative procedures, medical diagnoses, welfare institutions, professional specialisations and business interests. In Europe and North America, disability is a political privilege entitling one to financial support and a series of services. The state assigns to physicians the task of determining who is entitled to those rights. In this way, the political issue of redistribution, which involves separating the deserving from the undeserving, becomes a clinical problem. (Ingstad and Whyte, 1995)

Starting in the 1960s, changes in policy and professional practice aimed at moving disabled people from residential institutions into the community led to some rethinking. Vic Finkelstein has provided a fascinating account of the development of a new Open University course in Britain in the 1970s (Finkelstein, 1998). The initial aim of the course, he explains, was to help professionals improve their professional and social skills 'in order to assist handicapped people to achieve maximum autonomy.' A professional dealing with disabled people would be taught to 'examine [his or her] professional role and ideology.' The various course components that were being developed raised issues that were totally absent from the normal education of therapists and medical professionals. For the first time, disabled people were specifically recruited as colleagues when preparing educational materials at university level. (Vic Finkelstein himself, trained as a psychologist, was one.) The course was called 'The Handicapped Person in the Community'. Through the late 1970s and early 1980s, as disabled people and organisations acquired more influence, its focus changed. Increasingly, the emphasis came to be placed on the 'disabling barriers' that society placed in the way of people with impairments, and on how these could be overcome.

Gradually, a few disabled scholars, most of them in Britain and the United States, began to develop a more radical critique of the dominant conceptions of disability, in which medicine played a central role. For example, in 1990, Michael Oliver, a disabled British sociologist, published a book in which he analysed the ways in which disability was defined as a problem of the individual, subject to the authority of medicine (Oliver, 1990). At the same time, he questioned the failure of the social sciences—sociology and anthropology—to address critically what this medical understanding of disability meant, and what it excluded from consideration. Out of the research and writing of critical sociologists in Britain and in the U.S.A. (where Irving Zola was a key figure) emerged what is generally called the 'social model' of disability (see Part 1).

Over the past twenty years these perspectives have generated a substantial literature, much of it making use of the methods of qualitative social research. Narratives and life histories produced by disabled people themselves have a central place in this literature (see the Introduction to Part 2). A number of excellent introductions to what is today generally called Disability Studies have appeared, and the field has its own journals, professional societies, and university courses and departments (see, for example, www.disstudies.org, www.disabilitystudies.net and www.disabilityworld.org). This work has major implications for professionals in the rehabilitation field, for the social sciences, and—the ultimate goal—for the full integration of disabled people into society. However, almost all of it focuses on the traditions, practices and dilemmas of northern countries. There have been few attempts in southern countries to draw on this work, or to establish related traditions of emancipatory research.

DISABILITY AND REHABILITATION IN ASIA

The proportion of the population of Asian countries said to be in some way impaired or disabled has been estimated at anything between 1 per cent and 10 per cent. Many impairments are birth-related, either congenital or acquired in early childhood, or are caused by industrial and traffic accidents. There are major differences between countries. Fortunately, few countries share Cambodia's terrible legacy, with something like 40,000 people, mostly young, having lost a leg because of land mines. In Thailand, 1.8 per cent of the population is estimated to live with some kind of disability. This statistic comes from a national household interview survey which is conducted every five years. The reliability of the survey is now being questioned, since this figure has been stable for two decades, while many epidemiological studies have shown increasing prevalence of disabilities of all types. The disability definition and the survey method used may be key issues here. From 1986 to 2002, people with disabilities were noted in the surveys by their impairments, particularly visible ones, and the main focus was on access to basic welfare services. Only in the last survey, in 2002, were people asked about their capacity to perform the activities of daily life. The *International Classification of Functioning, Disability and Health* of the World Health Organisation, which is based on a socio-medical model of disability (see, for example, Bickenbach et al., 1999), may have played a role here.

In traditional Thai society, powerfully influenced by a Buddhist worldview, most people with disabilities are supported by their families and by a number of charitable organisations. But they have to live their lives quietly, with little social integration. Reflecting Buddhist belief in merit-making and the theory of karma, people with disabilities are turned into objects of charity rather than being permitted to make merit actively by themselves and so escape from their karma of being disabled. It is significant, and quite contradictory, that people with disabilities (particularly deaf and blind people) are not allowed to be ordained. They sometimes live their quiet lives in a temple, not as ordained monks but as objects of mercy. Similarly, there is no obligation to report the birth of a disabled child to the authorities. A family stricken by the birth of a disabled child does not want to face the shame of announcing this fact in public. But without an official certificate, people with disabilities are not full citizens and have no legitimate place in society.

This view of people with disabilities as pitiable, as objects of charity, as existing on the margins of society, is reinforced by their representation in Thai novels, television dramas and films. The stereotypical disabled person depicted there is usually crippled, and socially excluded or hidden in the limited space of a house. Such persons have to be good, polite and voiceless. They must demand nothing but pity, since they are repaying for their past karma. At the end of the story, they might escape from their karma by becoming normal or accepted by their loved ones. In popular Thai culture, disabled people are often used as moral indicators. Just as litmus paper can distinguish acid from alkali, so can disabled people show the difference between the good people who help them, and the wicked people who despise or mistreat them. All this has its roots in the karma theory within the patronage relationship characteristic of Thailand's collective society. However, in the last decade we see the beginnings of change. In some novels, people with disabilities are now represented differently. More novels use the real life-stories of people with disabilities as their main plot, pointing to their human dignity and physical potential. The equalisation of opportunities in society is becoming a focal issue.

Alongside the traditional Buddhist perspective, new scientific knowledge has also helped shape the lives of people with disabilities. Since the middle of the nineteenth century, Thailand has been engaged in a process of modernisation that has had major implications for the country's educational and medical systems. When the International Society for Rehabilitation of the Disabled (later Rehabilitation International) was established, Thailand joined as a member country in 1945. Yet the new understanding of disability, embodied in new practices and technologies, could not easily be integrated holistically into the everyday lives of disabled people, because local social and cultural contexts were ignored or considered irrelevant.

In the verbal-visual world of modernity, deaf and blind people were left far behind as human communication became more expressive and dialectical. Sign language for deaf people and Braille, a printing system for the blind, seem to be irrelevant for the rushed world of today. Parents who can hear still do not understand why their deaf children prefer to go out with deaf friends or hang around in some particular public places. As for the blind, little effort has been made to provide information in Braille. People who are deaf or blind have limited access to the knowledge needed to function in modern society, including knowledge of health risks and their prevention. They are at greater than average risk of succumbing to various health problems.

In Thailand, as in most of Asia, the field of disability continues to be dominated by the biomedical model. Thus, 'disability' was defined as an incurable chronic illness, and increasingly became an object for medical diagnosis and investigation. As disabilities were more and more medicalised, the role of being 'sick' was imposed on those with disabilities. They were exempted from regular duties, but at the same time their human rights were usually ignored. Although disabilities were perceived as diseases, the modern healthcare system provided little in the way of encouraging answers or choices for those with them.

As part of the flux of western knowledge, many modern assistive technologies have been introduced. Following western rehabilitation discourse, these technologies are claimed to improve the quality of life of disabled people. In making these claims, much is forgotten. Wheelchair technology has been imported for people with restricted mobility, but little thought has been given to environmental barriers to wheelchair use. The concept of universal design of the physical environment has not really been understood. Hearing and visual aids have been made available for people with reduced hearing or vision. But little thought has been given to how their use might affect the personal—including the social—lives of people with sensory disabilities. The need to evaluate or problematise these technology-driven rehabilitation programmes, the focus of much recent critique in the west, has not been appreciated in Thailand.

The United Nations Year of People with Disabilities (1981) was followed by the Decade of People with Disabilities (1981–91). Particularly during the Asia Pacific Decade of Disabled Persons (1993–2002), much changed in Thailand. We have already referred to changes in the social representations of disabled people in Thai novels and films. At the political level too, long discussions over the need for legislation guaranteeing rights to disabled people reached fruition in this period. 'Rehabilitation' gradually came to be viewed as a process of personal empowerment. The Rehabilitation Act of 1991 was a major social tool for gaining access to social services, which were regarded as basic human rights. Gradually, many disabled-people organisations (DPOs) have redefined their roles, and have joined hands to protect the rights of those with disabilities. These rights were universally defined in terms of access: to medical and educational rehabilitation services; to vocational rehabilitation training and job placement; to the physical environment; and to other forms of social support. Based on this 'rehabilitation-oriented' model, the former patronising and charitable approach of DPOs has gradually altered to that of promoting self-help or independent living.

Although these changes contribute greatly to the improvement of certain aspects of the lives of people with disabilities, it is doubtful whether such an approach can achieve much more than the improvement of physical functioning. Moreover, employing a universal single-operation model without taking into account local cultural contexts runs the risk of imposing upon the ways of life of those with some kinds of disability.

Thus, the disability-development programme in Thailand has continued to rely heavily on a quantitative approach and on biomedical concepts. Policy formulation and decision-making processes have been based on quantitative information gathered from the five-yearly national household surveys. As we pointed out above, the concept of 'disability' and of the 'need' employed in the survey were narrowly and medically defined.

Surveys showed that physical and mobility impairments constituted 47 per cent of the total, while hearing and seeing disabilities accounted for 22 and 11 per cent, respectively. Mental and learning disabilities shared about 27 per cent of the total. In the last twenty years, quantitative aspects of disabilities have been rather well studied, and the planning and evaluation of rehabilitation programmes have also depended largely on quantitative indicators. However, such measurements cannot adequately reflect the social and cultural dimensions of the everyday life of people with some kinds of disability. Most of the studies provide rather technical knowledge from which people with disabilities themselves can benefit only indirectly. No research criticises or problematises the concept of the quality of life of people with disabilities, or tries to take their point of view. There is little or no attempt to gather and synthesise the experiences and knowledge, that people with disabilities themselves can use, either individually or collectively.

In the Asian context, Thailand is not unique. Despite many positive developments, little convergence between disability politics and practice on the one hand, and sociology and anthropology on the other, seems to have occurred in any of the Asian countries (with the exception of Japan). Surveying the international literature on disability and rehabilitation, we find that many studies emerging from Asia are designed to measure the extent of (unmet) needs, or the impact of services or attitudes to disabled people. Few of the published studies make use of the innovative, usually qualitative, approaches developed in western countries over the past twenty years.

With this book we hope to introduce Asian readers to the recent disability literature of the west. We also hope to inspire new thinking among social scientists, rehabilitation professionals and organisations of disabled people themselves that could lead to a multi-disciplinary approach to Disability Studies. The book has been supported by the Thai Health Promotion of People with Disabilities Programme, which is an active participatory programme involving health and social professionals, people with disabilities, and some non-governmental organisations in Thailand. One of us (W.R.), who has a background in rehabilitation medicine, is the manager of this programme. The programme aims to change the societal attitude to the terms 'disability' and 'people with disability', and thereby bring about a social structure more supportive for people with disabilities. It makes use of a number of strategies, including research, knowledge management, social communication and stimulating the formation of social movements involving crucial change agents. This programme has been in operation since 2004 and is funded by the Thai Health Promotion Fund. The first (one-year) phase has ended and the programme has entered its second (three-year) phase (2005–8). The responsible agencies include the Sirindhorn National Medical Rehabilitation Center, the Research Institute on Society and Health, and the Health System Research Institute of the Ministry of Public Health, Thailand. Major partners are disabled-people organisations for five types of disability and some non-governmental organisations.

The Thai Health Promotion of People with Disabilities Programme contracted with the Innovia Foundation to produce this book. The latter is a virtual research institute, established in the Netherlands, whose objective is 'to facilitate a socially optimal development and deployment of new healthcare technology through multi-disciplinary studies and related activities which focus in particular on the individual and collective experiences, concerns and aspirations of end users' (www.innoviafoundation.org). On behalf of Innovia, one of us (S.B.) approached a number of scholars with research experience in disability-related issues to serve on an editorial board. All accepted. Without the enthusiastic commitment, knowledge and experience of Renu Addlakha (then with the MacArthur Foundation in India, now with the Centre for Women's

Development Studies, New Delhi), Patrick Devlieger (University of Leuven, Belgium), Osamu Nagase (Research Centre for Advanced Science and Technology, University of Tokyo, Japan), and Myriam Winance (Centre de Recherche sur Medicine, Santé et Société, Paris, France), this book could not have been produced.

We hope that this book will encourage and inspire disabled people and their organisations, service providers and researchers from many disciplines to work together. We hope that it will help build a bridge across which knowledge and power can flow. The ultimate objective is to strengthen and empower people with disabilities in all corners of the world, to liberate their potential and help others do the same.

References

Bickenbach et al. 1999. 'Models of disablement, universalism and the ICIDH', *Social Science and Medicine*, 48: 1173–87.

Finkelstein, V. 1998. 'Emancipating disability studies', in Tom Shakespeare (ed.), *The Disability Reader*. London and New York: Cassell.

Gritzer, G. and Arluke, A. 1985. *The Making of Rehabilitation: A Political Economy of Medical Specialisation, 1890–1980*. Berkeley, Los Angeles and London: University of California Press.

Guyatt, M. 2001. 'Better legs: Artificial legs for British veterans of the First World War', *Journal of Design History*, 14: 307–25.

Ingstad, B. and Whyte, S.R. 1995. *Disability and Culture*. Berkeley: University of California Press.

Oliver, M. 1990. *The Politics of Disablement*. London: Macmillan.

Stiker, H-J. 1982. *A History of Disability*. Ann Arbor: University of Michigan Press.

Stone, Deborah. 1984. *The Disabled State*. Philadelphia: Temple University Press.

PART 1

Disability in Medicine, Culture and Society

Introduction

Myriam Winance & Patrick Devlieger

'**D**isability', 'handicap' or, to start with, the more neutral term 'impairment', has always demanded a response from society. But the ways in which societies have reacted to impairment have differed over time and between one society and another. In any society, shared representations of the person and of the world influence the identification, definition and social responses to impairment. Impairment is both constant as well as culturally and socially shaped. This means that social and cultural dimensions shape how impairment is perceived and how it is responded to. They also influence what a person with an impairment can be or do in any particular society. Depending on those dimensions, impairment gives rise to 'abnormality', 'disability' or 'handicap'. In the same way, a 'person with an impairment' was once viewed as a freak or monster (in old Greek society), or as 'crippled' or 'infirm' (in old western society). Today he or she is perceived as and considered 'a disabled person' or 'a person with a disability' (in contemporary Anglo-Saxon usage), or 'a handicapped person' (in contemporary French usage). The treatment of impairment varies accordingly: it can be social, political, medical, religious, ethical, or something else.

The first part of this Reader will introduce some of the social and cultural dimensions that shape impairment, and will provide resources with which to analyse those dimensions. The chapters in Part 1 will make clear that impairment cannot be reduced to a biological reality, that it is also a social and cultural reality. In other words, they will show that impairment gives rise to different realities depending on the historical and geographical contexts in which it appears. It is important to keep in mind that disability is shaped by culture and society (of which therapy and rehabilitation are also part) while studying disability or working with disabled people.

A second aim of Part 1 is to present different ways of conceptualising disability. During the last thirty years, two models of understanding disability have been hotly debated in the west. The debate, and the fact that it has emerged, is itself a cultural characteristic of rapidly changing societies. The first model, which dates back to Enlightenment ideals, is usually called the 'medical' or 'individual' model. It explains disability as caused by a disease or a bodily disorder. A person is disabled because he or she is or has been ill, or because he or she has suffered a trauma. This model was embodied in the classification of impairments, disabilities and handicaps developed by the World Health Organisation (WHO) in 1980. It has been criticised for reducing disability to a particular individual's problem, and as leading only to medical action (treatment and rehabilitation). Against this model, some activists have developed what is called the 'social' model. According to this, disability is created by the social, cultural, architectural and economic barriers set up by a society designed for non-disabled people that forgets people with impairments. The social model defines disability as exclusively a political and social problem, to be analysed as the result of oppressive relationships. It is not medicine that is needed but the transformation of society. Between these two opposed models, intermediary models have been developed. One of these, the Quebec approach, defines disability as produced by an interaction between individual factors and environmental factors that lead to restrictions on daily routine and behaviour.

Much of the debate regarding these models took place in the 1980s and 1990s, and was particularly centred on the process of revision of the WHO classification. The resulting new classification (the International Classification of Functioning, Disability and Health), produced by the WHO in 2001, is no longer about the consequences of disease, but about health, functioning and disability. This is a major change. Functioning and disability are considered and analysed as the two sides (positive and negative) of health. They are defined as an interaction between a health condition and contextual factors. This model is presented as integrating the medical model and the social model into what is called a bio-psychosocial model. It is supposed to offer a synthesis of the different dimensions of health: biological, individual and social. It not only describes deficiencies, but also aims at being a universal description of human functioning and participation. In other words, it claims to provide a universal and transcultural model and language that go beyond cultural and social specificities and can be applied in any country. But this claim has been criticised, and the new classification is also considered as reflecting western representations of disability. Though these criticisms, and some others, are justified, the new classification and the debates it has raised show that much progress has taken place. They bear witness to: the growing involvement of organisations of disabled people in debates concerning them and in disability policy (see Part 5 of this Reader); the transformation of the definitions of health and disability; and the acknowledgement of the role of social, cultural and physical environments.

These developments have given rise, in particular, to studies of the historical developments and situational contexts of disability, and have required multiple methods of research. Histories and ethnographies of disability are especially valuable in clarifying the very different relationships that societies and cultures have developed with people with disabilities. They can provide answers to questions about the status and daily lives of disabled people, and about the rituals and representations that regulate this status. They enable us to see to what extent they are excluded or included, and what sense they have of a unique identity and culture. Histories and ethnographies of disability cannot avoid critical reflection on societies and cultures. It can therefore be said that disability also provides a lens on society and culture.

The papers selected for this first part of the Reader clarify what we mean by the social and cultural dimensions of disability. They also introduce the different ways in which disability can be conceptualised and researched. The paper by Ravaud and Stiker shows the need to put current debates on disability into historical context. Doing this helps us see that societies throughout history have been challenged to formulate ethical responses to the tension created by the choice between exclusion and inclusion of persons with disabilities. An understanding of the social and political processes through which this tension is temporarily resolved is important for researchers and policy-makers alike. The article by Patrick Devlieger emphasises the importance of language. It analyses the shift from the word 'handicap' to the word 'disability' that occurred in the U.S. during the 1980s. This shift had important consequences for both individual experience and for collective action. The paper by Miles deals with the transplantation of western concepts and practices of disability into Asian contexts. This transplantation has often failed to take specific Asian contexts into account, with unfortunate consequences. The author highlights the specificities of disability issues in Asia and the unbalanced relation with western countries. Miles stresses the need to develop disability services based on Asian disability histories and representations. The last paper of Part 1, by Rioux, makes explicit the idea that there is a link between conceptual approaches to disability and practical and political consequences. Her paper does not only discuss theoretical issues, it also has important things to say about doing research on disability. Rioux argues that research on disability is never simply a matter of turning up the facts; that it always embodies unconscious or buried judgements about the causes and meaning of disability; and that these judgements have practical and political consequences. Acknowledging that these judgements are present and important will help to conduct research that avoids reducing the disability question and experience. Sensitive research of this kind will also help transform the situation of disabled persons.

1

Inclusion/Exclusion: An Analysis of Historical and Cultural Meanings

Jean-François Ravaud & Henri-Jacques Stiker

Questions regarding the inclusion or exclusion of disabled persons cannot be separated from questions related to the global processes of social cohesion or social dissociation. The way in which a society situates and treats its disabled is not independent of the way in which it constructs social bonds or dissolves them. However, each society (and, in a broader sense, each culture) has its own fashion of integrating or excluding certain categories or certain subjects, that is, of creating social links or denying them. We must thus expect the meanings of words and practices not to remain the same over time (in the history of societies) or across space (the synchronic diversity of cultural eras). There are numerous ways of posing and answering the question of social bonds, and thus of addressing inclusion and exclusion. There is not just a single set of problems concerning the inclusion and exclusion of disabled persons.

Consequently, our objective in this chapter is to avoid being restricted to a single, reductive vision of the problem, whether this perspective is

---

Ravaud, J-F. and Stiker, H-J. 2001. 'Inclusion/exclusion: An analysis of historical and cultural meanings', in Gary Albrecht, K. Seelman and M. Bury (eds), *Handbook of Disability Studies*. London: Sage Publications, pp. 490–512.

French, British or North American. We shall strive to reveal the different historical and cultural facets of inclusion and exclusion and show their origins and effects, which are both diverse and, most often, ambivalent. This sociological and historical observation raises a conceptual problem. The terms 'inclusion' and 'exclusion' operate in tandem, and can be understood only in relation to one another. For any definition of inclusion, there is a corresponding definition of exclusion. This means that it is necessary to determine who are affected by exclusion and inclusion; what aspect disabled persons are excluded from or what they are included in; and how and to what degree they are in or out at different times and in different social groupings.

Now that the general framework of our approach is set out, we shall proceed as follows. Starting from some major theories of the social bond, we will show the difference between societies that could be called pre-modern and those we recognise as modern. The aim of this distinction is to reveal that our present societies are continuously in search of processes and procedures; that is, they are unable to maintain a stable state inherited from tradition, but swing ceaselessly between different models. We will lay out the structure of these models and the mechanics of these global processes using a sociological inquiry.

From the perspective of the consequences of this state of affairs in our societies, we will illustrate current forms of exclusion and inclusion and establish a typology of praxis. This typology will, in turn, illuminate our premise that the modalities of inclusion and exclusion are variable, ambivalent, and often connected, in that some of the modalities of pre-modern societies still crop up in modern societies.

Returning to the way in which the question of inclusion or exclusion is generally posed today, we will show the relevance and value of this historical and sociological distancing for the future of advocacy and action in the sphere of persons with disabilities. Today's problems can be profitably illuminated by a consideration of the problems of every society, even though the contemporary situation is a specific one, and history does not offer lessons.

THE FUNDAMENTAL SOCIAL PROCESSES OF EXCLUSION AND INCLUSION

Mechanical Inclusion and Organic Inclusion

These terms are derived from Durkheim. This French thinker, one of the fathers of sociology, saw clearly that in modern societies of increasing complexity, one of the central phenomena is the division of labour or, in a broader sense, social division (Durkheim, 1930). Unlike Spencer, who analysed this fact from the perspective of the utility that could be gained thereby, Durkheim called attention to the increase in 'the social and moral density of societies', in other words, 'the number of persons who are in effective relations with each other, with the same population volume' (Durkheim, 1930, p. 214). With such an augmentation, the system of social roles becomes increasingly differentiated, and entails constant shifts in the system of norms and values. An evolutionary process is thereby initiated, in the sense that the fundamental forms of 'mechanical' or 'mimetic' solidarity, which were those of traditional societies, give way more and more to forms of solidarity that are 'organic' or 'complementary'. But the latter entail increasing individualism, which conflicts with the priority that had traditionally been given to the social whole.

Durkheim's distinction is pertinent on several counts. It permits us to emphasise the dynamic character of contemporary societies as well as the permanent challenge that confronts them. On the one hand, we can stress the risks of social dissociation, which are greater than in traditional societies; on the other hand, we note the possibilities societies have, by virtue of their organic nature, of increased integration of the new and the alien.

A second reason to cite Durkheim is to alert us to the fact that, in the present global space, social groups may still proceed from a mechanical form of solidarity, or at least be caught between a modern dynamic and powerful tradition. This is not to say that all trace of the 'mechanical' is absent today, even at the very heart of our globalised western world, where exchange is continuous and rapid and technology is dominant. We will do well to recall that these are processes. To the extent that the ruptures are not absolute, we could interrogate African and Asian societies. We are not sufficiently competent in these matters, but there are enough indications that in the above examples the pre-modern and the modern are interdependent and connected.

A third point of interest in Durkheim's distinction is that it assists us in seeing the difference between exclusion *from* a society and possible exclusion *within* society. Societies founded on mechanical solidarity are indeed strongly integrated, but they are not able to admit 'foreign bodies'. When they exclude, they do so in radical fashion, and are often incapable of assimilating the new. Modern societies have a very great capacity for inclusion but, on the other hand, are in danger of getting pulled apart by the creation of enclaves within themselves.

Before turning our focus fully to contemporary societies, we will briefly describe those societies that proceed from mechanical solidarity.

Early Societies

In societies characterised by mechanical solidarity, which can be compared to the holistic societies of Louis Dumont (1966), or what Tönnies (1979) called the *Gemeinschaft*, the individual is a constituent of an irreducible whole. The individual has his or her fixed place, determined at birth, and in this sense is completely integrated. The individual is a cog in a set of gears. There is no question of changing one's place; it would jeopardise the global mechanism, leading to severe sanctions against the cog that no longer performs its function. In such societies, persons with infirmity may be integrated and may have a definitive and entirely predetermined place, but without having any claim to free participation in society. This was the case of crippled buffoons at princely courts: the role that was devolved onto them also enclosed them. Take the example of the dwarf Joseph Boruwlaski (1788). At the height of the eighteenth century (the threshold of the modern era), he illustrates the kind of inclusion of which we are speaking. In the society of the *ancien régime*, he had his place as a Polish princess's Joujou, her pet and entertainer. He was integrated—on the condition of not trying to leave his situation, which was fixed once and for all. The day he laid claim to love, marriage and an independent life, he was rejected and condemned to wander through Europe. Nothing had been foreseen in social terms that could assist his emancipation. Today, persons of short stature are still subject to deprecatory representations, but the right to live and work among others is no longer denied them. On the other hand, if they want a place, they have to struggle for it, for although society is legally 'open', all of its spaces are conceived on a scale dictated by the average stature of its citizenry as a statistical norm:

transportation, public counters, equipment, and the layout of controls. It is here that the issue of accommodation arises. The gap between the dwarf Joujou and persons of short stature today is great because we have passed from a society with mechanical solidarity, which assigned an invariable place to its members and thus included them in a certain fashion, to a society that *works* for their integration but scarcely succeeds, because it has surrendered its social mechanics in favour of organicity.

Thus, we can establish a first meaning for the concept of integration in the following terms: a place, a single and fixed place in a whole that has no intention of modifying itself. A person who does not have a place of this kind is literally not part of society. He or she may be a stranger whose assimilation is problematic and presupposes, when it possibly occurs, recognition of similarity and partial integration by means of a subgroup (Simmel, 1908). Most often, however, one cannot say whether the individual is excluded or included, because he or she cannot enter into the society, being so completely 'other'. This person is excluded through negative rather than positive action. Barbarians could not become Romans, foreigners could not become citizens of Athens (except through a very special procedure), and so on.

A positive act of exclusion, on the other hand, can occur when an individual raises the issue of his or her 'integration'. In some cases we could use the term 'disintegration', in the sense that the disruptive element will be destroyed. (The death penalty imposed in some societies for certain kinds of behaviour can be explained in this way.) The typical example is antiquity's treatment of infants born deformed. Their strangeness, referencing a divine warning, and a fear of deviance within the species and of more or less imminent misfortune, led to the well-known 'exposure' beyond the social space. We are dealing with a society, however capable it was of strongly integrating its citizens, which could not tolerate the 'stranger', who is then excluded from society. In this kind of mechanical solidarity, a term such as *inclusion* is inadequate or, at a minimum, too weak. One has one's place or one does not, but there is no real process of 'being included'. When solidarity is of the mechanical kind, belonging is a factor of the idea of community. One must be similar, a relative or a neighbour. Nor can we speak of exclusion within society, for these societies, however hierarchical they may be (and thus encompass the status of the privileged as well as the status of the pariah), assign each group and each individual a place. Even if the superior 'castes' are not mixed with the inferior, all social strata are integrated into the whole.

Today, there remain only a few societies that exhibit pure mechanical solidarity. Colonisation, economic development, the international doctrine of human rights, and democratic trends have all combined to produce many mixed-culture environments, positioned between centuries-old tradition and modernisation at work. The inclusion that we have called mechanical is now, in global terms, behind us. However, we would do well to bear it in mind, for societies cannot be voided of their holistic character; they are always something more structured than a myriad individuals or even a sum of individuals. Even when the whole no longer exclusively directs the collective arrangements of a society, there still exists an imperative for cohesion and minimal conformity.

Modern Societies

In societies characterised by organic solidarity, which may be compared to the individualistic societies of Louis Dumont or the *Gesellschaft* of Tönnies, there is a tendency for the individual to be isolated. What must be emphasised here is that these societies have to construct their solidarity and their modes of integration. They cannot fall back on the idea of a place for each determined by tradition and culture. They are under pressure to offer each individual a place that allows evolution. Integration is a long road, and there is a reiterated obligation to make new advances, because the division of labour and social division entail the constant introduction of new procedures (legislative, institutional, financial), so that individuals are not left to the rigours of competition and isolation. In other words, in modern western societies, we are moving toward the idea of a *process of integration*, and are no longer focused on places and statuses that are determined once and for all. When these processes loosen, individuals are at risk of being left adrift, subject to what Durkheim (1930) called *anomie*. There are no longer sufficient common arrangements to sustain the social bond. Moreover, on the global level, there must be sufficient commonly shared mental representations that these processes can be maintained. This is what Durkheim called the collective consciousness. This notion is one of Durkheim's most contested ideas, but it indicates that societies are made up of representations as much as concrete practices. Sociology has developed these ideas at considerable length, as has the

Chicago school with Goffman (1963) and Becker (1963), particularly with reference to persons with disabilities.

It is useful to ask why modern societies are thus simultaneously engaged in the task of inclusion and at risk of disaggregation. Societies displaying mechanical solidarity, almost completely holistic, are also societies that may be qualified as religious, in the sense that they conceive of themselves in relation to an exteriority or believe that their foundation and fundamental rules are derived from elsewhere, in the divine. These are heteronomous societies (from *heteros* = other, and *nomos* = law), in the sense that laws are based on a radical alterity. In all traditional societies, the way to address the question of disability is to maintain a connection with the transcendental, with the beyond, and with the gods or the dead (Stiker, 1982, 1999). Western societies, on the other hand, are characterised by having broken with the notion of heteronomy. They base themselves on their own immanence. They have become autonomous. Theories of the social contract, whatever the manner of conceiving this contract, are theories of society's autonomy. This is because the origin of civil society, in contrast to the state of nature, derives from a 'contract' on which humans have agreed in order to secure their existence and raise the possibility of living together. Admittedly, not all theories of the social contract lead to the establishment of democracy. There is a huge gulf between Hobbes and Spinoza. Yet all of them institute society on an immanent foundation. Even the absolute monarchies of seventeenth-century Europe, although they were regimes more onerous in terms of subjection than many others, inaugurated this new way of conceiving society (Gauchet, 1985). This passage from heteronomy to autonomy is not the only product of the new political thought first evidenced in the early seventeenth century. It is also referred to as the birth of scientific thought, in which people could think and know the world by its own means, without recourse to revelation. Galileo's famous 'But it does move,' when he compared his discovery to dominant theological discourse, is significative of emancipation from collective reference to an exteriority. To this must also be added the individual's conquest of autonomy, not only that of society. This affirmation and claim had their specific origin in the Reformation, which permitted each individual conscience to interpret scripture independently of established religious authority and dogmatic definition. The autonomy of the individual also includes the capacity to be an economic agent and to create one's own place and role, as Max Weber (1920) has emphasised.

All these factors then contributed to the emergence of societies that, relying only on themselves and on the strength of constituent individuals, are entirely responsible and accountable for people living together. This equally explains why they are vulnerable, and why the risk of marginalisation, even social abandonment or exclusion, is so great. This is the greatness and weakness of democracies that are all continuously working at the process of integration. Here we distance ourselves from the thesis that emerges from a reading of Michel Foucault (1961, 1975). He describes exclusionary measures that take the form of confining the insane or incarcerating the criminal. In so doing, he gives the impression that, ever since the seventeenth century, western societies should be characterised only by exclusion. This fails to take into account the very powerful revolutionary movement toward political equality. This is not the place for the full discussion of Foucault's thought that would be needed to explore all its contrasted aspects. What is certain, however, is that since the end of the eighteenth century, western societies have experienced a thrust toward inclusion because they were obliged to do so by virtue of their very founding principles (Gauchet, 1995). Let us explore in greater detail this idea of society as a 'construction site for democracy', illuminating clearly the nature and degree of the inclusion or exclusion of persons with disabilities in our contemporary societies.

Constructing Inclusion in Modern Societies and its Contradiction

The Normalisation Process

One of the major procedures in the attempt to integrate is normalisation. Let us be sure we have an exact sense of this concept. It is not a question of leading all members of a society to an ideal model of humanity, as was the case in certain earlier philosophies or religions. Stoicism and the imitation of Christ may serve as examples. It is a question of defining the mean, comparing deviations from this mean, and trying to diminish such deviations to bring individuals closer to the mean.

Our societies no longer have a single ideal for a human being or a citizen, any more than they have one conception of a fixed and definitive form for the social order. As a consequence, a system of reference that permits minimal conformity and basic social cohesion becomes the effective mean in practical terms. Society's approach is based in statistics and probability theory.

This manner of inclusion is clearly illustrated in the case of persons with disabilities. For children with mental retardation to be admitted to school, they need to be able to follow lessons and thus reach the required level of competence. If they fail to reach this level, they are placed in separate institutions, which are supposed to bring them (back) to the norm. In the event of impossibility, they risk being segregated for almost their entire lives. For disabled adults to have access to employment in a business environment, they must acquire the equivalent autonomy and vocational competence, and these too must match the mean. These unquestionably beneficial efforts to re-educate the body and mind are also aimed at reducing the gap between disabled and able-bodied individuals. To be, to do 'like others', is the objective of such rehabilitation. In addition, it is on this idea of deviation from the norm that the notions of the notorious *International Classification of Impairment, Disability and Handicap*, proposed by the World Health Organisation (WHO) in 1980, are founded. Disability is equated to any restriction on or lack of ability to perform an activity in the manner, or within the range considered normal, for a human being. (Which human being is meant, if not the one taken as the reference?) A handicap is in turn defined as a disadvantage that limits or prevents the fulfilment of a role that is normal (depending on age, sex, and social and cultural factors) for a given individual. The normalisation imperative could not be more evident. We would do well to recall Goffman (1963). In humorously describing the average American by showing that anyone found at odds with one of his or her characteristics was considered deficient and more or less to blame, Goffman analysed the power of the statistical norm with acuity. He wrote:

> For example, in an important sense there is only one complete unblushing male in America: a young, married, white, urban, northern, heterosexual, Protestant father of college education, fully employed, of good complexion, weight and height, and a decent record in sports. Every American male tends to look out on the world from this perspective, thus constituting one sense in which one can speak of a common value system in America. Any male

> who fails to qualify in any of these ways is likely to view himself—during moments at least—as unworthy, incomplete and inferior; at times he is likely to pass, and at times he is likely to find himself being apologetic or aggressive concerning aspects of himself he knows are probably seen as undesirable. The general identity values of a society may be fully entrenched nowhere, and yet they can cast some kind of shadow on the encounters encountered everywhere in daily living. (Goffman, 1963, pp. 128–29)

Similarly, Norbert Elias (1965) shows that between the *established* and the *outsiders* the distinction is based less on problems of characteristic features than on the disparity in credo, values and established *habitus*. It is racism without race. If there is still a problem of identity, there is first and foremost the difference with respect to accepted norms.

The will toward normalisation must be referred to another force that permeates our contemporary societies: the appeal of the universal. Modern western societies, driven by the necessity of establishing the conditions of inclusion on their own to further cohesion and reduce inequalities, think their forms of sociability are the most advanced. In this they pursue, perhaps without being too aware of it, the Christian universalism that formerly justified the conversion of nations and the wholesale imposition of Christian civilisation. However, this is clearly not our present problem. What is certain is that democratic principles (the celebrated notions of liberty, equality and fraternity) seem destined to rule the world, just like our production modes, with free trade, salaried employment, and all the other components of industrial society. Topping it all, the individualism of success, performance and pursuit of well-being also seems universal. The assimilation model is suited to summarising a powerful thrust in our societies, and is a model that plays a determining role in the social treatment of disabled people.

The Assimilation Model

The point of departure is the undeniable universality of humanity. The human species is a unity. The other can only be another 'I'. In principle, there are no limits to the rights of human beings as such. This is the great triumph of the democratic revolutions, both French and American. Yet we move very quickly from recognition of equality to a desire for sameness. The other is destined to become like me, for I represent the universal human. In concrete terms, this slippage from the universal to pseudo-universalism is frequent, whereas the universal ought to remain only a regulating idea. This was the temptation of many an empire: one way of life or one ideology is raised to the status of universal, seeking to impose itself against an insurmountable diversity. The former Soviet Union is an obvious example. The Stalinist mould sought to impose uniformity, and after its failure, nationalities and nationalism were instantly reborn. The temptation is a constant one; it is seen in the pretension of western nations to be the guardians of an order that is above all their own, and also in that of certain Middle Eastern countries to impose their own politico-theological conceptions.

In more empirical fashion, the assimilation model generates more or less this discourse: there are common values, common objectives, canons of conduct, and a mean that we must strive to approach. The task consists of doing everything to rejoin this consensual and homogenising communality. There is a kind of French-style republicanism here. The republic defines its points of reference and its criteria, often enviable or even grandiose: secularism, social rights, an educational system, public morality, and equality of rights. In turn, one must agree to live according to these norms, and this kind of republican environment then becomes 'blind to differences'.

In such a model, we are on our way toward forceful integration. Each element must conform enough to assume its place in the good order of the whole. In return, the powerful denial of anything 'other' keeps us in check. The other can be annulled. In its fullest expression, this model leads to the rule of 'in-difference'. Concerning persons with disabilities, this model seems to account for such an orientation as positive discrimination. This statement may appear paradoxical, because such a measure isolates and stigmatises. One has to be labelled 'handicapped' to benefit from the special measures reserved for this population. A legislator has foreseen a series of aid measures (financial) and special means of training or work (sheltered institutions of all kinds) in consideration of the fact that people in difficulty due to an impairment constitute a vulnerable population for which special dispositions are required so that it can 'catch up with the rest' and not be left adrift. We can clearly see how this perspective leads social environments to become disinterested, and view themselves free from the day-to-day integration of disabled persons.

Compensating for disability sometimes entails social isolation, rehabilitation, training and work, all of them under the rubric of *adaptation*. However, what must be emphasised is that this segregating effect is first and foremost the consequence of a will toward assimilation. This discrimination, which we will metaphorically and euphemistically call a *detour*, has as its objective a return to ordinary life or, if this is really not possible, at least a behaviour and mode of life close to the average citizen's. If it were not for the attraction of these norms and common *habitus*, many of these efforts would not be sustained.

Let there be no misunderstanding about our analysis. Our purpose is not to discredit this pull toward conformity or the assimilation of disabled persons into the mainstream. The assimilation model is a powerful stimulant toward equality and integration. We seek only to point out that it is one of the points of reference that has a pronounced effect on attitudes toward persons with disabilities. The critical point is the following. If we go too far in the direction of assimilation and thus fall into what could be called 'assimilationism', we will end up rejecting the other in his or her irreducible difference, in the right to be as he or she is. We will end up rejecting the richness of the multiple ways of being human. We will end up being drawn into what psychoanalysis knows so well—denial. Denial is always dangerous, for what is denied surges up again, and can at times advance its claims with violence. An example is the former proscription of deaf sign language. It has returned in full force, but not before the deaf community had to 'bang on the table'.

Contradictions

The will to assimilate, which finds its major process in normalisation, entails a series of contradictions, and runs up against phenomena that are moving societies in a quite different direction. The normalisation process collides with the increasing complexity of our societies. Regarding disabled persons, we may have succeeded in eradicating certain impairments or diseases such as poliomyelitis (at least in the west), but we have seen quadriplegia increase, brain injury become a major cause of disability, and are now confronted with instances of multiple disability. These examples permit us to pinpoint two facts. Society, by its very development, multiplies risk, and medical technology saves and prolongs 'cases' that otherwise would have disappeared. Moreover, the risks are due as much to evolution in behaviour (e.g. sexual risk) as to technological evolution (traffic accidents, among others).

We must also point to the innumerable consequences of lengthened life. Here, too, we confront problems in the sphere of disability that were unknown a few decades ago. We have won many additional years of life for those with Down's syndrome or muscular dystrophy, but we must now face the problems that accompany their reaching adulthood, such as their employment and, later, the complex problems of adequate services in their old age.

In short, present-day society can no longer lay claim, as it did more easily in the case of victims of accidents at work or wounded veterans, to an inclusion or even an erasure of the consequences of these deficiencies. However, this is not the essential point. We must analyse the new processes of social exclusion in wealthy societies and the rising tide of claims to identity.

When the Social Bond is Broken

From a functionalist perspective, exclusion results in dysfunctionalities in a society whose norms bar the way to integration for populations that do not correspond to the norm or do not do so sufficiently. The new phenomenon is that, for the last twenty years or so, western societies have found themselves in the paradoxical situation of continuing to produce great wealth but no longer having the means to ensure sufficient employment. The production of wealth (material goods, services, financial products) occurs more and more without labour resources. Unemployment has become endemic, as if it were one of the preconditions for society's functioning. In addition, habits and customs have changed (divorce, single-parent families, substantial vocational mobility), and a considerable number of people no longer find a sufficient foundation in human relationships. Economic instability and the fragility of relationships rise in tandem (Castel, 1995). Clearly, the loss of revenue, to the point of having no revenue at all, and the degeneration of relationships, to the point of complete isolation, are processes; as a consequence, they can come to a halt and even recede. This is why public policy, thanks to more or less shifting measures, occasionally succeeds in maintaining these populations in social inclusiveness. Yet, at other times, and quite frequently, there is precariousness, a kind of social sub-status. The affected populations are continuously in the process of losing and regaining income or relationships. Unemployment, like employment, is intermittent. If this prevents people from falling into absolute, permanent poverty, it does not permit true integration, in the sense of lasting participation in the enjoyment of material and cultural goods. When the two processes—unemployment and loss of relationships—come to a head, then the fundamental social bond is breached, even lost. Then one receives little or nothing from society, while no longer contributing to its wealth and social development. One is finally supernumerary and superfluous. In historical terms, it is not carved in stone that such a situation cannot change or be reversed. The exclusion of today, as it is historically situated, is not a fixed destiny. The problem of exclusion today is much more a problem of the social bond than a problem of poverty. Substantial populations are at constant risk of finding themselves removed from what constitutes the very basis of social belonging, that is, exchange. Exchange is what Marcel Mauss (1923) analysed so well in the category of gifts. The degradation of the social bond, for a considerable percentage of the population in the so-called advanced societies, foils the work of inclusion, which is nonetheless inscribed in the ongoing democratisation that characterises them.

Are disabled persons affected by these processes of social dissociation, which the French sociologist Robert Castel (1995) calls 'disaffiliation'?

When there are no specific measures (special programmes such as affirmative action), there is a great risk of seeing those struck by illness or accident being drawn into the vortex of exclusion, in the sense in which it has been analysed above. This is less true when public authorities direct specific attention to them, in the form of allowances, institutions, and human and technical assistance. Yet no one is free from being swept away by the processes we have described. When this happens to disabled persons, the situation is aggravated by the usual barriers that block their route and by their lack of access (physical, psychological, cultural) to social spaces. We should stress the difference between exclusion in the socio-historical sense described above, in which the future may well change even if the end is not presently in sight, and exclusion from certain goods, places or services. This non-accessibility has a dimension that is more constant, but it is also more commonplace, because it is the lot of a great number of citizens—in fact, of everyone at one time or another. The social barriers are certainly more numerous and more insurmountable in the case of deficiencies, but they are determined to a greater extent by the political will for accommodation, which can be achieved successfully if we persevere and bring appropriate technologies into play. In any event, this type of exclusion is not dependent on the central mechanisms that are part of the world economy and established customs, as is the type we have called disaffiliation. We prefer to call it segregation, because it entails moving people to the side, and is also an obstacle to the full participation of citizens.

Identity Traps

We called attention to another factor—that of claims to identity. Our perspective will be from those with profound deafness. Let us summarise the argument of the deaf community. First, we are speakers like other speakers, and we have a language. Admittedly, it is a language of gestures and signs, not of sounds and words, but it is a whole and distinct language. We also have, through this medium, a way of thinking, of situating ourselves, of being in the world. In short, we have a culture. Our 'inferiority' is nothing other than oppression, and can be compared to that of minority cultural communities, either in the simple numerical sense or because they are too alien to the dominant and dominating culture. From this position, we easily see how the notions of disability and impairment begin to withdraw, become a secondary feature, or are completely dropped.

Second, the deaf are in fact deaf, just as some people are black, white, male or female. To wish to transform this condition is as absurd as wanting to make a white person black or a woman a man. One part of the eugenics movement, fearing the evolution of a 'deaf race', proposed forbidding marriage between deaf people, and called for sterilisation (Bell, 1883). The condition of deafness entails a mode of communication and signifying of its own, namely sign language, and also a specific and original culture. Withdrawing a deaf child from his or her natural community is an inadmissible violation. In *Mask of Benevolence*, Harlan Lane writes:

> Even if we could take the children destined to be members of the African-American, or Hispanic-American, or Native American, or Deaf American communities and convert them with bio-power into white, Caucasian, hearing males—even if we could, we should not. (Lane, 1992, p. 237)

The possible is not the desirable. The ethical debate over cochlear implants proves the topicality of the question. Nor should we ask a deaf person to express himself or herself in oral speech like hearing people. Deafness is not a limitation; it is a biological characteristic that has given rise to a specific culture (Lane, 1984). This position reflects a vision of identity that can be translated into the notion of minority. The sociological concept of minority, in fact, stresses the ethnic and cultural aspects of difference well beyond the question of number. Minorities are composed of individuals who have a common history and culture (and often a common national origin), who transmit their membership along lineage lines, who are in a position to demand signs of loyalty from some of the members, and who are in a relatively disadvantaged position in society. (Goffman, 1963, p. 145)

From this background, we can understand why deaf people and other kinds of disabled people have formulated slogans such as 'deaf pride' and 'disability pride'. It is a matter of pride to belong to a cultural minority, to a group that not only has nothing to be ashamed of but can also make valid claims for its own characteristics. The characteristics of the deaf community lend themselves well to the American 'culturalist' interpretation of the situation of blacks, women and Hispanics. The question of the deaf can be taken as symbolic of a broad range of problems, joining those of cultural communities and, more generally, of different identities in a society that cannot allow itself to fragment but then ought also to be capable of creating social bonds, cohesion and integration. Our modern societies are thus confronted with the question of managing differences.

The Differentiation Model

In contrast to the assimilation model discussed above, a model based on differentiation has been formulated. One form of the differentiation model is called *hierarchical*. This sub-model seems more obvious in European history than in that of North America, but it is, on the other hand, very close to many holistic and religious societies. Specificity and difference are recognised and may even be accepted. However, following the scheme of species within a genus, a common human genus is defined, and within it a series of points of view are situated that correlate with at least one distinctive feature. Thus, from the reference point of sex, the distinction would be man/woman; from that of biological conformity, the distinction would be able/disabled; and from the reference point of appearance, the distinction would be white/person of colour. Yet, once these 'species' are established, they are not thereby all considered equal. They are situated on a scale of positions and values. This is one means of integrating differences, for they are made to hold together in a coherence that is at the same time a system of subjection and submission. For example, man and woman represent two ways of being human. Yet man will dominate woman, because the social roles attached to these 'species' result in one having a greater precedence, dignity and importance than the other (political role vs. domestic role, productive role vs. nurturing role, authoritative role vs. affective role). In his *Souci de soi* (*Concern for Oneself*), Michel Foucault (1984) shows that relations between the sexes in ancient Greece, as also the relations between adult men and younger men, for that matter, were dictated by social position, which determines rights and liberties. This is a kind of cohesion through hierarchy. The Roman Catholic Church has offered us the purest model of this conception. The clergy are different from the laity but enjoy a dominant position. Christian people form a genus, but within this genus there are two great species: clergymen and laymen. In each of these species (which can then in turn play the role of genus), there are sub-species. The clergy is divided into bishops and priests, the laity into consecrated laymen (men in orders who are not priests) and laymen in secular life, and the latter group can be divided into men and women. A fine pyramid is created, from the summit where the clergy is to the base with its simple lay people. This grand terrestrial hierarchy must then correspond to a no less grand celestial hierarchy. All differences have a place on a scale of values. The common and equal nature of people as children of God in no way precludes different situations that are differently valorised.

Since the above example may appear Eurocentric, and Roman Catholicism is not a universal reference point, we will also illustrate the hierarchical model by Indian caste society. The massive social hierarchy created by means of the caste system is too well known to need retelling. We should, however, stress that it is only from a basis in diversity and differentiation that national integration is possible. The caste system is not by itself antidemocratic. India is a democracy, a very specific one admittedly, but a real one. The hierarchy of status, inegalitarian in its very essence, does, however, leave room for the autonomy of the individual will. Each person is responsible for his or her acts. The principle of caste, like that of 'states of life' in Catholicism, neither isolates nor encloses in a group that dictates decisions to all its members. It opens onto a network of possible relationships in which each person must constantly take initiatives to improve or maintain his or her status, gain influence, build personal prosperity, and ensure survival. This manoeuvring space around hierarchised positions introduces a real possibility for participation in a common life. On the other hand, the hierarchical model, because it has its point of departure in difference, is not incapable of permitting a modern form of integration and inclusion.

The example of India also permits us to comment on a point made earlier. Louis Dumont (1966) put the caste system beside holistic societies, which we in turn compared to those displaying mechanical solidarity. We said that this solidarity was characteristic of ancient societies. Yet it should be noted that the lines of reality are not so sharply drawn. It is not only that India's holism is in evolution, for we are witnessing a living, contemporary society, but also that holism is not entirely synonymous with mechanical solidarity. There can be mixed forms and also very original forms of conceiving inclusion and possibly producing exclusion. We note this in support of our intention to make a number of distinctions in a subject as complex as that treated here.

The hierarchical model makes it possible to suppress differences by an initial acceptance of similarity, although one that is strictly controlled. This is, of course, a means of consolidating differences that already exist. Here we link up with the analysis of Robert Castel (1995), who shows that throughout European history the categories of 'handicapology' are constant. There are always groups that, unable to meet their needs through their labour, are legally exempted from such labour and are assisted. The disabled have always been seen this way. Even when they are not excluded, they have a well-established inferior position. Even if it is not impossible to break out of the category of the permanently assisted, both mental and social structures are, in practical terms, opposed to it.

Still, in the universe of differentialisation, we meet a second model, that of *juxtaposition*. It is, no doubt, most frequent in countries with a British heritage. This is a model with a degree of tolerance, in the sense of accommodation. They are what they are, and we are who we are; their culture is that way, and ours is this way. We have no cause to subjugate them or render them inferior, but we really have nothing to do with them. The recognition of difference is pushed far enough for each person to exist on his or her own, a stranger in the midst of a group of strangers. There is a certain kind of nationalism reflected in this model. Foreigners have the right to exist as long as they stay out of our space. There is no integration. The result is a jigsaw puzzle, a mosaic, both from the international point of view, as it rejects any kind of transnational organisation, and from a state's internal point of view, as it leads to fragile unions (Yugoslavia). This model can be wedded to a form of democracy, as we see in the multi-culturalist thought of the United States, but left to its own logic it destroys all common space and could destroy a nation's foundations. Federalism attempts to surmount the disadvantages of this model, from which, in a certain sense, it issues. When groups, classes or cultures are in simple juxtaposition, an opposition of values necessarily arises which will hamper the social order and, above all, reinforce the pre-existing social structure.

This model is more reflective of a possible tendency in the treatment of persons with disabilities than a policy that has been applied in the past. Yet the tendency may be in a direction one could call the 'Indianisation' of disabled persons, referring to the reserves set up for Native Americans. Fortunately, the extermination of Native Americans has come to an end. This was a policy that placed them in a situation of radical difference, of terminal exclusion. But now they are situated apart, a sequestration in the very name of their difference. There are a number of people who would not be unhappy to exploit this form of segregation if it led to the purification, a purging, of their group space.

In its most extreme form, which we will call *differentialism*, this model states: you are other and you will have nothing to do with me, unless it is to submit to placement on a scale of values where I am more perfect than you. Let us make no mistake. Juxtaposition, like hierarchy, is a way of putting some people at the top and letting it be thought that they alone represent the universal. Misfortune always follows when a social group (or a state or a nation) believes itself to be the sole realisation of the universal, when the universal is a panorama, all of whose aspects are singular. There can be only parts of the universal. Once a people or an ethnicity takes itself for the universal, perversion is at work and can lead to the worst consequences.

Returning to the question of the deaf, a surplus of identity could result in exacerbated differentialism. The reasoning of the deaf, when taken to extremes, reflects the juxtaposition model, but in a radical form that mixes two approaches that are not comparable. Deaf culture exists, but it has been forged, like all cultures, in the historical process. It is not a 'natural' fact. On the other hand, being deaf, like being black or white, being a man or a woman, is a natural fact. Can we draw cultural consequences from a natural feature? Doing so is risky, for we recognise that this kind of confusion has served as the basis for so much exploitation and racism. 'They' have natural features of such a kind that they can have no part in our evolved white culture! The act of locking a group into its natural features amounts to establishing it in a closed specificity, and preparing the ground for all the extreme forms of cultural identity, ultraculturalism, and even group fanaticism. By virtue of wishing to affirm our own identity—however undeniable it is—we risk being enclosed in our own ghetto and finding ourselves excluded at the very interior of the society to which we, by our own logic, belong.

To conclude our discussion of the contradictions and tensions of normalisation and of the models of assimilation and differentiation, let us summarise the different senses of inclusion and exclusion that we have met. Doubtless, the most dynamic notion of inclusion leaves room for an effort toward adjustment, acceptability, acceptance and social participation. The notion of integration presupposes conformity and alignment, which are always experienced as domination, or even oppression, by the group that defines the norms, or by the majority over the minority. Being included may represent a situation in which you are a part, in an organic way, without necessarily being forced to conduct yourself according to a rigid norm. Otherwise, inclusion (or *insertion*, as it is sometimes called in French, with a rather different thrust) can prove to be weak, a synonym for simply being present, being admitted, and being tolerated. One can be supported without being recognised. One can be received without being incorporated. We have seen that the semantics differ according to the sociological and linguistic contexts. Being fully recognised as an equal, a partner, or a participant, with the same dignity and of the same quality as any other, is called *integration* rather than *inclusion*. Yet these are translations of French terms, and what is true of one language is not true of all. We must perhaps resign ourselves to the impossibility of translating terms that are charged with such historical and cultural weight.

In inverted fashion, exclusion in contemporary societies designates several phenomena: radical exclusion from society; segregation within a society; discrimination, also within, as concerns access to social goods and spaces; and disaffiliation and withdrawal from social exchange. Historically and in practice, inclusion and exclusion may take on differing significations. They are not univocal or unambiguous terms, and are not historically fixed. There is diversity in exclusion and diversity in inclusion. We will illustrate this diversity, and show the indivisible relationship between the two aspects, by establishing a typology. To one form of exclusion there corresponds another form of inclusion or, at a minimum, a tendency toward inclusion. This typology is necessary to do justice to a whole series of practices that we have thus far not been able to mention.

A DRAFT TYPOLOGY OF EXCLUSION AND INCLUSION

In the first part of this chapter, we saw the multiple facets of inclusion and exclusion, both processes and states. The analysis of different models has made it possible to view these notions in the context of other theories of the social bond and its possible dissolution (marginality, deviance). Anthropologist Robert Murphy (1987) employs the concept of liminality to express the fact that in all societies disabled persons live in a state of social suspension. They are neither ill nor well, neither dead nor alive, neither really excluded nor really included in society (Murphy, 1987).

These failures of inclusion or integration that may be experienced by disabled people translate into loss of, or difficult access to, a place in society, a permanent move to the sidelines. Studies of the historical treatment of disability (Stiker, 1982, 1999), as well as anthropological studies on the same theme (Ingstadt and Reynolds Whyte, 1995), show that the exclusion of disabled persons through time and across civilisations has assumed, and still assumes, extremely diverse forms within the host society. We shall therefore try to draw up a typology of different forms of exclusion, whether they are social, geographical, economical, cultural or judicial, while comparing the forms of inclusion that seek to offset them.

From radical forms of exclusion such as extermination or abandonment, there is a continuum of exclusion *from* society to diverse forms of exclusion *within* society, through segregation, marginalisation or discrimination. We observe that each of these types of exclusion, even if it was characteristic only of an ancient society, nonetheless displays some survival in our contemporary western societies. Moreover, it appears possible in such a typology to establish correspondences between each form of exclusion *within* society and a form of inclusion in it.

Exclusion through Elimination

The most extreme form of social exclusion, and one of the first types of exclusion that can be identified, is exclusion through elimination. The elimination of disabled persons can be effected in a direct way by putting them to death, or indirectly through abandonment or the deprivation of care. We may also remark that elimination, not of disabled persons but of the disability, may be considered before life. This raises topical questions regarding termination of pregnancy when a deficiency is identified in the foetus before conception using the latest developments in genetic engineering. Eugenics theories show a possible link between the practice of elimination in ancient societies and the application by contemporary societies of the most recent technological developments.

This radical, ultimate form of exclusion of persons with disabilities is situated at the level of the most fundamental principle, that of life itself. In Greco-Roman antiquity, the practice of exposing deformed infants offers an example. The fear of seeing the species deviate from its true course (that is, eugenics) was projected onto deformed births, even if the deformation was, to modern eyes, quite minimal. Such births were interpreted as a baleful sign sent by the gods that must be officially expelled from the social space and returned to its senders (Stiker, 1997, 1999). Infants who came into the world with deformities were left outside inhabited space, on fallow land, in a rut, or along a stream. In short, they were not socialised. Although they were not sacrificed in a formal manner, they were ritually abandoned. The practice of exposure, which we are not encouraged to believe was ever implemented on a massive scale, is a form of elimination, given what we know of the cities of antiquity, even if we could in one sense connect it with abandonment. The myth of Oedipus, one of the founding myths of the west, certainly constitutes one of the best illustrations of the ancient practice of exposure. However, it is probably Nazi Germany that offers the most extreme example of the extermination of disabled persons. Some 200,000 people (in particular, those with a mental illness or congenital malformation) were exterminated in hospitals and death camps because of their disability (Burleigh, 1994).

From another perspective, the ethical debate over euthanasia or assisted suicide deserves to be mentioned here as representative of the current way of posing again the question of the elimination of disabled persons. 'Quality of life' has become a key notion in public health, and some economists go so far as to speak of the 'price of human life'. The value accorded to human life is conditioned by social representations of disability, and, in our western societies, is influenced by the existence of severe forms of impairment. The value of a person's life may be judged negatively, with life under certain conditions deemed not worth living, which then justifies a certain number of medical practices that surround the beginning or end of life. On such a basis, it becomes possible in some countries to put a person to death in fully legal fashion. What is under discussion here is not, of course, the freedom of individual choice of life or death for a severely impaired person, but the fact that social pressure, by reducing disability to a kind of personal tragedy, makes it acceptable to accommodate disabled persons in their desire for death. Death, in this sense, is qualified as 'natural', whereas for persons who are not disabled, everything will be done to convince them of the transitory nature of a wish to die, and thereby prevent an attempt at suicide. In other words, the latter group is considered depressed and treated as such, while members of the former may well be offered in suicide the help that they were unable to obtain in daily life.

Even though they are interventions before birth, medical measures that aim at precluding the birth of a disabled child can be included in this discussion of exclusion through elimination. These methods share the radical nature of the foregoing, and raise the question of the very humanity of disabled persons. A decision to terminate a pregnancy through medical means can be taken after prenatal diagnosis, or a strong presumption resulting from ultrasound detection of a foetus' anomaly or risk of birth as a disabled child. With new genetic techniques and pre-implantation screening, it has become possible to identify a certain number of genetic diseases even before pregnancy. The question of elimination can be raised in these terms, and we could then speak of the eradication of Down's syndrome or muscular dystrophy, for example. Thus, we could see societies emerge that have been 'cured' of certain genetic diseases, but achieving this prospect will be attended by concern over the limits that will have to be put in place to regulate such an evolution. Associations of persons with disabilities may speak in this context about genocide and crimes against humanity. The eugenics perspectives opened up by the possibility of genetic screening are certainly among the most difficult ethical problems that democratic societies will have to face in the near future. Lastly, the sterilisation of mentally disabled women, which has occasionally been practiced, although often illegally, can also be associated with measures addressing procreation.

Exclusion through Abandonment

Abandonment can be distinguished from elimination by the fact that it does not entail death, or at least not in a direct fashion. Practiced in antiquity, exclusion in the form of abandonment recurs in a contemporary form of social death, namely social abandonment. There is no lack of examples of the practice of abandoning people: children who are born deformed, victims of multiple injuries, and very dependent elderly persons. Abandonment can take different routes: transferring parental authority to another agency; leaving in God's hands the fate of a newborn; or the more modern fashion of anonymous delivery with a view to adoption. Abandonment, then, is not something specific to ancient societies. A French study has shown that, parallel to the increasingly widespread success in the prenatal diagnosis of Down's syndrome, the number of such infants who are abandoned at birth has increased in France in recent years (Dumaret et al., 1998). The hypothesis can then be advanced that more widespread prevention methods have been accompanied by a decrease in the social acceptability of this type of disability. To abandon something or someone is to cease to be concerned with it, to deprive it of care. Here we return to the question of passive euthanasia, which consists of no longer providing all possible care to a newly born infant, an accident victim, or an elderly person who is considered too severely disabled or at risk of becoming so.

The surplus population thesis has been advanced as one of the chief explanations of exclusion by abandonment (Oliver and Barnes, 1998). The evolution of European thought in the nineteenth century—the emergence of liberal utilitarianism and social Darwinism—raises the question of the place of individuals who are too weak, too dependent, or incapable of meeting their needs without assistance. Decisions like not attempting resuscitation and disconnecting life-support systems represent the modern face of this form of abandonment, which quite simply consists of ceasing to look after someone. We can also see that the duties and responsibilities of family and of society may diverge here.

Exclusion through Segregation or Differentiated Inclusion

Segregation and the various practices of sequestration constitute one of the most widespread forms of exclusion. This *geographical* exclusion, in the generic sense of the word, can be found, with immediate topical relevance, across eras and cultures. This is also a form of social treatment that, by clearly setting out an inside and an outside, is very close to the basic meanings of inclusion and exclusion. The point here is that this separate treatment does not necessarily occur outside the community but frequently at its very centre. Lastly, we may note that this kind of segregation may be more or less constraining, and may entail a greater or lesser deprivation of personal freedom.

In his *L'histoire de la folie a l'âge classique* (*A History of Insanity in the Age of Reason*), Michel Foucault (1961) describes in convincing detail what he calls, after the creation of the *Hôpitaux Généraux* in France in 1662, the 'Great Confinement' of the seventeenth century. Most European countries have known a parallel evolution; for example, Britain had its workhouses. The first institutions for disabled people were often intended for the deaf and the blind. The confinement of the mentally ill or deficient against their will (legislated in 1838 in France and 1845 in Britain) is a particularly characteristic example of the kind of social control that would henceforth be imposed on this population through the power accorded to physicians. In western European countries, this movement toward the institutionalisation of disabled persons would last until the 1970s.

In the sphere of disability, the term *institution*, which we relate to the concept of segregation, refers to a kind of establishment that is most often structured to treat, train and intern disabled people on a residential basis. Thus, it has been possible to speak of 'total institutions' (Goffman, 1961). The institutions created by the first educators in the domain of persons with infirmity are of this type. The Abbé de l'Epée (1712–89) founded a school for the deaf, with whom he learned to make himself understood by means of sign language. Valentin Haüy (1745–1822) founded an Institution for Blind Children (*l'Institution des Jeunes Aveugles*) in Paris, and conceived of letters printed in relief that would permit the blind to read, before Louis Braille (1809–52), a blind teacher, devised the systematic code that still bears his name. In the same period, Jean Marc Gaspard Itard (1774–1838) tried to educate a feral child, Victor of Aveyron. His failure in this attempt did not prevent Edouard Seguin (1812–80), his successor, from inventing a pedagogy designed for mentally retarded children. His special establishments, which Seguin promoted in America since he was poorly received in France, were based on the segregation model, despite their creator's passion for education in the broadest sense of the word. Similarly, Philippe Pinel (1745–1826), well known for having freed the insane from their chains, affirmed the curability of the 'mad', and laid the basis for modern psychiatry. However, he did not envisage his famous 'moral treatment' other than within the sequestering walls of a hospital. In our time, the greater part of treatment, placement, training and education is still done within the framework of institutions. Severely criticised by the anti-psychiatry and de-institutionalisation movements, such as at Basaglia in Italy, the institution has also been the object of heated criticism on the part of numerous organisations of disabled persons. Thus, in Great Britain, the Union of the Physically Impaired against Segregation (UPIAS) describes the segregated residential institution as the 'ultimate human scrapheap'. It adds:

> Thousands of people, whose only crime is being physically impaired, are sentenced to these prisons for life.... For the vast majority, there is no alternative, no appeal, no remission of sentence for good behaviour, no escape, except the escape from life itself. (UPIAS, 1976)

One of the constant features of the institutionalisation of disabled people has been the separation of the sexes. This repression of sexuality, thus precluding all procreation, can be associated with the practice of sterilisation and the eugenics issues treated above. It must be stated that the theories of degeneracy that were developed in the nineteenth century envisaged a major solution to 'degeneration' in the barring of disabled persons from reproducing. If the decline of institutionalisation was furthered by strong advocacy based on humanistic arguments, it is probable that economic arguments and the waning of the welfare state really precipitated this evolution. However, this segregating institutional environment was part of the matrix that generated the movements of rebellion and protest by disabled people against these structures, which they considered primarily responsible for oppressing them and their will to gain control over the services that mattered to them. This form of exclusion through segregation may also affect other aspects of social life, such as education, employment and transportation. Thus, there are specialised schools for disabled children, sheltered workshops for disabled workers, and specialised forms of transportation for persons with disabilities.

One of the paradoxes is that segregation (e.g. in the form of temporary separate schooling) is often presented as a 'detour' that has integration as its ultimate goal. In fact, such segregation is today most often conceived of as a provisional bypass to regain the mainstream, to participate more fully in society, even if it should happen that this detour never does come back around. Thus, the intention is not to exclude but to include at a future date. The goal of sequestration is no longer confinement, as in the seventeenth century, but a mediated inclusion.

Exclusion through Assistance or Conditional Inclusion

The reference to employment and productive capacity permits us to address another form of exclusion, namely, exclusion through assistance, an 'economic' form of exclusion that has permeated the entire question of social policy since the end of the Middle Ages. In fact, the lot of the crippled was linked to the social treatment of poverty during the entire medieval period.

The distinction erected in the countries of western Europe since the Middle Ages between the meritorious poor, who included persons with deficiencies, and the able-bodied indigent, sought to distinguish those who were exempted from work and those who were obligated to it. For the former, recognition of incapacity would open the way to the possibility of being assisted. Measures to combat begging condemned the second group to repression: deportation, forced labour, and the banishment of vagabonds.

Assistance is a form of close-up protection, intended, for example, for other inhabitants of the village, and concerns those who, by virtue of their inability to work, cannot meet their own needs. Christian values, including charity, dominate what we may call the Christian West. Disability recalls the suffering of Christ, and the charity that it stimulates enables practicing Christians to atone for their sins. The church plays a major role in the development of individually targeted assistance, initially through the intermediary of its convents, monasteries and other religious institutions, and then through specialised institutions such as hospitals, hospices and orphanages. This protective role of the church was also an aspect of its power. Until the French Revolution, the church may be said to have been the principal organ for the provision of assistance. The counterpoint to this aid was that disabled persons were obliged to show complete humility toward their benefactor. Welfare activity and good works marked the history of the social treatment of disability until the twentieth century. If the relationship to work is a determining factor in understanding the economic role of disabled people, work represents, beyond its connection with production, a justification for inscription in the social structure. Thus, failure to participate in any productive activity, and isolation from other human relationships, combine their negative effects to generate exclusion, or rather, disaffiliation (Castel, 1995). Inversely, the combination of stable work and solid functioning relationships creates conditions for integration. Between the two lies a zone of social vulnerability. Assistance is a form of economic exclusion that defines those who are 'useless to society'. It also introduces a relationship of subordination and dependence between those helped and their benefactors. The individual so aided is divested of all responsibilities, such as that of working, in exchange for submission to a status of inferiority. This surrender of obligations, or 'irresponsibility', is a source of marginalisation; it calls the very idea of citizenship into question.

Some theorists of disability regard exclusion from the world of work as the ultimate cause of other, different forms of exclusion that disabled people experience (Oliver and Barnes, 1998). Some among them argue that criteria for citizenship cannot be based on social usefulness. The passage of assistance into the secular sphere did not resolve this inequality of position, which is now being challenged from the perspective of civil rights. On the contrary, present-day dissociation from systems of economic production often entails exclusion from systems of compensation and social protection. Assistance or, inverting the terminology, social security and welfare are admittedly weak forms of participation in society. They confer a social sub-status. Yet, to assist is not to exclude, because those who are helped are part of society by the very fact that society is concerned about them. At times, as during the medieval period, this sub-status is necessary even for the well-to-do, because it offers them the opportunity to win eternal salvation. However, those helped are part of society only on condition that they stay in their place. Georg Simmel (1908) has clearly shown that poverty does not mean being without resources; it means being assisted, with such assistance being the very means of ensuring social cohesion on this level. Assistance is basically a sociological relationship, and it has an indispensable function. This is why the objective of social assistance policies is not the elimination of poverty, as one might believe, but its integration into the system, to the benefit of the latter.

Exclusion through Marginalisation or Inclusion through Normalisation

In the precise sense of the word, *marginalisation* is the process of moving a person to the side as a consequence of that person's refusal to accept, or impossibility of accepting, currently recognised rules of operation. The marginalised are defined by transgression of, or protest against, the values and constitution of the community. Whether a person (e.g. a criminal or panhandler) puts himself or herself outside the boundaries, or is someone rejected by the dominant group (e.g. a prostitute or a teenager forced into delinquency by his or her parents' oppression), marginality is always characterised by a lifestyle that cannot be accommodated within the behavioural norms that are in force. Its origin may lie in a conflict over rights (both rights recognised and rights denied); in the absence of rules (total permissiveness on the part of parents, leading youngsters to set up their own rules); or in a conflict of values (such as a person who no longer wants to live according to the law of consumption and goes into self-imposed exile to lead an autarkical way of life). Disabled persons who reject norms that are applied to them, or who are rejected for not 'playing the game', are susceptible to being drawn into this process of marginalisation. Yet this is not the general case, because their desire to integrate into society often makes them accept the common rules. The fundamental problem is that of norms. To be included, you must accept and achieve a certain degree of conformity. The key concern of rehabilitation (called *réadaptation* in French) is to reduce deviation from the norm. Action on the individual who is to be reintroduced into the mainstream is accompanied by the desire to efface any differences. The individual must act 'like others', even if this requires technical aids, various devices, or prostheses. However, this same concern to reduce deviance laid the groundwork for the kind of normalisation procedures developed by Wolfensberger (1972) for mentally retarded persons.

Exclusion through Discrimination or Progressive Inclusion

The last type of cultural or juridical exclusion that must be addressed is exclusion through discrimination. To discriminate is to single out, put a social group to one side, and restrict its rights. When made in social life at the expense of disabled persons, these distinctions may be judged unacceptable because they violate social norms and the principle of equality before the law, even if in other societies and at other times they are or were current. To define *discrimination* as the act of treating equal individuals inequitably shows to what extent this concept is tied to modern society, which puts equality at the centre of its code of values. In societies based on differences in status or caste, discrimination is a neutral, descriptive notion, devoid of the pejorative connotations we in western societies would ascribe to it.

With the development of civil rights, most modern democracies instituted judicial protection against negative discrimination based on criteria related to the impairments of an individual. If the intentional discrimination of individuals is therefore proscribed in the United States, Great Britain, Australia and New Zealand, this does not preclude, in these very same countries, the existence of statistical discrimination at the level of the population of disabled persons. It has been shown (in France) that, despite a law that uses an obligatory quota system for both private and public sectors to promote the employment of disabled workers, disabled persons continue—all other things being equal—to experience discrimination in their search for employment (Ravaud, Madiot and Ville, 1992).

However, discrimination may also be positive, and have the restoration of equality as its goal. It is interesting for French researchers to note to what extent the current English phrase *affirmative action* differs in this respect. Positive discrimination can be effected by social assistance measures in cases determined according to extrinsic characteristics (tied to income, for example). It can also be ensured by authoritarian measures (which raises the question of personal freedom), or by preferential measures (e.g. policies of employment quotas favouring disabled workers, women or certain ethnic minorities). It may also be conceived of as a compensation measure, and justified on the basis of distributive justice, which is not without its paradox, because it is not the injured individual who benefits from the compensation (Auroux, 1990). It has an inherent defect: since it necessarily takes place only after negative discrimination, it must temporarily violate the principle of equality on which it is based. It can thus be defended for reasons of social utility; for example, the employment of disabled persons may at times be part of a company's communications and public-relations policy. We can see the contradictions inherent in the principle of non-discrimination, which tends to be too generalised. In the struggle against negative discrimination, it makes vulnerable the systems that are based on protective and compensatory measures.

The principal question that is posed today in western countries is the nature of the citizenship that disabled persons may enjoy. Modern politics excludes the possibility of distinguishing among different categories of persons in the public sphere. Behind these questions of discrimination and exclusion, we discern the principle of equality of citizens before the law as the moral ideal of a democratic nation. We will do well to state precisely the limits of this equality before the law: right to identical treatment, right of access, right to equal opportunities, and right to an identical quality of life. We can see to what extent, in a society that has become segmented, the perspective we assume will depend on our conception of justice and social inequalities.

Summary

The typology given above is of course quite schematic, and there are numerous intermediary forms between each of these modalities of exclusion and inclusion. Thus, the very act of judging people to be socially and economically useless is deeply interwoven with eugenicists' notions of elimination. Discrimination is not just cultural or judicial exclusion but also economic exclusion. However schematic, our typology makes it possible to identify differences in the reactions of cultures to anomalies such as impairments: reduce them, control them physically, avoid them, catalogue them as dangerous, or adopt them as rituals—as described by Mary Douglas (1966).

Exclusion needs to be examined from a global perspective that encompasses the view of the excluded and that of the entity that rejects him or her. This is because, contrary to contemporary representations, exclusion is not an abstract, inexorable phenomenon, without actors, nor is it ultimately an inevitable consequence of entering the new global economy. As Norbert Elias (1965) illustrated in his study of the logic of exclusion, it is clear that exclusion is also inscribed in a society's power relationships.

Lastly, the tension between the two approaches to disability policy that we have characterised as differentialist and universalist is not without consequences for the social situation of disabled people. The first calls for a right to difference, for specificity, even a minority-group identity; the second invokes the universality of human rights, and rejects all particularism. The former carries the latent risk of segregation, the latter of inequalities.

A CHALLENGE TO DEMOCRATIC SOCIETIES

The models of exclusion and inclusion that we have reviewed, as well as the multiple forms of integration and segregation, raise the fundamental question: what form should true democratic inclusion take? According to us, addressing this question offers a real prospect, a real future, for a just stance on the issue of disabled persons. The word *just* must be understood in its two senses—justice and justness; that is, it covers what is theirs by right and what is right for their specific case.

We shall base our discussion on two thinkers who have recently sought to conceive of a way beyond the opposition between the policy of assimilation (whose proponents are called 'liberals' in the United States) and the inward turn to group-identity issues or communitarianism. Kymlicka (1995), who we would qualify as a moderate liberal, attempts to find room for expressions of collective identity, taking as point of departure the irrefutable principles of individual citizenship. Charles Taylor (1992), on the other hand, who could be called a similarly moderate communitarian, looks for ways to publicly recognise specific cultures without neglecting the equality of citizens. We shall not develop these lines of thought here, centred as they are on the problems of cultural communities more or less located within the North American context. Yet it is important to see how the search is being conducted—by Michael Walzer (1988), for example—for a differentiated citizenship, a democracy of participation, the conjunction of individual citizenship with a policy of support for minorities and singular identities, in short, for a democratic pluralism.

It seems that, to a greater or lesser degree, these forms of relating to the 'other' have, in turn or at the same time, been able to influence the way the disabled are treated. Their lot seems to have always swung between subjection, indifference or denial. Denial is apparent in the older forms of radical exclusion or in more modern forms of direct segregation, but also, very subtly, in the form of a passion for assimilation through normalisation at all cost. Subjection is shown when the crippled serve some 'other purpose': offering salvation to those being charitable to them; playing the fool; being exhibited as freaks; or in more contemporary terms, partaking of policies for population management and business, or justifying the existence of a service industry for the disabled. Indifference is shown when the disabled are placed in what Murphy (1987) calls liminality; they are neither included nor excluded, neither rejected not accepted. Either the disabled are left to the care of the welfare establishment in accordance with a roundabout principle of non-discrimination, or they are protected and assisted according to the arrangements of a compensatory discrimination that are not brought to their full conclusion.

The positions adopted by disabled persons themselves may favour one model or another, and entail the perverse side effects of each. Minority activism at times takes on the trappings of overdriven differentialism, as discussed above. Will Kymlicka's (1995) idea, according to which the recognition of separate collectivities is not unconditional, and according to which the individuals of a group ought to be free to both enter it and leave it, is to propose a kind of communitary extremism.

Inversely, one form of discourse on the abolition of differences and the claim to be like others may derive from an assimilationist model that is not just euphoric. It is a way of putting emphasis on the 'social model', but this has its drawbacks. The social model has become the means of referencing a train of thought that tries to examine disability from the side of the social barriers of every order that constitute it, by abstracting its corporeal and individual dimensions (Barton and Oliver, 1997). It is the state of society alone that creates disability, its material and mental states. Even if the diffusion of this model has the undeniable pedagogical merit of throwing into relief dominant social praxis, the risk now is of 'disembodying' disability by neglecting its corporeality and the dimension of individual experience. Once the social barriers are abolished, what is left of disability are banal differences—moving in a wheelchair instead of walking, not recognising certain communication signs but having others in their place. To approach disability from the direction of impairment is to see it upside down and to attribute difficulties to the individual, which, when we think about them, have to do only with the management—'in the act'—of the environment. If we follow this logic to its end, we would come to a common space that could, metaphorically, be called de-sexed, one where all expressions of particularity, including cultural ones, are swept away. In the name of individual citizenship, there would no longer be any collective identities. In fact, even the assertion of a disabled identity with a view to abolishing social barriers presupposes a certain collective identity, because otherwise there is only a swarm of individuals. Under which flag would people then gather? It seems that it is impossible to disregard the fact that two poles have to be maintained: civic universalism, on the one hand, and groups and differentiated individuals, on the other. What is fundamental in the struggle to abolish social barriers, and in advancing the claim to be like others, is to reassert the need to create a truly common social space and truly common access—a universal design. What is fundamental in the affirmation of a certain specific identity is to require this social space, which will never be an incarnation of the universal, to compensate, on an ongoing basis, for the weaknesses of certain people by putting at their disposal what they need to occupy, just as they are, this common space.

To take the example of schooling, disabled children would have their specific needs met, but within the framework of regular classes and classrooms, and with all the necessary support. As Stainback and Stainback write:

> Full inclusion does not mean that special educators are no longer necessary; rather, it means that special educators are needed even more to work with regular educators in teaching and facilitating challenging, supportive and appropriate educational programmes for all students. However, special educators do need to be integrated into, and, in effect, become 'regular' or 'general' educators in the mainstream, who have expertise in specific instructional, curricular and assessment areas. (Stainback and Stainback, 1990, p. 4)

This school example clearly shows a concrete application of what we have formulated in a more abstract fashion. We could go on with examples from the business world and daily life. Imagine if we introduced a sufficient number of professionals trained in disability *into work environments*, so that accessibility became total. Then all the structures of sheltered employment would become useless. What is necessary to achieve this vision is the conversion of corporate officers; but having a utopia before one's eyes does have an effect, as history shows us. Let us imagine that in city neighbourhoods, 'social workers' are present on a daily basis, discussing and working with all the vital resources (associations and various service agencies) and with all those who are active there (storekeepers, tradespeople, professionals). Many disabled persons could then maintain themselves and live among others. Daily democracy has a fine, wide path ahead of it. The necessary precondition for the progressive realisation of such a utopia is the existence of political will. The role of the citizen is indispensable here in influencing elected representatives and administrative officers, and also in convincing groups of disabled people to move openly and boldly in this direction. We are well short of the mark, so it is all the more reason to get started.

In the meantime, many efforts already begun must be reaffirmed and amplified: the creation of services to accompany children and their families throughout the schooling process; the development of ergonomic services (in the widest sense of the term) to adapt urban spaces, transportation and work stations; the training of public health and social work professionals in the issues of disabled people; public advocacy campaigns to combat stigmatisation, prejudice and stereotypes; and the presence of well-informed persons at the moment of birth of a disabled child. This is not an exhaustive list.

This model is a challenge for what we, as French speakers, would call a truly republican, truly democratic space: to establish relationships that presuppose and respect particular terms of existence, invent various combinations of such terms, and take into account all forms of alterity. If we wanted an image for such a model, we could find it in language where all the differences (since that is all there is) oppose and interconnect with one another to constitute meanings—meanings that are always open, since the combinations are infinite. In turn, each language, however alien to the others, can still to be translated into another language, not completely transferred but translated, with some of the inevitable betrayal of original meaning. Disabled persons cannot be reduced to a social identicalness (the deviant, the marginalised), or to an identity based on 'able-bodiedness'. Their existence in the world is singular (and singular in differing ways, depending on the persons and their impairments), but they can translate our experience into theirs and vice versa.

It should be possible to install a common, shared space where there would no longer be any hierarchy, but where we would no longer be separated without being reduced. This is what Diderot envisaged in his famous *Lettre sur les aveugles à l'usage de ceux qui voient* ('Letter on the blind for the use of the sighted', 1749), when he shows that Saunderson, or the celebrated blind man of Puiseaux, was an 'anthropological variety'. The following is what a literary critic, well experienced in disability, expressed at the end of a conference devoted to the topic of disability in literature:

> In light of all this, it should be evident that traditional literary images of the afflicted contribute little or nothing toward creating attitudes which might make possible in actuality a society in which the disabled would be recognised as representing not some absolute, unendurable Other, but one pole on a human spectrum, in which differences of perception and agility separate not merely one individual from another, but one stage from another in each individual's life: from the total dependency of infancy to the gradual crumbling of our powers in old age.... In such a utopian society, worked for, as well as dreamed by, committed professionals and amateurs of goodwill, all means of information retrieval and transport would be

> redesigned to accommodate such differences. And on a psychological [level], even the most debilitating handicaps would be perceived as constituting not a departure from but another assertion of the almost infinitely varied human 'norm'. Even pain and early death would come to be faced head-on, tragically and joyously, rather than sniggered at in embarrassment, turned away from in terror, or denied in pity. (Fiedler, 1982, pp. 68–69)

CONCLUSION

We have chosen to address the question of exclusion and inclusion as evidenced in the principal forms of 'relationships with others' in our organic societies, which are societies which must create their own processes for cohesion and social equalisation. If we had limited ourselves to what could be called the primary degree of opposition between exclusion and inclusion, we would have only skimmed the surface of the attendant phenomena. Evidence supports the notion that every citizen—and certainly even more a disabled citizen—is excluded from some places, from some social goods, and even from some *rights* (to culture, leisure, education), at least in part. Intolerable as this may be, it is proof that society is not egalitarian. This is the rationale that justifies the present claims, and the concrete action proposed for their realisation. Persons with a 'disability', more than any others, are living proof of iniquity and inequality. On this level, the specifics of inequality between the able and the disabled are of degree and not of nature. We are all targets for inequitable and unjust treatment, disabled people often to a greater degree than others. Still, the struggle of disabled people is of the same nature as of all those who do not have access to the social goods that are their due. It is the social dimension of citizenship that is called into question.

The most serious question is to ask whether rights—to free expression, to freedom of movement, to the vote, that is, the universal rights of human beings—are being denied to the disabled. In certain countries perhaps they are, but doubtless because they are also being denied to all individuals. In countries where citizens have rights, these specific rights are not being denied to disabled persons, even though certain guardianship systems could be criticised from this perspective. The disabled are not excluded from 'political' citizenship. Analysis does not support a brutal assertion to the effect that 'disabled people are excluded people', because exclusion itself is a process. It can take different forms, always relates to a social context, can be effected by degrees, and can be common to many other individuals and groups.

On the other hand, situating the issue of disabled people by means of models, schematics, reference points, the principles of a given society, and so on, has the advantage of greater intelligibility. This is the case not only because, as in the preceding instance, persons with disabilities are situated in a global movement of which they are the symptom, but still more because neither their singularity nor their quality as citizens is effaced.

References

Auroux, S. 1990. 'Les notions philosophiques', in *Encyclopédie Philosophique Universelle.* Paris: Presses Universitaires de France, p. 669.

Barton, L. and Oliver, M. 1997. *Disability Studies: Past, Present and Future.* Leeds: The Disability Press.

Becker, H.S. 1963. *Outsiders.* New York: Free Press.

Bell, Alexander G. 1883. *Memoir upon the Formation of a Deaf Variety of the Human Race.* New Haven: National Academy of Sciences.

Boruwlaski, J. 1788. *Mémoires du célèbre nain Joseph Boruwslaski, gentilhomme polonais.* London.

Burleigh, M. 1994. *Death and Deliverance: Euthanasia in Germany, 1900–1945.* Cambridge: Cambridge University Press.

Castel, R. 1995. *Les métamorphoses de la question sociale: une chronique du salariat.* Paris: Fayard.

Douglas, M. 1966. *Purity and Danger.* London: Routledge and Kegan Paul.

Dumaret, A-C. et al. 1998. 'Adopting and fostering babies with Down syndrome: A cohort of 593 cases', *Prenatal Diagnosis,* 18: 437–45.

Dumont, L. 1966. *Homo Hierarchicus: le Système des Castes et ses Implications.* Paris: Gallimard.

Durkheim, Émile. 1930. *De la Division du Travail Social.* Paris: Presses Universitaires de France.

Elias, N. 1965. *The Established and the Outsiders.* London: Sage.

Fiedler, Leslie A. 1982. 'Pity and fear: Images of the disabled in literature and the popular arts', *Salmagundi,* 57: 57–69.

Foucault, Michel. 1961. *L'histoire de la folie à l'âge classique.* Paris: Pion.

———. 1975. *Surveiller et punir.* Paris: Gallimard.

———. 1984. *Le souci de soi. Histoire de la sexualité 3.* Paris: Gallimard.

Gauchet, Marcel. 1985. *Le désenchantement du monde.* Paris: Gallimard.

———. 1995. 'Pour une autre histoire de la folie', publishèd with Gladys Swain in Gauchet Marcel and Gladys (eds), *Dialogue avec l'insensé: essai d'histoire de la psychiatrie*. Paris: Gallimard.

Goffman, Erving. 1961. *Asylums: Essays on the Social Situation of Mental Patients and Other Inmates*. Harmondsworth: Penguin.

———. 1963. *Stigma: Notes on the Management of Spoiled Identity*. Englewood Cliffs: Prentice-Hall.

Ingstadt, B. and Reynolds Whyte, S. 1995. *Disability and Culture*. Berkeley: University of California Press.

Kymlicka, Will. 1995. 'Multicultural Citizenship', in Will Kymlika (ed.), *A Liberal Theory of Minority Rights*. New York: Oxford University Press.

Lane, Harlan. 1984. *When the Mind Hears: A History of the Deaf*. New York: Random House.

———. 1992. *The Mask of Benevolence*. New York: Knopf.

Mauss, Marcel. 1923. 'Essai sur le don. Forme et raison de l'échange dans les sociétés archaïques', *Année Sociologique*, Seconde série, t. 1. Reprinted 1950 and 1983 in *Sociologie et anthropologie*. Paris: Presses Universitaires de France.

Murphy, Robert. 1987. *The Body Silent: A Journey into Paralysis*. New York: Holt.

Oliver, M. and Barnes, C. 1998. *Disabled People and Social Policy: From Exclusion to Inclusion*. London: Addison-Wesley.

Ravaud, Jean-François, Madiot, B. and Ville, I. 1992. 'Discrimination towards disabled people seeking employment', *Social Science and Medicine,* 35(8): 951–58.

Simmel, G. 1908. *Der Arme*. Munich: Duncker and Humblot.

Stainback, William and Stainback, Susan. 1990. *Support Networks for Inclusive Schooling: Interdependent Integrated Education*. Baltimore: Brookes.

Stiker, Henri-Jacques. 1982. *Corps infirmes et sociétés*. Paris: Aubier. (1997) Revised edition. Paris: Dunod.

———. 1999. *A History of Disability*. Ann Arbor: University of Michigan Press.

Taylor, C. 1992. *Multiculturalism and 'the Politics of Recognition'*. Princeton: Princeton University Press.

Tönnies, F. 1979. *Gemeinschaft und Gesellschaft: Grundbegriffe der reinen Soziologie*. Darmstadt: Wissenschaftliche Buchgesellschaft.

Union of the Physically Impaired against Segregation (UPIAS). 1976. *Fundamental Principles of Disability*. London: Author.

Walzer, Michael. 1988. *Sur la tolérance*. Paris: Gallimard.

Weber, Max. 1920. *Gesammelte Aufsätze zur Religionssoziologie*. Tiibingen: Mohr.

Wolfensberger, W. 1972. *The Principle of Normalisation in Human Services*. Toronto: National Institute of Mental Retardation.

World Health Organisation (WHO). 1980. *International Classification of Impairment, Disability and Handicap: A Manual of Classification Relating to the Consequences of Disease*. Geneva: WHO

2

From Handicap to Disability: Language Use and Cultural Meaning in the United States

Patrick J. Devlieger

INTRODUCTION

Language is a powerful instrument. How something is called has important implications for the way it is spoken about and how it is handled. When people in the United States talk about their 'car', 'automobile' or 'vehicle', they can in these three cases speak about the same object, but the meaning of each of these words becomes clear only when the situational context of the word's use is known. This context is indicated by the nature of the story or conversation in the situation in which these develop. The use of a car, the maintenance, the purchase, and the sale are examples of situational contexts.

Users of concepts are not always aware of their language use. Many Americans use, for example, the terms 'handicap' and 'disability' concurrently, and are confused by the possible differences between the terms. In such cases, the view of the anthropologist as outsider can be useful in understanding the differences by interpreting them. Cultural sensitivity for the differences in language use is important for a correct understanding of a phenomenon. In working with people of a different

---

Devlieger, Patrick. J. 1999. 'From handicap to disability: Language use and cultural meaning in the United States', *Disability and Rehabilitation*, 21: 346–54.

cultural background, a different cultural content of the phenomenon of 'disability' might be communicated. Such a cultural content has an impact on the way messages are communicated and on their understanding.

This chapter examines an important shift in American terminology use and the way it figures in societal discourse. For Foucault, discourse is a vocabulary which is created to maintain certain forms of social domination. This vocabulary is not a 'list of words' but a complex combination of language uses and practices, professional qualifications and practices, which concurrently sustain a system of social control. Foucault describes in his book, *Madness and Civilisation*, the development of the ways in which people talked about so-called 'mad people'. He describes the development of a new profession, psychiatry, which constructs a certain vocabulary, and acquires the power to declare people mad and, even against their will, send them to clinics for therapy. According to Foucault, the power of psychiatry lies in its discourse, in the vocabulary which is invented to 'sell' its statements to outsiders and to sustain its authority (Foucault, 1965, 1966, 1972).

Cultural sensitivity to the differences in language use is important for a just and accurate understanding of a phenomenon. In cross-cultural work, both in a national context with people of different ethnic backgrounds and in an international context, a different cultural content of the phenomenon of 'disability' will be apparent. This cultural content always has an impact on the way we communicate and the way in which messages can be understood. Recent developments in American society serve to illustrate the implications of changes in language.

FROM 'HANDICAPPED' TO 'DISABLED'

The shift from 'handicap' to 'disability' in American language use largely took place in the mid-1980s. The use of the term disability has consolidated after a period of mixed use of disability and handicap. The term disability is now consistently being used in official documentation about persons with disabilities (Boston, 1992). In new legislation, the term handicap is no longer used (Pope and Tarlow, 1991). In professional literature, the term is only sparely used to describe barriers to certain activities, and not to refer to a certain group. 'The handicapped' exist no longer, but 'the disabled' and, more recently, 'people with disabilities' are recognised and discussed. The term disability has become part of authorised language, in the sense that 'language represents, manifests and symbolises power' (Bourdieu, 1991). Despite this obvious external influence, held in place by the rules and communication networks of politically correct language, there is a historical and social-cultural development in society by which language terminology incorporates connotations that become a match or mismatch to larger societal developments. Semiotics is the science that is interested in the value of signs (such as words) in a sign system (for example, the literature), and in the relation between a sign and that which it signifies. In applying a semiotic approach to the shift from handicap to disability, the author is situating these words as signs in the larger historical and social-cultural context of the United States.

In this analysis, the author does not share the point of view of the World Health Organisation (WHO, 1980), nor of Nagi (Nagi, 1965, 1969, 1991), that disability (and impairment) can exist in a social-cultural vacuum, while handicap supposes a social-cultural reality (Dijkers, 1995). Both handicap and disability are terms which, in daily usage, cannot exist without being assigned a meaning which is historically and culturally determined. The purpose here is to uncover this meaning. A language-historical approach to shifts in usage of terminology provides a partial insight into the real meaning, but it is still insufficient for an anthropological approach. A more complete picture is obtained when language shift, in this case from handicap to disability, is tested against the concrete experiences of individuals with disabilities in society. To this end, the changes in the life-course of the generation of American youth with mild mental retardation who were born around 1970 will serve to illustrate historical significance. Their historical lot was that, for the first part of their lives, they were labelled as handicapped, but as young adults they were gradually introduced with the label disabled. This leads to a central point in the anthropological study of disability: namely, to confront the discourse of disability with the personal experiences of individuals with disabilities (Reynolds Whyte, 1995).

MESSAGES FOLLOWING THE AMERICANS WITH DISABILITIES ACT (1990)

Customers of grocery stores in Illinois could, in 1995 and 1996, see a sign at the entrance that said: 'Handicapped or disabled customer, please contact store manager for assistance.' The message is clear: people with disabilities are customers, they have the right to make purchases like anyone else, and the staff at the store are available for assistance. The message has also seeped into the world of advertisement, which now addresses people who use wheelchairs, or people with other visible disabilities. The sign at the entrance was a concrete result of the Americans with Disabilities Act of 1990. This law prohibits discrimination, and therefore requires reasonable accommodations to meet the needs of persons with disabilities. The law is an extension of integrative thinking and policy since the 1960s. The vision is that the 'difference' of persons with disabilities needs to become unnoticeable. In this sense, the law reinforces a flattening modernist thinking, by which differences constitute barriers and need to be made invisible. This development is not yet completely concluded. The next step is already recognisable: there are already organisations of people with disabilities that demand recognition of their uniqueness. This is most prominent in the community of the deaf, which emphasises its own cultural identity based on a unique, owned, language usage. But other groups of persons with disabilities have also begun emphasising their uniqueness.

The message 'handicapped or disabled customer' in the store signs also expressed that there is confusion in thought and practice regarding a phenomenon, which has led to the introduction of new understandings that need to be communicated to the larger public. The replacement of the term 'handicap' by 'disability' occurred in the mid-1980s. After a confusing period during which both terms get used concurrently and parallel with each other, it may be expected that the term 'handicap' will disappear. Disability activists, as one primary consumption group of this terminology, have been struggling through this confusion. Some persons use the term 'handicap' to identify with the disability movement, while others use it to indicate a functional limitation. The term 'handicapped' is also used in different ways by different persons. Some disability activists may be comfortable saying, 'I am disabled because I have paralysed limbs, but I am not handicapped, because I have a job and a family.' For the same circumstances, others might say, 'I am handicapped because I have paralysed limbs, but I am not disabled, because I can move around quite well in a wheelchair' (Pfeiffer, 1993; Omansky, Gordon and Rosenblum, 1997).

This confusion is still sorting out in different arenas of public life. For example, in 1995, signs at the entrance to some stores changed to 'Persons with disabilities please contact service desk for assistance.' This sign indicates two important changes: the term 'handicap' has been replaced, and the impact of people-first language is present, meaning that disability is only part of identity. In 1997, the sign 'handicapped parking' was gradually replaced by 'disabled parking'. It can be expected that the term's use will continue to diminish, but the possibility should not be excluded that it will be reclaimed by certain groups in the future. Recently, some disability activists have reclaimed the outmoded term 'cripple', which has a history of slowly being replaced by the term 'handicap' in the period between the turn of the twentieth century and the 1950s. They did so for purposes of personal identification and social movement.

The signs in stores or in their parking places are not a reflection of charity, but an implementation of legal changes, as well as the interest of stores to build a positive image and find an edge in the game of competition. The Americans with Disabilities Act requires that barriers that make participation impossible or difficult be taken away. In the case of stores, it means making available accessible parking, automatic doors, wheelchairs, and sometimes personal assistance with shopping. The emphasis is on accessibility. The business world translates the requirements of the law in policy and advertisement, and tries to use them to compete, as can be seen in the speed with which the new requirements are implemented. Stores such as Walmart use persons with disabilities in their television advertisements to communicate their care for the customer and for customer service, and to emphasise their correct interpretation of the pluralism in American society. While the history of racial integration still serves as the model, there is an effort to add a person in a wheelchair or a person with Down's syndrome. The person in the wheelchair brings the image that persons with disabilities can work and shop like anyone else, and that neither costs nor effort will be spared to provide customers with the best service. The use of persons with Down's syndrome in advertisements adds the quality 'cute' to goods being sold.

The reaction of stores to the ideology which has been building up surrounding disability has another dimension: one of potency. Disabled people represent a market; they are people who work and contribute to society, and, ultimately, they are people, to be addressed in people-first language. Ironically, the term disability also expresses the opposite, the negation of ability. The 'disability ideology' has, for the business world, many recognised characteristics, because it is part of the mainstream ideologies that sprouted in the 1960s out of the civil-rights movement. But the consequences of this disability ideology for the personal lives of people with disabilities are hard. Disability is in essence about ability. There is no avoiding physical or mental limitation, and the ideology of charity or of equal chances has become too weak an argument with which individuals with disabilities can ask for solutions to the real problems that are inherent in the experience of a disability. In a sense, by moving the person to the forefront in the 'person with a disability' expression, the possibility of real problems has been diminished. The problem is characterised as no longer in the person but in the environment. Disability advocates are already seeing the danger in overemphasising the problem of disability as environmental, and have started to define disability identity in terms of 'ambiguity', recognising the danger of 'disability as social construction', which ignores real problems (Gill, 1997).

HANDICAPS DO NOT EXIST

One can question the fact that persons with completely different bodily or mental impairments, such as deafness, blindness or mental dysfunction, are categorised together as 'handicapped' or 'disabled'. These terms do not respond to an observed impairment, but need to be understood as a social reality, the result of an interaction at the level of society in which the needs of that society are expressed. It is interesting to note that in African languages, both contemporary or in proto-Bantu languages, there is no equivalent for the word 'handicap'. This indicates that the term has an important western influence. Terms for lame, deaf and blind are available in African languages because they respond to an observable reality. The necessity for a generic term does not seem to present itself. The development of local generic terminology is sometimes delayed, partly because such terms are adopted from colonial languages. Where an African language is the official language of the country, for example Kiswahili in Tanzania, such generic language development may occur faster. One stage in generic language development, for example in the Shona language of Zimbabwe, may be that the term for 'physical disability' or lameness may be adopted as a generic category (Devlieger, 1998).

A policy toward people with disabilities can be connected to the need for cohesion in times of danger, or the need for unity in times of confusion. Such a need gets translated in an ideology on the position of persons with disabilities, and finds an entrance in language use. Generic terms such as 'handicap' or 'disability' are therefore good instruments for anthropological research on the ways societies handle impairments. Such ways are always connected to a certain historical period and culture. To research them, cross-cultural and historical work is necessary. For example, the connections between the term 'invalidity' and war experience are: to have become 'invalid' because of war, the societal position of the veteran, and the societal response in terms of insurance. Equally, the term 'mentally defective' is connected to war experience; only, here it is connected to being unsuited for participation in war. The term was developed to suit the testing of recruits.

The development of generic terminology is also culturally inspired. There is a strong field of tension in American culture between the recognition of individuality and the effective participation of individuals in society. An analysis of these tensions is outside of the purpose of this article, but the fundamental reason needs to be sought in the Protestant ethic and the history of the United States as a country of immigrants.

The tension between an emphasis on individual differences on the one side, and societal control on the other, has historically had an important influence on attitudes and expectations toward persons with disabilities. The tension aids in clarifying some radical points of view toward persons with severe mental retardation in American society: from sterilisation in the 1920s to creating the possibility and the obligation to work in the 1990s.

Radical viewpoints in the official debate get reduced in the daily use of language concerning the life of persons with disabilities. Also, the official and scientific terminology that reflects a phenomenon never provides the totality of thought. Names of organisations often change only after a certain terminology has been used in daily, official and scientific language. A good example is the name change from 'American Association for Mental Deficiency' to 'American Association for Mental Retardation', which took place in 1980, long after the term 'mental deficiency' had been discontinued.

HANDICAP AND DISABILITY IN A SEMIOTIC SQUARE

In a semiotic square, it is possible to embed a term in a basic opposition derived from antonyms. For example, the antonym of 'beautiful' is 'ugly'. The purpose of constructing such a square is 'to see the deep logic of the whole, which always exists from fundamentally opposed concepts. The value is less in the opposite terms than in the opposition itself. Its power is to show the logical path [of conceptual development].' (Stiker, 1987, p. 166; my translation.) The semiotic square is based on two semantic axes. The first is one of contrariety, and is composed of an assertion and a negation on the horizontal axis. For example, there is only meaning in the term 'life' because of its contrary meaning in the term 'death'. The diagonal semantic axes represent contradiction, that is, the presence or absence of meaning. For example, there is only 'life' if one can conceptualise the absence of life. The result is a four-term constellation in which a new type of semantic relation, implication or complementarity, appears—'life' implies 'non-death', 'death' implies 'non-life' (Nöth, 1990, p. 318–19). It is important for the social scientist to understand the logical cohesion of concepts such as handicap or disability, well knowing that this logic is cast in a socio-cultural context.

Figure 2.1 is a semiotic square of the term 'handicap'. The basic opposition is between 'normal' and 'handicapped'. 'Normal' is the absence of deviation. In policy-directed thought, 'handicap' is equalised with 'lack of chances'. Being normal is the consequence of not being handicapped,

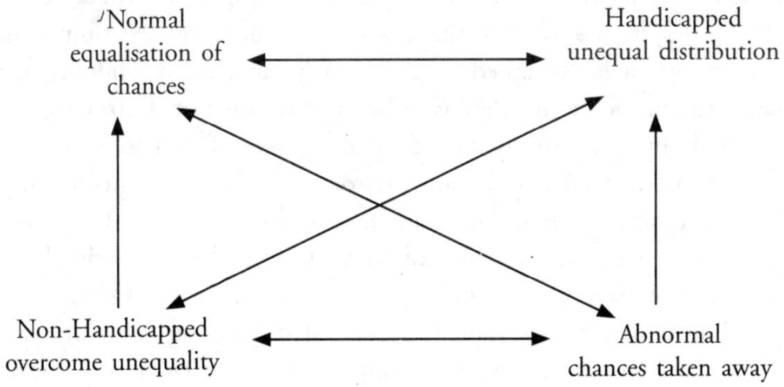

Figure 2.1. The Meaning of the term 'Handicap'

a situation in which the inequality of chances is undone. In other words, an inequality of chances which is undone leads to normality, a logic that makes sense in the United States of the 1960s and 1970s. 'Handicapped' refers to unequal distribution of characteristics in a group of people, and is the result of the 'abnormal', which represents a situation where chances were taken away. In the logic of handicap there is some optimism. Potential is ascribed to a change in action that is based in the calculable lot of chances. The optimism in the logic of handicap goes back to the 1950s, with high points in the 1960s and 1970s, but diminishing its force in the 1980s and 1990s.

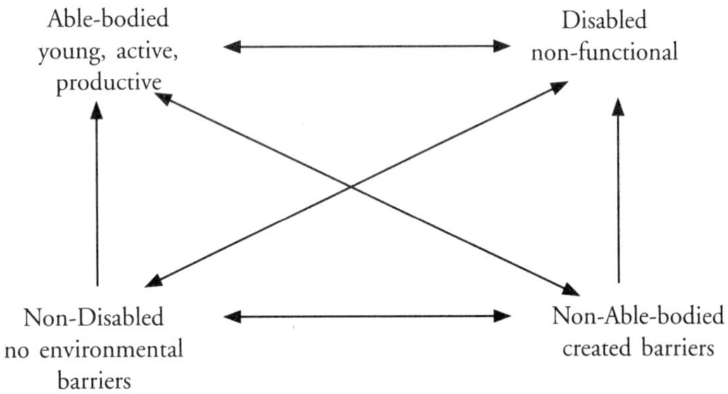

Figure 2.2. The Meaning of the term 'Disability'

Figure 2.2 is a semiotic square of 'disability'. It appears that the deep logic is totally different from the logic of handicap. The term *disability* was chosen despite the fact that the new term includes the negation of *ability*. The image of 'able-bodied' is of being 'young, active and productive', while the image of 'disabled' is of being 'non-functional'. In language use on disability, the issue is not of equal chances offered to an individual, but of barriers created in an environment. When someone disabled 'cannot function', it is the result of a relation between that individual and his or her environment, not from the fact that the individual does or does not have the capability. In other words, when someone with a physical or mental deviation is successful in meeting culturally valuable expectations, such as having a family, buying a car or having a job, that person is not 'disabled'.

That the origin of non-functioning does not necessarily need to be sought in the individual but in the poor adaptation of the environment is a very important shift. The implication is that when the environment is adapted to a deviation, there is no excuse for the person with a disability to not answer the expectation of being 'young, active and productive'. This is the underlying meaning of the current legislation pertaining to persons with disabilities in the United States, and some of its important shifts in service delivery. In this context, it needs to be noted that both 'handicapped' and 'gifted' are sometimes put in the same category. The largest and most prestigious organisation that represents special education, the Council for Exceptional Children, represents both groups.

HISTORICAL BACKGROUND OF THE SHIFT FROM 'HANDICAPPED' TO 'DISABLED'

Biklen and Bogdan claim that the term 'handicap' is derived from the fact that persons with disabilities were begging, cap-in-hand (Biklen and Bogdan, 1977). The historical evidence for such a claim needs to be produced. Rather, it seems that the authors produced a plausible explanation in support of a case for overall dismissal of negative attitudes toward persons with disabilities. An exploration of the historical emergence of the term handicap in the United States is beyond the scope of this article. The gradual replacement of the term 'handicap' by 'disability' in the United States was initiated by emphasising the negative connotations of the term 'handicap' and labelling the use of this term as medical and limiting. It also implies that there is no connection with the social and physical environment of the disabled individual (Pope and Tarlow, 1991; Brown, 1993).

There is, however, an important aspect of handicap that remains unaccounted: namely, the fact that handicaps provide access to services. Parent associations and the civil-rights movement have made very significant contributions to increasing such access. For example, access to education was strongly supported by parent associations, in preparation of legislation (Education of All Handicapped Children Act, P.L. 94–142 of 1975), as well as in the implementation of service provisions. The principle of 'equal access' was strongly supported by the civil-rights movement and its call for equal rights for every citizen. Historically, the civil-rights movement ignored persons with disabilities, but many groups, including people with disabilities, benefited from its principles.

Once access to the school system was obtained, the parent associations lost a great deal of their motivational strength. This development was enhanced as more professional support for service provision became available. The civil-rights movement measures 'normal' according to the outcomes of chances and rights. In order words, 'normal' is a matter of proportion and statistical expectations; it evolves from a discrepancy between reality and what can be expected as the result of pure chance. Someone belongs to the category 'normal' when a personal situation is the result of access to equal chances and rights; or, in other words, where a person's outcomes do not deviate beyond what would be ordinarily expected, a statistical mean. Handicapped persons were labelled 'abnormal' in the 1970s because they were not offered access to equal chances. The social status of a handicapped person was the result of the creation of a situation of unequal chances. While this was interpreted for many years as that person's 'rightful place', the civil-rights movement made it possible to interpret lack of access to equal chances as discrimination.

HANDICAP AND DISABILITY IN THEIR SOCIETAL CONTEXT

The validity of a semiotic analysis of the terms handicap and disability needs to be tested in the societal context and in relation to the personal experiences of young persons with disabilities. This two-fold test needs to form the basis of the analysis. Without such a test, a semiotic analysis is too far removed from reality. People who were born in the 1970s with disabilities did not have, in comparison to earlier generations, an experience of institutionalisation; they were not housed in separate institutions. The deinstitutionalisation of persons with mental retardation since the 1960s has been changing the nature of the social stigma that these persons have carried: normality is something that is feigned; people with disabilities 'pass'; the ignoring of difference is a new game that is played by both persons with mental retardation and other persons in their daily environments. Edgerton described the process of 'passing', and clarified the role of a benefactor in making the process possible (Edgerton, 1993). His analysis was embedded in the symbolic interactionism of Goffman, in which the concept of 'stigma' is central, and the influence of culture and history are marginal. It is only since the 1980s that anthropologists have started to analyse disability in the United States in terms of culture (Groce, 1985; Langness and Levine, 1986; Murphy, 1987; Philips, 1990).

American youngsters with mental retardation, who became adults in the 1990s, were educated until the age of 18 or, depending on specific state legislation, up to 21 years of age. This life experience is the result of a particular historical period, beginning in the 1920s and culminating with the efforts of parents of children with disabilities in the 1950s, and ultimately resulting in the Education of All Handicapped Children Act of 1975. This law ensured that children with disabilities obtained access to education in public schools.

The implementation of this law encountered uneasiness in both teachers and regular students. Teachers saw the decision as a threat to the level of education, and as a form of protection for students with mental retardation. The majority of students may have stayed indifferent, but some did develop teasing or even antagonistic behaviour. In such situations, students with mental disabilities had to maintain themselves. The stigmatisation of young adults with mental retardation in the 1990s was the one immediate outcome. Positive in this development is that there is now a place for persons with disabilities in the world of adults, supported by the protection of parents. On the other hand, there are considerable problems in relationships with peers (Devlieger, 1995).

It is important to understand that stigmatisation is historical, not a static given. This is illustrated by the names that were applied to persons with mental retardation in the United States during the nineteenth century: idiot, feeble minded, defective, deficient, mentally subnormal, mentally deficient and mentally retarded. The term *mental retardation* as it is currently used must be regarded as an American development. It has a negative connotation in many English-using areas outside of the United States (Fernald, 1995). The changes in terminology need to be connected directly to the social-political climate in the United States, and support the position that 'to be mentally retarded' is being constantly reinterpreted in the course of time (Lea, 1988; Trent, 1994). In the person who carries the label of mental retardation, the societal and ideological ideas of historical time are reflected. The historical development of the conceptualisation of mental retardation is reflected in the fact that the nineteenth century was characterised by a search for a term that was sufficiently positive. In this sense, it can be argued that mental disability is continuously being reinvented, both to avoid negative historical connotations and to adapt the new term to a new social and cultural context.

EXAMPLES

Young people with mental retardation who have completed secondary education since the mid-1980s belong to the half of American youth for whom college education is generally not an option. They belong to a 'forgotten half' (Glover and Marshall, 1993), in the sense that the ideal of obtaining a college education or exercising a profession is not an option. Some become strongly immersed in the world of mental retardation and the variety of programmes that are geared towards different age groups.

Sami (a fictitious name) is a 20-year-old Indian-American man who is mentally retarded. His mental disability does not allow him to have a simple conversation. He is also physically disabled, and can only walk with difficulty, using crutches or, most of the time, a wheelchair. Sami can do simple tasks at a photocopying machine. However, these tasks cannot be done independently.

Steve, 21 years old, has no physical limitations, and can understand and engage in a conversation, follow rules, and execute tasks on an assembly line. His abstract thinking is limited, and his reading and writing skills are limited for his age. He struggles most to maintain social relationships, especially with his peers.

Both men, while they are identified as mentally retarded and have strongly different intellectual and physical capabilities, are also the reflection of a particular historical development. Both were born in the 1970s as 'handicapped', and both became adults as 'disabled persons'.

Sami lives at home and makes photocopies three mornings a week at a research institute of a major university. He has a personal assistant, who is paid by Sami's father and who is supervised by an adult agency for persons with mental retardation. The system is known as supported employment, which means that persons with mental retardation receive personal assistance, making work in an ordinary job and circumstances possible. For lay people who are not familiar with the ideological background, the system seems somewhat absurd, because the work of one person is now being performed by two persons, and the possibility that Sami will ever do the work independently is rather slim. However, because of budgetary arrangements that support the system, and because advocates argue that such a system is more cost-effective than maintaining special institutions and work environments, the implementation of such programmes makes sense. Sami's life is couched in cultural programmes and projects such as supported employment, which are derived from a mainstream ideology in which paid work in the community is considered extremely important. From the perspective of persons with mental retardation, supported employment can be a step in a career of decreased support and, ultimately, independent work. Programmes such as supported employment are part of what makes a culture of mental retardation: the development of a specific, historically determined, long-term plan, with different steps for different life-course developments. In its implementation, such a plan is the result of negotiations between families and adult agencies, against the background of socially important ideals, such as 'independence' in American culture.

What for a lay person may seem an absurdity must be understood, from an economical point of view, as a radical reinterpretation of *ability* as the result of a successful interaction between a person and an environment. Only, the accent is shifted toward a restructured environment. Sami's personal assistant is part of a restructured environment which enables Sami 'to work'. Within the ideology of handicap, Sami would not 'work', but would be involved in an institute, a day centre or a protected workplace, where he would have been largely the receiving party. In a very radical way, access to services is being transformed by the disability ideology to an access to services that enable Sami to be a giving party. At the workplace, this is recognised regularly by emphasising the work that Sami does. Within the disability ideology, and the available legislation and funds, there is no longer the excuse that persons with disabilities, irrespective of the severity of disability, cannot work. Sami lives at home and goes to work as an expression of a societal development which transforms the disability of his handicap into ability.

Steve reflects the shift from 'handicap' to 'disability' in a very different way. As a white youngster born in a rural town in the 1970s, his mental retardation was translated not to life in an institution but, rather, to access to an ordinary public elementary school, followed by education in an ordinary high school, from which he exited with a high school diploma. It was in many instances a hard experience, because both teachers and students had limited experience with students with mental disabilities. Steve remembers very clearly the kind and amount of teasing by other students, the uneasy reaction of the school administrators, and the role of his parents in mediating conflicts. But he also remembers the assistance and support of certain teachers, and of a small group of students that would take his side. Steve's experiences were especially hard because he was one of the first students with mental limitation at his high school, and served in this sense as a test case.

The ideology of disability that Steve experienced after high school was no less hard. Steve's parents did not have the option to refer him to an institution, but needed to find a solution for his ability. In coordination with the high school and an adult agency for persons with mental retardation, they decided that Steve would have to make it on his own, since such a decision would have to come sooner or later. The responsibility for Steve's independence was transferred from his parents to the adult agency, which adopted Steve in a group home and enabled him to work in a sheltered workshop. Group homes are regular houses in which a number of adult persons with mental retardation live together. Each group home has a staff that carries responsibility for the supervision of house chores, recreation, and division of other group-home tasks. The adult agency is obliged by law to arrange work for Steve, because a person who lives in a group home cannot reside at home during the day without having been involved in an activity outside of the house. In other words, the ability of Steve is regulated by law. For Steve this means that every workday he takes a bus to work at the sheltered workshop. Steve's perspective on life is the result of an imposed need to grow in independence, at the level of both living and work. He hopes within the near future to move out from the group home and to live in a supervised apartment that is managed by the same adult agency. In terms of his work career, he hopes to follow the path of some of his peers, who ultimately obtained a minimum-wage job in the city, such as work at a fast-food restaurant.

The examples of Sami and Steve allow us to see how mental retardation has developed historically from 'handicap' to 'disability'. It is interesting that it is not the degree of mental limitation that ultimately provides direction to the lives of these young men, but more the influence of their environment and of the way a society constructs the phenomenon of disability. In the case of Sami, the support of his father was crucial; and for Steve the policy and a variety of services were crucial. In both cases, the ideology of ability had an important role.

DISCUSSION

Research on the cultural meaning of terminology is essential in the study of daily language use and the discourse surrounding a particular phenomenon. The shift in American language use from 'handicap' to 'disability' has important cultural and historical backgrounds. Both terms have cultural and historical meanings which makes their use in changing societal circumstances impossible. Certain terms become obsolete. The internal logic of terms is more than the accumulation of negative connotations, which is often advanced as a reason for a change in terminology. A semiotic analysis makes the internal logic of terminology visible.

What has remained undeveloped in this article is an analysis of the distribution of terms between daily language use and discourse. For example, the term 'handicap' is still part of daily American language use, but it has disappeared in discourse. The use or lack of use of certain terms in different arenas, and the influence of the media on the process of terminology distribution, need to be part of a separate study.

It has been emphasised that an anthropological study of disability cannot be limited to an analysis of concepts and terms without testing them against the life-course of real persons to whom the term 'disability' can be applied. Having a disability is a complex phenomenon, because the entire life of a person (learning, education, work, marriage, family, division of work and economy) is being influenced. Because of this holistic nature, the phenomenon of 'disability' and the way a society handles the phenomenon are unique opportunities for social scientists. There are several reasons why such a development has largely not occurred. The first needs to be sought in the development of disciplines, and the way subjects for study have been partitioned and claimed. Anthropological research has taken the cultural and social dynamics of *groups* to explain variation and typical patterns of behaviour. Second, the intersection with societal and ethical considerations regarding disability has distanced the phenomenon from social-science research. Certain western ideologies, for example those that prescribe different forms of charity, alienate social-science research endeavours. Third, disability is often seen as an epiphenomenon of social and cultural dynamics, and for this reason it is dismissed as an avenue for social-science research. However, it is from its unique vantage point that disability research provides a unique critique of culture and society.

The study of the logic inherent in terminology use and its impact on real lives is important. Professional groups are usually the first consumers and implementers of shifts in discourse. Becoming more clearly aware of the logic in terminology and its impact may contribute to the practice of professionals and consumers in the rehabilitation process. Such a consciousness may explain the fact that rehabilitation processes occur in the context of a societal discourse of disability. A historical awareness among professionals and its communication to consumers may add a human dimension to the rehabilitation process. In social terms, it may imply that people with disabilities are more centrally located in a society's political process. However, professionals and people with disabilities should also be aware that such a discussion may also lead to displacement and alienation.

References

Biklen, D. and Bogdan, R. 1977. 'Media portrayals of disabled people: a study in stereotypes', *Interracial Books for Children, Bulletin 8.*

Boston, B.O. 1992. 'Portraying people with disabilities: toward a new vocabulary', *The Editorial Eye*, 15: 1–3, 6–7.

Bourdieu, P. 1991. *Language and Symbolic Power.* Cambridge: Harvard University Press.

Brown, S.C. 1993. 'Revitalising "handicap" for disability research', *Journal of Disability Policy Studies*, 4: 57–76.

Devlieger P. 1995. *On the Threshold of Adult Life: Life-Course and Discourse of Mental Retardation in American Culture.* Doctoral dissertation. Urbana: University of Illinois at Urbana-Champaign.

———. 1998. 'Physical "disability" in Bantu languages: understanding the relativity of classification and meaning', *International Journal of Rehabilitation Research*, 21: 51–62.

Dijkers, M. 1995. Personal communication.

Edgerton, R. 1993. *The Cloak of Competence*. Berkeley: University of California Press.

Fernald, C.D. 1995. 'When in London: Differences in disability language preferences among English-speaking countries', *Mental Retardation*, 33: 99–103.

Foucault, M. 1965. *Madness and Civilisation*. New York: Random House.

———. 1966. *The Order of Things: An Archaeology of the Human Sciences*. New York: Vintage.

———. 1972. *The Archeology of Knowledge and the Discourse on Language*. New York: Pantheon.

Gill, C. 1997. Personal communication.

Glover, R. and Marshall, R. 1993. 'Improving the school-to-work transition of American adolescents', *Teachers College Record*, 94: 588–610.

Groce, N. 1985. *Everyone Here Spoke Sign Language*. Cambridge: Harvard University Press.

Langness, L.L. and Levine, H.G. 1986. *Culture and Retardation*. Dordrecht: D. Reidel.

Lea, S.L. 1988. 'Mental retardation: social construction or clinical reality', *Disability, Handicap and Society*, 3: 63–69.

Murphy, R.F. 1987. *The Body Silent*. London: Phoenix.

Nagi, S.Z. 1965. 'Some conceptual issues in disability and rehabilitation', in Sussman, M.B. (ed.), *Sociology and Rehabilitation*. Washington: American Sociological Association, pp. 100–113.

———. 1969. *Disability and Rehabilitation: Legal, Clinical and Self: Concepts and Measurements*. Columbus: Ohio State University Press.

———. 1991. 'Disability concepts revisited: implications for prevention', in Pope, A.M. and Tarlow, A.R. (eds), *Disability in America: Toward a National Agenda for Prevention*. Washington: Institute of Medicine, National Academy Press, pp. 309–27.

Nöth, W. 1990. *Handbook of Semiotics*. Bloomington: Indiana University Press.

Omansky, Gordon B. and Rosenblum, K.E. 1997. 'Ignoring disability: an impaired sociology', *Twenty-second Meeting of the Social Science History Association*, 16–19 October, Washington, DC.

Pfeiffer, D. 1993. 'The problem of disability definition', *Journal of Disability Policy Studies*, 4: 77–82.

Philips, M.J. 1990. 'Damaged goods: oral narratives of the experience of disability in American culture', *Social Science and Medicine*, 30: 849–57.

Pope, A.M. and Tarlow, A.R. 1991. *Disability in America: Toward a National Agenda for Prevention*, Washington: National Academy Press.

Reynolds Whyte, S. 1995. 'Disability between discourse and experience', in B. Ingstad and S. Reynolds Whyte (eds), *Disability and Culture*. Berkeley: University of California Press, pp. 267–91.

Stiker, H-J. 1987. 'Catégories organisatrices des visions du handicap', in J-M. Alby and P. Sansoy (eds), *Handicap: Vécu, Evalué*. Grenoble: La Penseé Sauvage, pp. 193–78.

Trent, J. 1994. *Inventing the Feeble Mind.* Berkeley: University of California Press.
World Health Organization (WHO). 1980. *International Classification of Impairments, Disabilities and Handicaps.* Geneva: WHO.

3

Community, Individual or Information Development? Dilemmas of Concept and Culture in South Asian Disability Planning

M. Miles

HISTORICAL BACKGROUND

In 1824, when Raja Kali Shanker Ghosal proposed opening an asylum for blind paupers at Benares, fears were voiced that it would attract

> … a Congregation at Benares of blind persons to such an extent as would be in many respects inconvenient and render the accommodation of them all in the Institution impracticable. Disappointment to many unfortunate objects would be the consequence and Benares and its vicinity would be crowded with applicants for admission on the occurrence of vacancies (India Office, 1826).

Modern tourists in South Asia are often warned that giving to one disabled beggar will attract 'swarms'. Quakers at Seoni in the 1890s delegated sheep-or-goat judgements to those with well-honed discriminatory faculties:

Miles, M. 1996. 'Community, individual or information development? Dilemmas of concept and culture in South Asian disability planning', *Disability and Society*, 11: 485–500.

> A crowd of halt and maimed and blind folks ... patiently await the arrival of the Mem-Sahib.... As only a fixed sum is given each month, and as this is known to the recipients, they themselves voluntarily arrange the matter of keeping out the undeserving. I pity the man who being able to work for his living sought a share of the weekly gifts; to raise the ire and start the tongues of the fifty old women I saw would be no trifling ordeal. (Pumphrey, 1900)

Many governments, welfare bodies or individuals faced with limitless numbers of 'needy and deserving' people go through moral contortions, and employ various filters, before fear of being 'swamped', or of pauperising the poor, hardens the heart.[1] At Benares in the 1820s, it was shown that most blind people lived within their families and would never wish to enter an asylum. Most could earn more begging than they would gain by asylum residence, where begging would be forbidden. Only the truly destitute would seek entry. An alternative proposal, that the Raja endow ophthalmological work so that less people would go blind, failed because existing hospitals were underutilised. The post-modern solution—changing the terminology so that problems disappear around the corner—did not occur to the Raja and his advisors. So the first disability institution in British India appeared. Later it hosted formal efforts to teach blind people reading and income-generating crafts (Shakespear, 1870). In fact, there were earlier asylums in South Asia dating back to 500 BC, efforts to teach disabled children from time immemorial, and creative activities by some disabled adults (Miles, in press). Yet, the Benares asylum is the first for which planning debates are extant, starting with the Raja's dismay at blind beggars' condition. To assess their needs, he commissioned a survey. Detailed discussion took place on the findings and their implications for the community at large, the public purse, the Raja's honour, and the moral fibre of the Empire (Miles, 1994).

South Asian disability-service planning has a past—though one barely known to modern planners. Some of the problems have changed little; yet, lacking a strong cultural-historical base, planners are vulnerable to western slogans of dubious cultural or conceptual relevance, compounding the

[1] Hodgkinson (1967) documents these processes exhaustively for nineteenth-century England. See also Ribton-Turner (1887) and Pullan (1994).

problems of decision-making.[2] Disability-service planning in nineteenth-century India, to the modest extent that it happened, was mainly done by westerners who lived in India and had to implement their own plans. There was then less disparity between disability provisions in India and England. For example, an occupational disability compensation fund existed at Madras as early as 1764 (Penny, 1904, pp. 385–89). By 1840, blind children at Calcutta were learning to read Lucas's new system imported from London (Annual Report, 1841, p. 11). An Idiot Asylum was separated from the Lunatic Asylum at Madras in 1841, before the first separate formal service for idiots at Bath in England (Crawford, 1914, II, p. 417; Editorial, 1847). The wretched disabled people observed in London slums by Hollingshead (1861/1985, pp. 26, 47, 78–79, 152, 169–70, etc.) could have come from any Indian city. Urban-rural differences, in terms of social organisation, were also smaller 150 years ago. Traditional communal care was stronger in villages than towns, but had not disappeared in the latter (Sanyal, 1977). By 1916, Jain, discussing begging, noted a decline in the joint family as 'welfare system'.

WESTERN TRENDS AND SLOGANS

Identifiable western trends and issues in the development of disability services have impinged on traditional Asian patterns of caring for, tolerating, ignoring or abusing disabled people. We will sketch recent trends of this kind, then some problems arising in the Asian disability

[2] The problems were experienced by the author and colleagues in the 1980s while developing disability centres in Pakistan as information and training resources for a community rehabilitation development project. A modest technical level of services and training was sustained, with information resources redirected more broadly to help local autonomous self-help organisations start services, each of which ultimately serves thousands rather than the hundreds served by a single centre. Other development agents planned 'centres of excellence' with trickle-down and outreach, rather than our modest 'centres of competence' aiming for low-tech multiplication; but few, if any, managed to provide both excellence and wide coverage. Many years elapsed before the problems of transferring knowledge and skills across not only cultural but *conceptual* boundaries fully dawned on us (Miles and Miles, 1993).

scene through the telescoped arrival of successive development waves. From the 1960s onwards, advocates for so-called 'community based' versus 'institutional' disability services battled in western countries, with associated slogans of normalisation, integration, demedicalisation and human rights.[3] Many 1970s slogans were exported to Asia in the 1980s without the context of the debates that accompanied them in Europe, and apparently with little awareness that their transplantation might be problematical (Kalayanpur, 1996). In fact, Asian disability services still suffer from western battles imported a century earlier, such as the Oral-Manual controversy in deaf education. Since then the Disabled People's Movement gathered strength in western countries, and efforts were made to define and give legal substance to disability rights. 'Social models' of disability were promoted (see the review by Oliver, 1986) which reallocated the 'problem' of disability to society, by analogy with women or blacks, i.e. 'There is no problem with women or blacks. Society has an oppression problem.' Similarly, one said there was nothing wrong with disabled people, who, like women or blacks, tended to be lumped improbably under one label. Society must change its attitudes and construct enabling, supportive, inclusive, people-friendly environments. These worthy ideals seem, however, to have had little impact on European mass perceptions. The unenlightened continue to think that if they have acquired an impairment resulting in the disability[4] of no longer being able to see their way around, or hear music, or stroll down to the pub, there must be something wrong with them, a personal problem for which society cannot entirely be blamed. Unenlightened employers continue to want smart, flexible, multi-purpose workers—if they cannot find suitable machines. Unenlightened politicians continue to ponder the cost of making Europe 'accessible'. Pfeiffer (1996), however, suggests some slow, but irreversible movement of opinion in North America.

[3] Some debates have been cyclical, as appears from nineteenth-century social history (see Moon, 1877; Report of the Royal Commission, 1889, *passim*; Rushton, 1988; Walmsley, 1990).

[4] The impairment-disability-handicap triad, devised in 1957–58 by Riviere (1970) and colleagues, aimed 'to re-orient professional attitudes and services towards individualised evaluation of the person as a human being, rather than the possessor of some detrimental condition' (p. 8).

There was some carry-through into international policy and planning for third-world disability services. From the 1960s on, 'community services' were experimented with. Segregated 'colonies' for disabled people fell into disfavour, for reasons ranging from ideological to economic. The term 'community-based rehabilitation' (CBR), borrowed from the American penal system, was given a new, cool, disability-friendly image, and is now in global use with at least six meanings:

1. Therapy or special measures given by families to disabled members in their homes, with some efforts made locally to change public attitudes and improve access to, for example, schools, public buildings and leisure facilities. The efforts may be supported by a paid worker or volunteers.
2. Therapeutic, educational, vocational or social *self-help* projects run by disabled people and their partners, whether in the home, centre or street, with or without external technical help.
3. An ideology whereby a nation's entire resources for medical and legal rehabilitation and social inclusion of disabled people (e.g. finance, skills, equipment, design and attitudes) are centrally planned and allocated equitably across the whole population. This promotes activities as in (l) and (2) 'at the community level', while noting that (1) and (2) are not the whole of 'CBR', which extends to the control of resources at district, provincial and national levels.
4. Projects where rehabilitation institutions or disability resource centres take knowledge and skills to rural or deprived communities. These are often called 'outreach' projects.
5. Externally-funded programmes in which networks of paid and trained 'CBR fieldworkers', without specific rehabilitation-centre bases, but with clear management structures, ongoing in-service training and negotiated referral contracts, undertake the mobilisation, training and public education tasks necessary before (1), (2) and possibly (4) can be expected to become self-sustaining.
6. A buzzword by which well-meaning people, not actively involved in community development, soften the contrast between their own access to professional services and the access of most of humankind; and by which aid agencies and institutions can appear to adopt the latest trend, while continuing their previous patterns of expenditure and service.

From about 1980 onward, largely monocultural western (or westernised) disability evangelists exported community slogans, muddled with the rhetoric of individual disability rights, to third-world countries having minimal formal service structures.[5] They found some willing converts and counterparts among western-educated Asians, and many countries happy to absorb 'soft aid' while deferring indefinitely the day when local budgets would take the strain. In many such nations, traditional *Gemeinschaft* caring continued in rural localities and kinship groups. People had few or no 'rights' as individuals, of the sort which they could 'claim' against state or society. But everyone was born into a network of relationships entailing mutual duties and obligations with a strong religious and economic underpinning.[6] Such networks have slowly evolved during the past century, under population pressure and mass-media cultural erosion, but they have been succeeded only minimally by voluntary organisations in which motivated citizens associate with like-minded strangers to demand their rights and assert their dignity under constructed identities such as 'Dalit', 'female' or 'disabled'.[7] Scotch (1988) notes that the construction

[5] See bibliographies in Werner (1987), and Thorburn and Marfo (1994); and references in Finkenflügel (1993), Zinkin and McConachie (1995), and Kalayanpur (1996).

[6] Hearing a lecture on the English Poor Law, Sir Subrahmanya Aiyar remarked, *without irony*, that the Laws of Manu had arranged such matters centuries earlier, so the topic had 'no practical importance in this country. ... Whether [Manu's provision] has been fully carried out or not, we may congratulate ourselves upon the fact that we have no Poor Law, and the poor are somehow or other maintained' (English Poor Law, 1910). India's ancient code of Brihaspati envisaged village welfare and relief societies (Jolly, 1889, pp. 346–50). There is little evidence of their practical functioning. Kautilya's *Arthashastra* (Rangarajan, 1992) allocated state handicraft work to disabled women (pp. 332–33) and recommended employing disabled people as spies (pp. 506–9). Implementation of these interesting policies is uncertain.

[7] By way of comparison, societies of blind people in China claim origins in antiquity, and certainly survived for centuries (Burgess, 1928, pp. 67–75, 117–18, 124), but these were united as occupational guilds with restricted entry, e.g. musicians and fortune-tellers (Burgess, 1928, pp. 159–60). In Japan, guilds of blind acupuncturists and of masseurs (who often doubled as moneylenders—a different kind of squeeze) flourished from the seventeenth century onward (Casal, 1962). Primary Health Care (PHC) boomed in 1970s

of the 'disabled' identity is hardly rapid or inevitable, even in western countries.

'Citizenship' as an identity entailing urban community responsibility is weak in much of South Asia, according to Ranganathananda (1995). He sees a continued hankering for responsibility to be shouldered 'by a king or *maharaja*,' the people 'being only *praja*s or subjects. *Praja* means offspring—children. As children, we have no responsibility.'[8] Furthermore, most people do not yet live in cities; and among those counted 'urban', the term hardly differentiates the minority with 'all mod-cons' from those agglomerated in shanty towns and overspills, lacking the benefits of either cities or villages. Vast numbers of people do not look to formal services for help, whether for disability or other welfare situations. They may be unable to look beyond their immediate kin, as so-called 'communities' become dysfunctional under growing pressures. A UN report noted:

> Many surveys and other research studies on all regions of the third world agree that deep and pervasive social, economic and political divisions mark the rural communities in which the majority often live a marginalised existence. (*Disability: Situation, Strategies, Policies*, 1986, p. 40)

Such thoughts underlie a deep scepticism about CBR among UN staff. Even if one believes that a margin of magnanimity is discernible in rural communities, it may vanish in periods of severe economic pressure. One analysis of CBR projects concluded:

> Where the primary focus of the family is on survival and overcoming poverty, involving the energy of both parents, commitment to the home management of disability is minimal. (Ganguly and Brar, 1993)

China, apparently preparing the ground for CBR development; but rural community participation in PHC collapsed in the 1980s (Cheung, 1995), leaving poor prospects for CBR. The urban CBR situation is also doubtful (Kwok, 1995).

[8] Ranganathananda's view is apparently more than a 'brown sahib' replay of colonial ideas of the 'native as child'. He searches the depths of Indian culture, finding *grihastha* (householder) virtues from which the modern responsible citizen can grow. The deficit of citizenship, if it is so, might well be connected (though causality would be hard to demonstrate) with the long subjection of Hindu populations under Mughal rule, followed by the painful reduction of the Mughal empire under the British.

The World Health Organisation (*Review of Primary Health Care Development*, 1982, p. 105), in a massive global review of more than 850 documents on Primary Health Care (PHC), earlier found that community involvement in PHC never begins effectively, in reality, prior to communities reaching a certain threshold in economic, social and educational development.

WHO's CBR strategy in the 1980s actually required communities to reach a higher threshold of development for CBR than for PHC, and a higher level than appears in many developing countries during the 1990s—a triumph of idealism over sober planning. From the mid-1980s, many disability institutions prudently began updating their image, to emerge as 'community centres'. There is also a growing realisation that CBR does not work without referral and resource centres. This was recognised in earlier WHO planning (*Community-Based Rehabilitation*, 1982, p. 9), but was played down for ideological reasons. It is now returning (Carpentier, 1994), though the blurring of boundaries infuriates CBR purists. Indeed, CBR in Oman is now described as 'Community Resource Centre-Based Rehabilitation' (Krefting, 1995).

SOUTH ASIAN MELANGE

Plans are needed for Asian populations, which include tens of millions who are technologically 6 months ahead to a year behind western consumers, and hundreds of millions who are technologically and educationally 20 to 200 years behind, those who Haywood (1995, p. 114) calls 'info-poor, underdeveloped and likely to stay that way'. Among them are many millions from every technological and educational stage who, despite pressures and economic stringency, are the equals or superiors of westerners in fulfilling traditional duties to close or distant relatives, and who are also equals or superiors in awareness of subtleties in human relationships and motivations, and in political sophistication. Across these populations there are also substantial differences of ethnicity, caste and religious practice, which may be recognised by differing laws applying to various groups within one nation, or which, if not recognised legally, may still constitute powerful obstacles to any unified policy. What is perceived as 'morally and ethically correct behaviour with disabled people' may vary sharply between three families on one street, who each belong to a different religious or cultural community. Furthermore, Ghosh and Talbani (1992) note:

> The basic values which underlie the current social order—liberty, equality, justice and fraternity—are not indigenous to Indian society.... India adopted a modern international ideology of equality and justice which was totally opposed to its traditions.

Whether wisely or hypocritically framed, the Indian Constitution of 1950 remains a dead letter for much of its population, especially its disabled people, when it concerns provision of meaningful education, health and welfare services. The government's colossal efforts since 1947 have been outstripped by the fecundity and increased survival rate of the populace.

INFORMATION APPROACHES

As an alternative to the culturally western 'rights' approach, disability-service development strategies may be re-conceptualised in information terms, broadly understood as *concepts*, *knowledge*, *skills*, *design* and *feedback*, and analysed as the flow and connection of these factors. This approach, which does not rely on vast and improbable ideological changes, is growing through the indirect influence of modern 'information societies'. Elsewhere, I have tried to indicate some part of its importance and relevance to Asian disability planning (Miles, 1990, 1993). Looking at different strategies in information terms reveals their complementarity, rather than pointlessly setting 'institution' and 'community' at odds. It also enables the planner to penetrate the jungle of existing buildings, technologies, professional privileges, political ideologies and time-worn practices, to review what the whole rehabilitation enterprise is supposed to be doing. Much has been learnt biomedically about various sorts of impairment and disability; and there is growing awareness of the ways in which impairments and disabilities become handicaps at the interface between individuals and society. Yet, this information is dispersed, and in third-world countries it is seldom focused effectively for primary and secondary prevention.

The total of disability-related information in a country, i.e. the available *knowledge* and *skills*, underpinned by various *concepts* and resulting in an array of *designs*, is distributed among professionals, clients, families, campaigning activists, associations and local networks, with certain nodal points and *feedback* mechanisms. How the information circulates, how it is applied and monitored, when and where disabled people augment or critique it, how it is studied by trainees, what feedback takes place, etc., are key issues which provide different perspectives for planning. In western countries, systems are highly complex and the amount of information is colossal. Studies have tended to concentrate on the use of various media to circulate bits and pieces of knowledge, without considering the underlying concepts or design applications. In most Asian countries, there is a much lower density of 'publicly accredited' knowledge, and one may trace more readily what is going on. But, as a corollary, there is less familiarity with concepts of information management, or with the idea that information is the new wealth, one that can be infinitely shareable and cumulative, rather than competitive and zero-sum. Access to Asian public-service systems is still highly personalised, i.e. dependent on 'connections', in contrast to the depersonalised 'supermarket-consumer' and 'batch-processing' style of western public services. Asian systems are dense with idiosyncratic 'human information', but are resistant to systematising in a way that could be modelled electronically, despite the efforts of modernising elites (see, for example, the uncritical approach to medical informatics in India by Indrayan, 1995). Modern technology vastly increases the *potential* for individuals and groups to acquire, appraise, use and disseminate rehabilitation information, making possible the self-empowerment of disabled people and families, forcing new roles for disability professionals as information guides and interpreters, and (possibly) shifting the attitudes of planners, designers, lawyers and broader communities. Yet, there are also drawbacks, presenting development planners with complex problems which have had little recognition or debate.

Incoming Disability Information has a Strong Western Liberal, Ideological and Conceptual Base

Such information may, for example, involve concepts of personhood, individuality, rights, relationships, etc., that differ substantially from those indigenous to Asian rural communities (Shweder and Bourne, 1982;

Hoch, 1993). Even with less clearly 'political' concepts such as those of 'teaching and learning' or 'the child', radical differences appear (Apte, 1961, pp. 152–92; Kakar, 1979; Misri, 1985). Yet these concepts are basic to transfer of knowledge and skills in special education and rehabilitation, to curriculum and programme design, and to the involvement of families and communities with disabled persons. Information mediators tend to be urban graduates, whose own education has been strongly western. There is a sharp split between the small 'modern sector' and the traditional masses. Some 'cultural' adaptation may be attempted, but it seldom reaches the conceptual level.

Efforts to transfer disability information do not lack all precedent. Similar convolutions were experienced when, for example, attempts were made to introduce kindergartens to India in the 1880s (Lamson, 1899). Kindergarten methods, which are relevant also to special-needs education, were subsequently promoted by the government of Bengal (Shahidullah, 1984). The new scheme came into effect in January 1901, and was intended to revolutionise Bengali school teaching by the introduction of a system under which 'children were trained but not taught.' The teachers themselves had not been trained before the launch of the scheme. After four years, 95 per cent remained ignorant of what they were officially meant to be teaching. Attempts to introduce a child-centred approach in Gujarat 80 years later followed a similar pattern of administrative bungling (Dyer, 1996).

Efforts to train Indian community-health volunteers in the 1980s, after sporadic experiments dating back to the 1840s, are similarly instructive. Their training was the most crucial moment in the implementation of the programme. This was where the much touted transfer of knowledge from professional institutions to community representatives was to take place. (Jobert, 1985)

What actually happened was a seriously flawed 'training of trainers', followed by compressed loads of knowledge getting dumped onto the community volunteers, with neither context nor reference to the social dimensions of health. These well-documented difficulties in introducing child-centred school practice and community-orientated health services to India over a period of 80 to 140 years cast doubt on the likely reception and speed of adoption in South Asia of western proposals in the much lower-priority disability field.

Developments giving Information Access to New Millions are Distancing them from the Hundreds of Millions who will Never Gain Access

Normally, 'development' cannot be expected to raise the poorest or reduce gaps—in practice; almost all 'development' *widens* the spectrum from 'have-nothings' through 'have-a-littles' to 'have-a-lots'. To give anything to those with nothing is difficult, since they usually lack storage capacity. Apart from what they consume hand to mouth, any surplus is quickly removed through various forms of exploitation practised by those who have a little, who are in turn exploited by the next layer up. An example of this process in disability-service development was denounced by Qamaruzzaman (1988) after studying a rural mental retardation project run under a Bangladeshi service organisation, which typically devoted most of its resources to a tiny minority of powerful urban families.

In theory, disability information should be transferable with less danger of early sequestration. What people know, if rooted appropriately in their concepts and language, cannot so easily be snatched; on the contrary, if they share it mutually, their knowledge should get enhanced. This was a principle of PROJIMO, the rural Mexican organisation in which the highly informative *Disabled Village Children* originated (Werner, 1987). Problems arise at an earlier stage, namely, of the capacity to receive and store. Packages of modern information contain a vast underpinning of concepts which are often hidden from the purveyors or are assumed (wrongly) to be universal. One such, in addition to the examples given above, is the idea that knowledge should be personally appropriated, tried out, questioned, tested and added to the individual learner's personal construction of the world (rather than being communally received and stored by community leaders). Without this individual-orientated concept and practice—absent from much of the world—the result of an offer of information is practically null. At best, some texts or a series of 'facts' may be memorised, with little or no internalised meaning.

Expansion of Information Enlarges Areas of Doubt where Specialists Clash, Forcing New Choices

The new choices, for which mid-level professionals feel as ill-equipped as clients, expose radical oppositions or discontinuities between modern, post-modern and traditional knowledge systems.

In traditional cultures, the 'smart cards' of illness and disability are held by deities and their local agents: the priest, shaman, hakim or vaid. The sick or disabled person's family presents him or her to this agent, who offers confident mumbo-jumbo, diagnosis, doses, prayers to say, and fees to pay. The information fuelling this system is limited, although some of it, such as the healer's knowledge of family psychology, may be perceptive; feedback and differentiation between successful and unsuccessful treatments is usually weak; and it is not for the family to question, or debate with, the practitioners. In the first flush of the modern system, basic sanitation and hygiene measures, antibiotics, immunisation, and nutritional knowledge are spread around confidently, whether or not the beneficiaries understand them. A more difficult phase follows, where health or rehabilitation measures are trade-offs between better and less desirable statistical consequences. The former practitioner assured clients that this injection, operation or gadget was undoubtedly the solution. Modern disability professionals or expatriate advisors cite risk figures and require a signed indemnity. Clients then seek further opinions. As disability information spreads, professionals tend to become guides rather than authorities.

In the disability-development field, the global polio eradication campaign illustrates some of the problems. To bounce governments into the substantial effort needed, much hype has been mounted, with the example of smallpox eradication as proof of feasibility. Yet there are major drawbacks 'known' but not discussed openly. Vaccination is a clean, technical solution, achievable by a military-style campaign, requiring minimal popular comprehension (Nichter, 1990). By contrast, polio is technically far harder to eradicate than smallpox. It requires a vast, improbable uplift of health care and autonomy among poorer South Asians. The failure of malaria control, rather than the success of smallpox, could be the pattern for outcomes with polio. Similar problems confront the (far less vigorous) campaigns against disabling iodine-deficiency diseases and lathyrism in South Asia. Though expertise is available, all three campaigns lack fire, partly because they hardly threaten the health of central planners or their children, whereas newly-resistant malaria and tuberculosis pose considerable threats. An opinion can always be found, from one expert or another, to justify reducing the priority of programmes that would benefit mainly disabled people or at-risk children living far from the capital city.

At the grass roots, there are problems even in giving information to families, especially the poorest, with a severely disabled infant. An honest prognosis, that with much family effort their child may gain the autonomy needed for basic daily living, though remain otherwise dependent throughout its life, is seldom accepted without prolonged and costly doctor-shopping. But once accepted, such a prognosis may precipitate a decision to 'let the infant go' (Scheper-Hughes, 1992). Infants are chattels still in rural Asia, mortality rates remain high, and autopsies are rare. If a counsellor deceives the family with unrealistic promises, a few years of life may be gained, although at some financial and emotional cost to the family, and perhaps the neglect of other children. Probably less than one in ten families, given the honest answer, would actually hasten a disabled infant's death. Yet, there is no shuffling responsibility off to 'social service provisions' or 'extended family networks'. The former are rudimentary; and the latter were never very reliable, and are crumbling.

Information Shock has Unpredictable Effects on Fragile People and Cultures Hooked to Electronic Networks

Large-scale disability information is a latecomer in the series of west-to-east information transfers and indigenous efforts. It coincides with the rise of immensely powerful media, whose impact as purveyors of disability information has been little studied in western countries (Brown et al., 1995; *Information Enables*, 1993). Western knowledge available by 1970 could probably have prevented half the impairments experienced in Asia now, and significantly changed the lives of millions of disabled Asians; yet the political will was lacking to disseminate this knowledge through the mass media in culturally appropriate forms. Momentum for better South Asian disability media began to grow in the 1980s, with some UNICEF pressure (*Childhood Disability and the Media*, 1984; Kolucki et al., 1988; Gill, 1990). Raina (1993) notes that by 1987 a Media Cell with regional task forces existed in India to enhance the role of the mass media in creating disability awareness. However, to be effective across the great range of disability concerns requires greater coordination than is common between government departments. Prasad (1994, pp. 47–71) lists the main information activities and media-production projects at national institutes. Non-governmental organisations continue to experiment with new and old media—whether puppet theatre, dance drama or printed cartoon strips—to communicate disability messages. But formal evaluations of the effects of disability information available through the mass media are rare. A meeting of Asian experts (Report, 1987) believed that 'Public information and awareness programmes had little impact among the rural populations, policy makers, employers, trade unionists and politicians' (p. 31). They could suggest only 'innovative media channels' to do better.

Apart from the lack of innovation and political will, one can no longer ignore the cultural devastation likely from being left out of the information explosion. The apocryphal don of Balliol College, Oxford, who intoned, 'I am master of this college; what I don't know isn't knowledge,' never logged on to electronic catalogues, networks or bibliographies. Modern postgraduates in the arts, science or philosophy from developing countries, who count as learned back home, are liable to humiliating encounters with this abundance when they pursue disability-related studies in the west. The total sum of formal, documented knowledge in their country can be balanced, like post-modern angels, on an electronic pinpoint.[9] Most of what is formally known about their countries has been published in English elsewhere. Since that data remains barely accessible, it has appeared without effective right of reply. Worldwide urban electronic networks are now delivering access, but we should not underestimate the damage to cultural confidence from the flood of electronic 'modern (= western) knowledge' into developing countries. A 'virtual brain drain' is occurring, of able people who remain physically in Asia but whose community and allegiance is to cyberspace, to the exciting, Anglophone Internet, a smarter universe than the dusty streets of Calcutta or Karachi.

[9] Macaulay (1835) notoriously found orientalists who valued 'the whole native literature of India and Arabia' no higher than 'a single shelf of a good European library.' After 160 years, Nobel Laureate Abdus Salam and Pakistani physicist Hoodbhoy are more scathing than Macaulay's orientalists in their estimate of the science, scientific publications and scientific mentality in Islamic countries. Hoodbhoy (1991) gives detailed evidence.

WESTERN INPUT?

Shifts from Tönnies' idealised *Gemeinschaften* to *Gesellschaften* (1955) have been happening over the past two centuries in Europe, whose masses are still adjusting to them as the information revolution generates new 'socioquakes'.[10] Asian societies are also undergoing several major shift patterns, but telescoped into decades. The social survival of disabled people in them has attracted little study. Westerners cannot be entirely neutral observers, since western economies generate many of the global stresses from which others suffer.

Many issues in disability development have had little serious discussion yet. In health development, prioritisation of child services over adult services is being questioned (Reich, 1995), but age issues seldom surface in the disability field. Several hundred thousand Asian children who suffer polio paralysis each year, and millions more who are at risk, while too young to make any moral choices, must compete for funding against highly vocal adults at risk from AIDS. The attraction of disability budgets to war zones has been little debated; media cameras follow war, funds follow the cameras. Men losing limbs in war are the most likely to absorb any available disability aid. Women and children suffering less heroic disabilities, and having minimal political clout, continue to rot. The ethical issues of relevance to disability that occupy the global stage are those that concern westerners: for example, bio-ethics, environmental pollution and disability-rights legislation. Yet the worrying biotechnology is available only in a few Asian cities, and hardly impinges on the masses preoccupied with day-to-day survival. Decisions that will generate disabling environmental hazards in Asia for the next twenty years have already been made, with minimal concern for such problems. South Asian governments may massage their international image with some modern-sounding disability laws, but lack the infrastructure and public support to give these more than cosmetic impact.

Is there any useful western contribution to these neglected Asian issues—or the reverse? Many westerners believe there is much to offer; fewer think there is anything to learn. Much recent western social science has generated and enhanced suspicion and mistrust: the semi-historical

[10] Bayley (1996) usefully analyses earlier South Asian information booms.

game of fingering the motivations of powerful groups; the exposing of conspiracies to dominate and oppress; the active fostering of resentment; and the promotion of criticism-struggle. These are luxuries affordable in western Europe, i.e. in societies that have begun to function with historically unprecedented levels of interconnectedness, public trust and cooperation. The latter factors have begun to be prized, and their fragility recognised, as the bleakness of a purely market-driven future becomes apparent. Yet the socio-political diseases of South Asia are the 'disconnections' of caste and the endemic mistrust towards anyone to whom one is not closely related. These add greatly to the time and energy costs of doing everything, whether buying a railway ticket, planning an accessible school, or motivating groups of disabled people. Such diseases are probably reinforced by western sociological imperialism, under which the efforts of health and rehabilitation workers, past and present, are rubbished by air-conditioned journalists and ivory-tower social scientists, those who seldom have personal experience of disability-service planning and delivery.

The inutility to developing countries of much western social science has been documented angrily by people who have tried it (for example, Pieris, 1969; Ake, 1979; Gardezi, 1993). Mshana (1992) insists on 'indigenous knowledge' as the only viable development base.[11] Doubtless, historical indigenous information is an illuminating starting point. The development of disability histories in South Asia is 'fundamental research' from which South Asians may more confidently develop culturally and conceptually appropriate disability services. Historical studies of South Asian disability information will also assist in evaluating western offers of knowledge, skills and design, revealing the points at which they may or may not fit indigeneous concepts. Some place exists for people, of whatever nationality, willing to undertake historical action research (Miles et al., 1995); listening long to the cultures and voices of Asian people; listening to disabled Asians; reflecting on disability ethics and choices with Asian colleagues; and strongly supporting those who are looking

[11] Mshana apparently defends the infanticide of disabled babies as a Tanzanian tribal custom and community decision (1992, pp. 117–20). Few westerners would follow him while memories linger of Nazi solutions. Poorer, more crowded populations may reluctantly participate.

deeper and taking the longer view. There is also a place for people who continue to take a friendly interest long after their suggestions have been ignored and the opposite done.

References

Ake, C. 1979. *Social Science as Imperialism.* Ibadan: Ibadan University Press.

Annual Report of the London Society for Teaching the Blind to Read. 1841. London: LSTBR.

Apte, D. 1961. *Our Educational Heritage.* Baroda: Acharya.

Bayley, C. 1996. 'Colonial rule and the "informational order" in South Asia', in Nigel Crook (ed.), *The Transmission of Knowledge in South Asia.* Delhi: Oxford University Press.

Brown, S., Roth, H. and Duncan, B. 1995. 'Searching electronic networks for information on disability', *International Rehabilitation Review,* 46 (1/2): 25–27.

Burgess, J. 1928. *The Guilds of Peking.* New York: Columbia University Press.

Carpentier, A-L. de. 1994. 'The role of institutions in community-based rehabilitation and in community-based special education', in *Making It Happen.* Paris: UNESCO.

Casal, U. 1962. 'Acupuncture, cautery and massage in Japan', *Folklore Studies,* 21: 221–35.

Cheung, Y. 1995. 'Community mobilisation and health care in rural China', *Community Development Journal,* 30: 317–26.

Childhood Disability and the Media: A Workshop Report, November 29–December 1, 1984. Bombay: UNICEF.

Community-Based Rehabilitation: Report of WHO inter-regional consultation, Colombo, Sri Lanka, 28 June–3 July 1982. Geneva: World Health Organization.

Crawford, D. 1914. *History of the Indian Medical Service 1600–1913.* London: Thacker.

Disability: Situation, Strategies, Policies. 1986. New York: United Nations Economic and Social Affairs.

Dyer, C. 1996. 'Primary teachers and policy innovation in India: some neglected issues', *International Journal of Educational Development,* 16: 27–40.

Editorial. 1847. 'Education of Idiots', *Chambers' Edinburgh Journal,* 8: 169–71.

English Poor Law. 1910. *Journal of the South India Association,* I (2 October): 186–218.

Finkenflügel, H. 1993. (ed.). *The Handicapped Community.* Amsterdam: VU University Press.

Ganguly, S. and Brar, B. 1993. 'CBR in India—some issues and reflections', *ActionAid Disability News,* 4 (2, Supplement): 17–20.

Gardezi, H.N. 1993. 'Academic sociology in Pakistan: a case of knowledge transfer across cultures', *Higher Education Group Annual 1992/1993*: 67–80.

Ghosh, R. and Talbani, A. 1992. 'Inequality and education in India: the case of the scheduled castes', in D. Ray and D. Poonwassie (eds), *Education and Cultural Differences.* New York: Garland.

Gill, R. 1990. *Preventive Health: Can We Improve our Communications about People with Disabilities?* Kathmandu: UNICEF.

Haywood, T. 1995. *Info-rich, Info-poor.* London: Bowker.

Hoch, E. 1993. 'Prevention and treatment intervention in the family', in M. Kapur et al. (eds), *Child Mental Health.* Bangalore: National Institute of Mental Health and Neuro Sciences.

Hodgkinson, R. 1967. *The Origins of the National Health Service.* London: Wellcome Historical Medical Library.

Hollingshead, J. 1861/1985. *Ragged London in 1861.* London: Smith, Elder; reprinted New York: Garland.

Hoodbhoy, P. 1991. Foreword by Prof Abdus Salam, *Muslims and Science.* Lahore: Vanguard.

India Office. 1826. Extract Public Letter from Bengal, 27 May. Boards Collections, Vol. F/4/955, Section 27109–27118.

Indrayan, A. 1995. 'Informatics: the key to efficiency', *World Health Forum,* 16: 305–11.

Information Enables: Improving Access to Information Services for Disabled People. 1993. London: Policy Studies Institute.

Jain, P.S. 1916. 'A preliminary note on pauperism in India', *Indian Journal of Economics,* 1: 351–68.

Jobert, B. 1985. 'Populism and health policy: the case of community health volunteers in India', *Social Science and Medicine,* 20: 1–28.

Jolly, J. 1889. *The Minor Law-Books. Part I: Narada, Brihaspati.* Oxford: Clarendon.

Kakar, S. 1979. 'Childhood in India: traditional ideas and contemporary reality', *International Social Science Journal,* 31: 444–56.

Kalayanpur, M. 1996. 'The influence of western special education on community-based services in India', *Disability and Society,* 11: 249–70.

Kolucki, B., Marchael, K. and Duncan, B. 1988. *How to Improve our Communications about People with Disabilities.* Islamabad: UNICEF.

Krefting, L. 1995. 'Oman adopts a community-based approach to childhood disability', *International Rehabilitation Review,* 46 (1&2): 20–21.

Kwok, J. 1995. 'The role of the family in disability-concerned policies and services: challenges for community-based rehabilitation in the Asian and Pacific decade of disabled persons, 1993–2002', *International Journal of Rehabilitation Research,* 18: 351–56.

Lamson, K. 1899. 'Kindergarten work in mission lands', in *Report of the Seventh Conference of the Foreign Missions Boards and Societies in the United States and Canada.* New York: Foreign Missions Library.

Macaulay, T. 1835. 'Indian education. Minute of the 2nd of February, 1835', in G. Young (ed.) (1967), *Macaulay: Prose and Poetry.* London: Hart-Davis.

Miles, M. 1990. 'Disability and Afghan reconstruction: some policy issues', *Disability, Handicap and Society,* 5: 257–67.

———. 1993. 'Service development by information, not ideology', in H. Finkenflügel (ed.), *The Handicapped Community.* Amsterdam: VU University Press.

———. 1994. 'Disability Care and Education in 19th century India: Some dates, places and documentation', supplement to *ActionAid Disability News*, 5(2).

———. (in press). 'Responses to mental retardation in South Asia: a 3000-year review', in G.D. Woodill and R. Hanes (eds), *The History of Disabilities: International Perspectives*. New York: Garland.

Miles, M. and Miles, C. 1993. 'Education and disability in cross-cultural perspective: Pakistan', in S. Peters (ed.), *Education and Disability in Cross-cultural Perspective*. New York: Garland.

Miles, M., Chandran, G. and Balasundaram, P. 1995. 'Mental handicap in Indian history: cross-cultural action research and communication', *International Journal of Special Education*, 10 (2): 12–21.

Misri, U. 1985. 'Child and childhood: a conceptual construction', *Contributions to Indian Sociology*, 19: 115–31.

Moon, W. 1877. *Light for the Blind*, 3rd edn. London: Longmans.

Mshana, R. 1992. *Insisting upon People's Knowledge to Resist Developmentalism*. Frankfurt: Verlag für Interkulturelle Kommunikation.

Nichter, M. 1990. 'Vaccinations in South Asia: false expectations and commanding metaphors', in J. Coreil and J. Mull (eds), *Anthropology and Primary Health Care*. Boulder: Westview.

Oliver, M. 1986. 'Social policy and disability: some theoretical issues', *Disability, Handicap and Society*, 1: 5–17.

Penny, F. 1904. *The Church in Madras*. London: Smith, Elder.

Pfeiffer, D. 1996. '"We won't go back"; the ADA on the grassroots level, *Disability and Society*, 11: 271–84.

Pieris, R. 1969. 'The implantation of sociology in Asia', *International Social Science Journal*, 21: 433–44.

Prasad, L. 1994. *Rehabilitation of the Physically Handicapped*. Delhi: Konark.

Pullan, B. 1994. '"Difettosi, impotenti, inabili": caring for the disabled in early modern Italian cities', in B. Pullan, *Poverty and Charity: Europe, Italy, Venice, 1400–1700*. Aldershot: Variorum.

Pumphrey, C. 1900. *Samuel Baker of Hoshangabad*. London: Hedley.

Qamaruzzaman, A. 1988. *A Survey on Mental Retardation: Nangalkot Rural Project*. Dhaka: Society for Care and Education of Mentally Retarded, Bangladesh.

Raina, R. 1993. 'Role of media in awareness creation on disability', in *National Conference on Welfare of the Disabled, Sept. 20–22, 1993*. New Delhi: Ministry of Welfare.

Ranganathananda, S. 1995. 'Enlightened citizen and our democracy', *Indian Journal of Public Administration*, XLI: 609–12.

Rangarajan, L.N. 1992. (transl. and ed.) *Kautilya: The Arthashastra*. New Delhi: Penguin.

Reich, M.R. 1995. 'The politics of agenda setting in international health: child health versus adult health in developing countries', *Journal of International Development*, 7: 489–502.

Report of the Regional Expert Seminar to Review Achievements at the Mid-points of the UN Decade of Disabled Persons, Bangkok, 2–5 June 1987. Bangkok: ESCAP.

Report of the Royal Commission on the Blind, the Deaf and Dumb, &c. 1889. London: HMSO.

Review of Primary Health Care Development. 1982. Geneva: World Health Organization.

Ribton-Turner, C.J. 1887. *A History of Vagrants and Vagrancy and Beggars and Begging.* London: Chapman and Hall.

Riviere, M. 1970. *Rehabilitation Codes: Classification of Visual Function.* Report to National Institute of Neurological Diseases and Blindness, U.S. National Institutes of Health.

Rushton, P. 1988. 'Lunatics and idiots: mental disability, the community, and the poor law in North-East England, 1600–1800', *Medical History*, 32: 34–50.

Sanyal, R. 1977. 'Indian participation in organised charity in early Calcutta, 1818–1866', *Bengal, Past and Present*, 96: 97–113.

Scheper-Hughes, N. 1992. *Death without Weeping.* Berkeley: University of California Press.

Scotch, R. 1988. 'Disability as the basis for a social movement: advocacy and the politics of definition', *Journal of Social Issues*, 44: 159–72.

Shahidullah, K. 1984. 'The new education in Bengal: the 1900 syllabus for the "kindergarten" and "lower primary" years and its problems', *Indian Economic and Social History Review*, 21: 215–47.

Shakespear, A. 1870. 'Annual report and accounts of the Asylum', in *Annual Report of the Dispensaries of the North-Western Provinces, 1869*, Appendix. Allahabad: n.d.

Shweder, A. and Bourne, E. 1982. 'Does the concept of the person vary cross-culturally?', in A. Marsella and G. White (eds), *Cultural Conceptions of Mental Health and Therapy.* Dordrecht: Reidel.

Thorburn, M. and Marfo, K. 1994. (reprint) (eds) *Practical Approaches to Childhood Disability in Developing Countries.* Tampa: Global Age.

Tönnies, F. 1955. *Community and Association (Gemeinschaft und Gesellschaft).* (transl. C.P. Loomis) London: Routledge and Kegan Paul.

Walmsley, J. 1990. 'Provision for the non-able-bodied poor in the eighteenth and early nineteenth centuries', *Local Historian*, 20: 9–19.

Werner, D. 1987. *Disabled Village Children.* Palo Alto: Hesperian.

Zinkin, P. and McConachie, H. 1995. (eds) *Disabled Children in Developing Countries.* London: MacKeith Press.

4

Disability: The Place of Judgement in a World of Fact

M.H. Rioux

INTRODUCTION

Two very different world views are reflected in the currently dominant research paradigm: one which is centralising and homogenising, and the other which stresses difference and diversity. In colloquial terms, these represent the 'melting pot' and the 'vertical mosaic'. These discrepant world views are particularly relevant when the issue is disability. The normative standard that ensues from either of these views has consequences in terms of both the importance placed on the abilities and disabilities manifested by people, and the social contribution made by individuals with disabilities. Empirical questions are driven by these implicit normative premises, despite the claims of objectivity so readily embraced by empiricists. Therefore, to some degree, the enterprise that we, as researchers, have to embark on is to uncover and disclose the premises of our research. I would argue that this is important because social, economic and political pressures are pervasive in research in this field. But I would also argue that it is a moral imperative to disclose the normative basis of the research in a field like ours, where the research affects the single most identifiably marginalised

Rioux, M.H. 1997. 'Disability: the place of judgement in a world of fact', *Journal of Intellectual Disability Research*, 41(2): 102–11.

class of people. Therefore, we ought to be more mindful of the potential value judgements and normative standards hidden in empiricism. Rather than simply engaging in a debate about one concept versus another, I want to step back and reflect upon the perspectives which underlie the various constructions of disability. It will then be possible to develop a methodologically rigorous and defensible approach to the way research is carried out in this field.

How disability is perceived, diagnosed and treated scientifically and socially is reflected in assumptions about social responsibility towards people with disabilities as a group. The assumptions or postulates about disability I will discuss are not mutually exclusive, nor are they chronological in time. Some disciplines have continued to characterise disability as a disease or a personal deficit, while others have adopted a framework in which disability is a social and political condition. There are any number of hybrids of these two major schools of thought. Consequently, policy, programming, treatment and care—both within the professional sphere and coming from government—reflect attempts to accommodate these shifting understandings of disability.

SOCIAL AND SCIENTIFIC FORMULATIONS OF DISABILITY

There are four social and scientific formulations of disability that can be identified, and they are reflected in the treatment of people with disability in law, policy, programmes and rights instruments. Two of these formulations emanate from theories that view disability as a result of individual pathology, and two from disability viewed as a result of social pathology (Figure 4.1).

Formulations that Focus on Disability as Residing in the Individual (Individual Pathology)

I am going to look at both the biomedical approach and the functional approach. These formulations have a number of common characteristics:

1. disability is approached as a field of professional expertise;
2. a positivist paradigm is used;

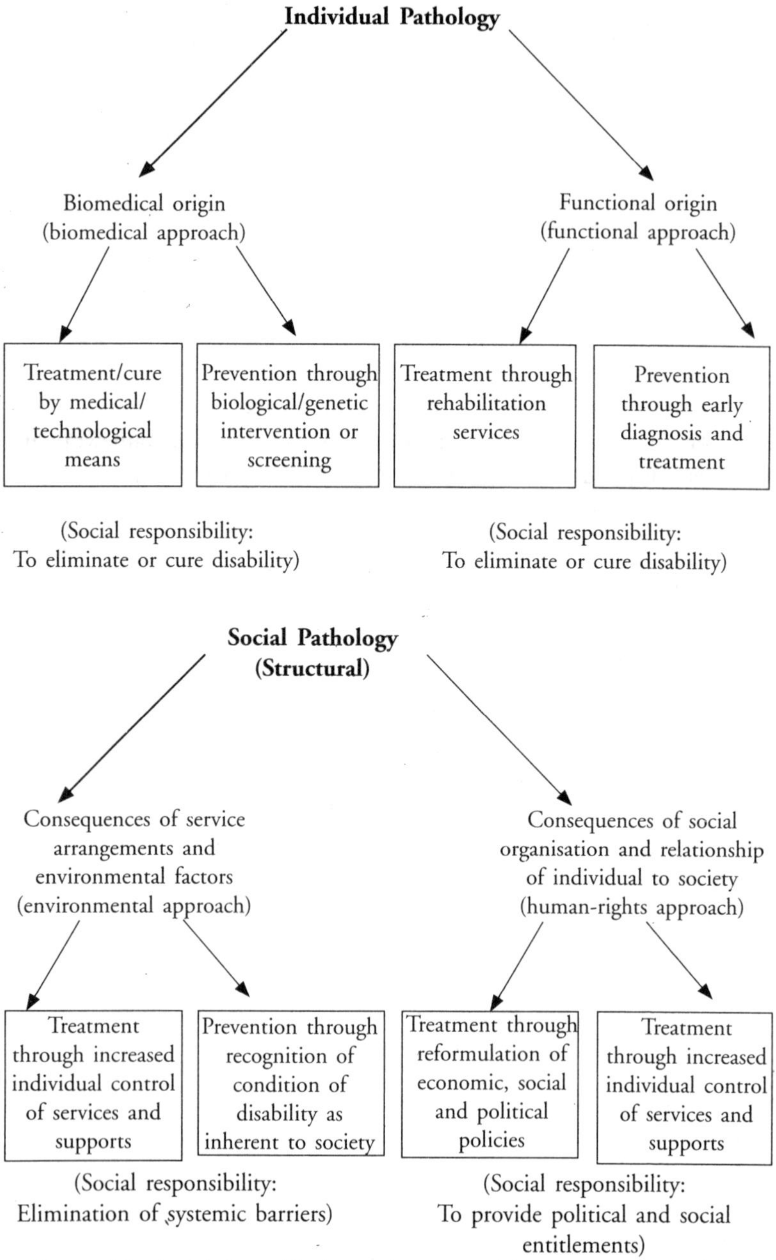

Figure 4.1. Social Scientific Formulations and Treatment of Disability

3. primary prevention, including biological and environmental conditions, is emphasised;
4. disability is characterised as incapacity in relation to non-disabled people, i.e. a comparative incapacity;
5. disability is viewed as an anomaly and social burden, including costs;
6. the inclusion of people with disabilities is seen as a private responsibility;
7. the unit of analysis is the individual; and
8. the point of intervention is the individual condition.

The Biomedical Approach

Of the two formulations of disability emanating from viewing it as an individual pathology, the first emphasises the biomedical origin of disability. The biomedical approach to disability research has been a powerful influence in determining disability policy and practice (Batshaw and Perret, 1981). Throughout the nineteenth and early twentieth centuries, infectious disease was the major cause of illness and death. The advent of the 'germ theory' of illness and disease facilitated the capacity to more correctly diagnose symptoms, and led to the pre-eminence of biological science as the basis for diagnosing disability, influencing treatments and guiding access to disability benefits. From the perspective of molecular biology and the attendant biomedical approach, it has been assumed that disability is caused by a mental or physical condition that can be prevented or ameliorated through medical, biological or genetic intervention. In such a characterisation of disability, the condition itself becomes the focus of attention. The aim of the professional or researcher is to decrease the prevalence of the condition in the general population. Treatment and prevention occur by means of biological intervention and critical care, including surgery, drug therapy, prenatal screening and genetic intervention. Therefore, the individual (or foetus) is commonly viewed as sick, injured or afflicted.

With the rise of institutional facilities and public benefits, medical science became established as the mechanism for keeping behind gates those who can be legitimately considered disabled. Assessments extend to various aspects of an individual's range of disability, such as: educational, training and work capabilities; fine motor skills and hand-eye coordination;

the need for financial benefits and mobility aids and devices; and access to rehabilitation. The biomedical model, with a focus on altering the biological condition, places less emphasis on the role that society plays in both limiting and enabling people.

The Functional Approach

The second of the two formulations of disability as an individual pathology can be called a functional approach. Like the biomedical model, the underlying presumption is that the deficit stems from an individual condition or pathology. However, this approach looks at ways of treating the functional incapacity through amelioration and by enabling strategies that will assist people to develop their potential. In the functional approach, the problems experienced by people with disabilities are interpreted as the results of a functional incapacity arising from an individual impairment. To treat this functional incapacity, services are made available to enable the individual to become as socially functional as possible (Wolfensberger, 1972; Meyer, Peck and Brown 1990). For example, the goal of rehabilitation is to increase an individual's range of skills and abilities so he or she can function more independently and become a productive member of society. The success of programmes is measured by how closely people who use services can approximate the lives of 'normal' people, and to what extent they can achieve the skills of able-bodied people.

Services developed from a functional approach (e.g. physiotherapy, occupational therapy, nursing and health visiting) have gone beyond therapeutic programmes associated with the biomedical model to include life skills, pre-vocational training, functional assessments, counselling and job training, as well as skills for independent living. Behaviour modification and developmental programming are also offshoots of the functional approach to disability. Behaviour modification uses a variety of reinforcement techniques to elicit individual behaviours that have been deemed socially desirable or useful (Koegel, Koegal and Dunlap 1996). The approach is also used to eliminate behaviours deemed inappropriate or ineffective for adjusting to the demands of everyday living. Developmental programming (Allen et al., 1994) targets the knowledge and skills that people usually acquire as they mature, identifies where and why individuals may be falling short of those benchmarks, and intervenes to assist individuals to maximise their developmental potential (Allen et al., 1994).

In placing the focus on the individual, a functional approach to disability can lose sight of environmental and situational factors that may limit individuals from achieving their ambitions. In targeting the individual for change, professionals operating on the basis of a functional approach run the risk of working with assumptions about the person's 'best interests' that may not always coincide with what that person wants for himself or herself. The way services are organised can also produce a power imbalance that creates tensions between people with disabilities and the professional community.

Formulations that Focus on the Socio-Political Nature of Disability (Social Pathology)

As well as the two formulations of disability based on individual pathology, there are two identifiable formulations based on social pathology. They start from a perspective that assumes that disability is not inherent to the individual. Rather, these formulations assume that the disability is inherent to the social structure. It is a structural approach rather than an individual approach. The identifiable pathology is that there is something wrong with society that we have to fix, rather than that there is something wrong with the individual (Rioux, 1995). These formulations have a number of identifiable characteristics:

9. disability is assumed not to be inherent to the individual and independent of the social structure;
10. priority is given to the political, social and built environment;
11. secondary rather than primary prevention is emphasised;
12. disability is recognised as a difference rather than an anomaly;
13. disability is viewed as the interaction of an individual with society;
14. inclusion of people with disabilities is seen as a public responsibility;
15. the unit of analysis is the social structure; and
16. the points of intervention are the social, environmental and economic systems.

The Environmental Approach

Advances in knowledge based on an understanding of disability as a social pathology have shown that personal abilities and limitations are not only the result of factors residing in the individual, but also of the interaction between individuals and their environments (Landesman-Dwyer, 1981). Increasingly, researchers are demonstrating that the failure of ordinary environments to accommodate people's differences exacerbates the impacts of disability. From an environmental perspective on disability, the research focus is placed on the way environments are managed (Bercovici, 1983). For example, research has shown that the absence of ramps into an office building creates an employment handicap for someone who relies on a wheelchair for mobility. It has been demonstrated that the lack of an ergonomically adapted work space makes it impossible for a person with limited upper-body movement to perform job tasks. Similarly, many research studies have shown that the lack of proactive hiring and employment-retention policies create disadvantages for individuals who require time away from work because of fatigue and other conditions caused by disability (Roeher Institute, 1993). An educational service disadvantages people with speech impairment where it fails to provide the opportunity to learn an alternative method of communication (e.g. through Blissymbolics or sign-language instruction).

Increasingly, research is showing that the impact of disability can be lessened as environments are adapted to enable participation. Building codes, principles of barrier-free design, adapted curricula, targeted policy and funding commitments are being shown in policy research to be useful tools to this end. Research shows that these tools enable modifications and supports to be made in home, school, work and leisure environments which increase the participation of people with disabilities in society and limit the disadvantages they otherwise would face.

The Rights-Outcome Approach

Another formulation of disability is based on the notion that disability has social causes; it is a consequence of how society is organised and of the relationship the individual has to society at large (Roth, 1983; Oliver, 1990; ICIDH, 1991; Barton, 1993; Beresford and Campbell, 1994; Rioux, 1994; Rioux and Bach, 1994; Ward and Flynn, 1994). Research based on a rights-outcome approach looks beyond particular environments to focus on broad systemic factors that keep certain people from participating as equals in society. This research approach holds that wide variations in cognitive, sensory and motor ability are inherent in the human condition, and that people with disabilities do contribute to society. It draws from a variety of disciplines (e.g. anthropology, sociology, economics and law), but it frames disability issues through the lens of human-rights principles (Veatch, 1986; Roeher Institute, 1995). It assumes that public policy and programmes should aim to reduce civic inequalities (Chappell, 1992) to address social and economic disadvantage. It also assumes that various supports (e.g. personal services, aids and devices) will be needed by some people in order to gain access to society, participate in it, and exercise self-determination as equals in society.

Research from a rights-outcome approach constructs an analysis of how society marginalises people with disabilities, and how it could be adjusted to respond more effectively to their presence and needs (Oliver, 1992). This approach focuses on the disabling aspects of society, on supporting human diversity, and on empowering disadvantaged individuals.

Social Obligation of Research

The social obligation of research from the rights approach to disability is to reduce civic inequalities. That is, social and economic disadvantages are addressed through providing supports, aids and devices that enable social and economic integration, self-determination, and legal and social rights. This is distinct from the social obligation of research grounded in individual pathology. Here, the goal of the biomedical approach is to eliminate or cure disability, and the functional approach has the social obligation of amelioration and the provision of comfort.

FORMULATIONS AND IDEOLOGY

Research from these social and scientific formulations of disability ascribes different attributes in terms of cause, prevention and social responsibility of the researcher, and of society, towards people with disabilities. These formulations also provide a mechanism to identify the way in which scientific ideology has provided the justification for particular treatment modalities, social programmes, laws and policies. Research from each of these formulations has an important contribution to make in ensuring that people with disabilities have the support services, social services, medical services and income they need. Because of differences in world view and fundamental assumptions about disability, each of these approaches leads researchers to have a different view of what is best with respect to disability. Even the understanding of what constitutes disability, disease, health, normality and abnormality is not shared across these approaches (Caplan, 1995; Hubbard, 1995; Whyte and Ingstad, 1995). Consequently, the formulation of disability leads to different ways of measuring and evaluating the success of what is accomplished.

All four approaches to research in disability can be critiqued on the basis of the degree of myopia caused by the disciplinary limits within which they deal with disability. Arguably, there is nothing wrong with any one of these formulations on its own; rather, the problem is the harm an approach may cause by claiming the field of disability as an exclusive domain. There are few other examples of a marginalised group of people having to cope with scientific hegemony to this extent.

FORCES THAT SHAPE RESEARCH AGENDAS

If these differences in approaches to disability research are not to dissolve into irresolvable conflicts, we need to understand the forces that shape research agendas in the field of disability. It is not good enough to critique the molecular-biological and biomedical approaches without recognising the social, economic, ethical and professional pressures that drive these research agendas. In the field of disability research, these pressures have driven research questions, findings and practice in a manner that has tipped the scales significantly in favour of information premised on disability as primarily an individual pathology. Therefore, research on policy, programmes and services that have an impact on individuals with intellectual disabilities have overly emphasised this perspective, to the detriment of the broader systemic conditions that disable people. There are a number of factors that are driving the research agenda in the disability field.

Neoconservative Economic Agenda

The first factor is the neoconservative economic agenda. In times like the present, when social policy is driven by economic neoconservatism

(Drache, 1995), funding is much more likely to be allocated to research that reinforces cost-savings. In a climate of scarce resources, if you assume that the individual is the locus of the problem, scarce resources are likely to be invested in lines of inquiry that establish the relative costs and benefits of some private and social investments over others in addressing individual impairment (Doyall and Gough, 1991). For example, there is a body of literature that provides rationales, using an actuarial approach, of the relative cost-savings of investments in techniques to prevent biological disability. This research favours interventions such as selective abortion and somatic germ-line therapy over the aggregate cost of supporting a person with a disability over a lifetime. There has been a critique of this position (Lippman, 1991; Waldschmidt, 1992; Asch, 1994). Other literature argues that the high cost of health care, and the probable increase in cost as treatments and technologies become more sophisticated, warrant rationing of health care based on reduced quality of life (Steel, 1995).

Another line of inquiry supported in the reductionism of the new economic environment is on research into ways to eliminate individual differences that cause inefficiencies and dysfunctions in the global economic system as it is presently constituted. Comparatively few resources are invested in research on how to reorganise economies to integrate human differences, to empower marginalised groups, and to ensure civic equalities (Bowles and Gintis, 1986). The political economy of research is such that well-endowed research projects tend to have an implied practical focus. Governments and private industry invest in research because they want to get something from it. In a neoconservative economic policy climate, researchers are pressured to look for cost-savings.

Utilitarianism as the Underlying Principle for Research and Professional Practice

The second major pressure on research agendas occurs when utilitarianism is the underlying ethical principle for research and professional practice. Ethical principles that underlie research have very different implications for deriving research questions, for methodology used, for the interpretation of research results, and for justifying the implied or explicit agenda that is the outcome as a basis for treatment, care and decision-making around disability. Utilitarianism has been the implicit moral/ethical premise for much of the biomedical and biotechnological research and practice in disability in western democracies. Health care, medical triaging and the allocation of services have tended to rely on the assertion of the principle of utility, i.e. in all circumstances, 'we ought to produce the greatest possible balance of value over disvalue for all people affected (the least possible balance of disvalue if only bad results can be brought about)' (Beauchamp and Childress, 1994). Beauchamp and Childress (1994) proffer that the refinement of the concept of utilitarianism, beyond its popular uses, is that it refers to:

> [the] moral theory that there is one and only one basic principle in ethics—the principle of utility. An ethical practice is consequently one in which a calculation is made which balances resources and compares the actual needs of everyone affected.

Utilitarians do not believe that this way of calculating imposes something alien or even unusual on the moral life. They think that utilitarianism simply renders explicit and systematic what is already implicit in ordinary deliberation and justification. The utilitarian believes that such reasoning is dominant, both in individual actions and in public policy.

We have seen in any number of examples how this translates into practice for individuals with disabilities. In a recent case in Canada, which is only an example of similar cases throughout the western world (and possibly elsewhere), a young man was refused a place on the list for a lung transplant on the basis of his having trisomy 21, a chromosome condition associated with Down's syndrome. In a time of scarce medical resources, the argument was made that there was a clear professional responsibility to give these resources to those who would benefit the most. This is a useful example of the way a utilitarian approach has filtered down from a philosophical system into practical policy-decisions affecting medical treatment.

Research on the human genome has been hailed as an important contributor to the advance of knowledge, to the prevention of disability and disease, and to improving the well-being of humankind as a whole (UNESCO, 1994). For a critique of that position, see the responses to the drafts of the declaration of the UNESCO International Bioethics Committee on the Protection of the Human Genome by Inclusion International (1995, 1996). Genetic screening has been made available for disabling conditions, which can then be identified and eliminated through abortion or non-conception. The decision has been made that there is a clear responsibility, in terms of the greatest good for the greatest number, to use biotechnology and research dollars to minimise the costs and risks of disabling conditions. The question that arises from the use of utilitarianism as a moral theory is: 'How do we determine what value could and should be produced in any given circumstance?' Most utilitarians would include health, freedom from pain, and the absence of disability as intrinsic values (i.e. things that are valued just for their own sake, not for something else they produce), but this is the fundamental problem with the hegemony of utilitarianism in the field of biotechnology research. At a recent seminar in Chicago, prenatal diagnosis and selective abortion were the topic of discussion among fifty genetic counsellors, researchers, disability-rights advocates, physicians and government officials. There was no agreement on whether the elimination of foetuses testing positive for Tay-Sachs disease and other such severe and life-shortening conditions could be argued to be of utility, either to society as a whole or to the potential individual.

The acceptance of utilitarianism as the underlying principle of medical and biological research generally has spilled over into research on disability, at least where disability is seen as residing in the individual. However, utilitarianism is only one model of moral reasoning (Drover and Kerans, 1993; Inclusion International, 1994). Within social formulations of disability, the moral principles that tend to be paramount are principles of justice, including either the Rawlsian notion of justice as fairness (Rawls, 1971), or the notion of justice as equality (Williams, 1962; Dworkin, 1981a,b). Principles of justice are reflected in research agendas and the funding of research, as well as in the social policy based on that research. As we shift from a utilitarian base to a justice base, tensions will arise, tensions that have, to date, been masked by the predominance of utilitarianism as the basis from which to view disability, undertake disability research, and formulate social obligation.

A Research Culture of Objectivity and Positivism

The third pressure on the research agenda is that driven by a research culture of objectivity and positivism. There is a strong cultural bias in industrialised countries towards scientific positivism in research and policy-making. Rationality and objectivity are valued as necessary conditions for the social and economic well-being of society. These cultural biases bring pressure on the research community to rely on strictly positivist criteria to judge the validity of research, and to be suspicious of more inductive and qualitative approaches. For example, there is an important and often debated issue around environmental therapy (and now prospective gene therapy) as compared to aversive therapy, in response to self-destructive and violent behaviour of people with intellectual disabilities (Lovett, 1985). At root, this debate is about the capacity to prove a valid and measurable stimulus-response effect of positive reinforcement. Stimulus-response trials are much simpler to carry out if the intervening variables can be reduced and clinical trials can be carried out in laboratory-type settings. For example, it has been possible to show that electric shock-sticks or the self-injurious behaviour inhibition system reduce particular behaviour manifestations, particularly in clinical or institutional settings. It has been far more difficult to show that particular changes in environment, programming, housing or social setting have reduced particular behaviours. Qualitative studies have been criticised for being unable to determine which of the environmental factors made the most significant differences, thereby limiting the presumed reliability and validity of the research results.

Therapeutic, molecular-biological and medical research, which lend themselves to this kind of empiricism, are much more likely to receive funding than research that relies on qualitative data, anthropological studies that emphasise the subjective experience of disability, or policy science that tries to deal with a myriad of interacting variables. Even though these types of studies may not receive much notice as a funding priority, work of this kind has nonetheless provided the field of disability with important new knowledge and analysis in, for example, educational research (Stainback and Stainback, 1984; Biklen, 1985; Gartner and Lipsky, 1987; Skrtic, 1987; Porter and Richler, 1991), research concerning the inclusion of people in the regular labour market (Roeher Institute, 1993), and in quality-of-life and health-promotion research, which sheds light on the dimensions of health for people with disabilities (Renwick et al., 1996).

The objectivity of research is sometimes justified by its disassociation from the use of the results. Thus, for example, there are claims made that pure research is socially useful in its own right and ought to be supported, in particular because it is not subject to special-interest group pressures. Research that investigates the impact of social, economic and political conditions is less likely to meet this type of test of objectivity on face value. Pressure for this type of objectivity and scientific positivism creates incentives for researchers to present their research designs and research methodologies in ways that mask the complexity of the experience and causalities of disability (Smith, 1993). There is a built-in bias against making explicit the potential consequences at both design stage and results stage, and in the carrying out of the research.

CONCLUSION

The research community in the field of disability has created a world of 'disability facts', but has been relatively unconscious about the judgements it has made in doing so. In creating the world of facts, we have assumed that the role of judgement belongs to the advocates, the policymakers, the politicians and the courts. I think that we need to reconfigure the role of judgement in the world of facts that we construct in the field of disability research. The judgements we make about the causes of disability, about the meaning of the concept, and about what factors to hold responsible for the experience of disability, have profound consequences for the directions pursued by advocates, policymakers, politicians and the courts. Instead of denying the place of judgement in our research, I think we can become conscious of it and begin to hold each other accountable for the judgements we make. To develop an international research agenda that is conscious of its own judgements, we need to recognise the very real forces that shape the questions we ask and the criteria of validity we adopt.

Uncovering the elements of various formulations and approaches to disability, the world-views that underlie them, as well as the social pressures to conduct disability research from the perspective of individual pathology, provide us with an opportunity to rethink the work in this field. Recognising the relative nature of disability as shown in the different approaches should provide an opportunity to address the reductionism common to disability research and scientific findings. We can make explicit the inherent biases in the linear and monolithic approaches found in research methodology and research findings. Instead of standing on the laurels of the research done in the field, we can work toward correcting the imbalance that has emerged because of traditional understanding of disability and social pressures on the research community and research funding. It is a challenge that will be difficult, but if the research we do is to benefit those who live with disabilities and future generations of those with disabilities, it is an imperative that cannot be ignored.

References

Allen, K.E. et al. 1994. *Exception Children: Inclusion in Early Childhood Programmes.* Ontario: Nelson Canada.

Asch, A. 1994. 'The human genome and disability rights', *The Disability Rag and Resource,* 12 January–5 February.

Barton, L. 1993. 'The struggle for citizenship: the case of disabled people', *Disability, Handicap and Society,* 8: 235–48.

Batshaw, M.L. and Perrer, Y.M. 1981. *Children with Handicaps: A Medical Primer.* Baltimore: Paul H. Brooks.

Beauchamp, T.L. and Childress, J.F. 1994. *Principles of Biomedical Ethics,* 4th edn. Oxford: Oxford University Press.

Bercovici, S. 1983. *Barriers to Normalisation: The Restricted Management of Retarded Persons.* Baltimore: University Park Press.

Beresford, P. and Campbell, J. 1994. 'Disabled people, service users, user involvement and representation', *Disability and Society,* 9: 315–25.

Biklen, D. 1985. *Achieving the Complete School: Strategies for Effective Mainstreaming.* New York: Teachers College Press.

Bowles, S. and Gintis, H. 1986. *Democracy and Capitalism: Property, Community and the Contradictions of Modern Social Thought.* New York: Basic Books.

Caplan, A.J. 1995. *If Gene Therapy is the Cure, What is the Disease?* Philadelphia: Centre of Bioethics, University of Pennsylvania Medical Centre.

Chappell, A.L. 1992. 'Towards a sociological critique of the normalisation principle', *Disability, Handicap and Society,* 7: 101–13.

Doyall, L. and Gough, I. 1991. *A Theory of Human Need.* London: Macmillan.

Drache, D. 1995. 'The eye of the hurricane: globalisation and social policy reform', in D. Drache and A. Ranachan (eds), *Warm Heart, Cold Country: Fiscal and Social Policy Reform in Canada.* Ottawa: Caledon Institute of Social Policy and Robarts Centre for Canadian Studies, Renouff Publishing, pp. 23–56.

Drover, G. and Kerans, P. 1993. *New Approaches to Welfare Theory.* Aldershot: Edgar Elgar Publishing.

Dworkin, R. 1981a. 'What is equality? Part 1: Equality of welfare', *Philosophy and Public Affairs,* 10: 185–246.

Dworkin, R. 1981b. 'What is equality? Part 2: Equality of resources', *Philosophy and Public Affairs,* 10: 283–345.

Gartner, A. and Lipsky, D. 1987. 'Beyond special education: toward a quality system for all students', *Harvard Educational Review*, 57: 367–95.

Hubbard, R. 1995. 'Transparent women, visible genes and new conceptions of disease', *Cambridge Quarterly of Healthcare Ethics*, 4: 291–95.

ICIDH, Canadian Society for. 1991. 'The handicap creation process', *ICIDH International Network*, 4: 1–2.

Inclusion International. 1994. *Just Technology? From Principles to Practice in Bio-ethical Issues*. Ontario: The Roeher Institute.

———. 1995. 'Respectful recognition: safeguarding the rights of persons with disabilities. Response to the documents issued until September 1994 by the International Bioethics Committee of UNESCO'. Unpublished paper available at Inclusion International.

———. 1996. 'Protecting human dignity and human rights. Response to the IBC Draft Declaration of September 1995 on the human genome and modifications'. Unpublished paper available at Inclusion International.

Koegel, L.K., Koegel, R.L. and Dunlap, G. 1996. *Positive Behavioural Support*. Baltimore: Paul H. Brookes.

Landesman-Dwyer, S. 1981. 'Living in the community', *American Journal of Mental Deficiency*, 86: 223–34.

Lippman, A. 1991. 'Prenatal genetic testing and screening: constructing needs and reinforcing inequities', *American Journal of Law and Medicine*, XVII: 15–50.

Lovett, H. 1985. *Cognitive Counselling and Persons with Special Needs*. New York: Praeger.

Lukes, S. 1980. 'Socialism and equality', in A. Sterba (ed.), *Justice: Alternative Political Perspectives*. Belmont: Wadsworth Publishing Co, pp. 211–30.

Meyer, L.H., Peck, C.A. and Brown, L. 1990. (eds) *Critical Issues in the Lives of People with Severe Disabilities*. Baltimore: Paul H. Brookes.

Oliver, M. 1990. *The Politics of Disablement*. London: Macmillan.

———. 1992. 'Changing the social relations of research production', *Disability, Handicap and Society*, 7: 101–14.

Porter, G. and Richler, D. 1991. (eds) *Changing Canadian Schools: Perspectives on Disability and Inclusion*. Ontario: Roeher Institute.

Rawls, J.A. 1971. *A Theory of Justice*. Cambridge: Harvard University Press.

Renwick R., Brown, I. and Nayler, M. 1996. *Quality of Life in Health Promotion and Rehabilitation* California: Sage Publications.

Rioux, M. 1994. 'Towards a concept of equality of well-being: overcoming the social and legal construction of inequality', *Canadian Journal of Law and Jurisprudence*, 7: 127–47.

———. 1995. 'Concepts of equality and intellectual disability'. Presentation to the International Symposium: *Should Difference Make à Difference*. New Haven: Yale Law School.

Rioux, M. and Bach, M. 1994. (eds) *Disability Is Not Measles: New Research Paradigms in Disability*. Ontario: The Roeher Institute.

Roeher Institute. 1993. *On Target? Canada's Employment-related Programmes for People with Disabilities*. Ontario: The Roeher Institute.

Roeher Institute and Partnerships in Community Living. 1995. *As If Children Matter.* Ontario: The Roeher Institute.

Roth, W. 1983. 'Handicap as a social construct', *Society*, 20: 56–61.

Skrtic, T.M. 1987. 'An organisational analysis of special education reform', *Counterpoint*, 8: 15–19.

Smith, D. 1993. 'Everyday world as problematic', in G.K. Drover and P. Kerans (eds), *New Approaches to Welfare Theory*. Aldershot: Edgar Elgar Publishing.

Stainback, W. and Stainback, S. 1984. 'A rationale for the merger of special and regular education', *Exceptional Children*, 51: 102–11.

Steel, K.O. 1995. 'The road I see: implications of new reproductive technologies', *Cambridge Quarterly of Healthcare Ethics*, 4: 351–54.

UNESCO International Bioethics Committee. 1994. 'Draft Declaration on the Human Genome and Human Rights'. Paris: UNESCO.

Veatch, R. 1986. *The Foundations of Justice: Why the Retarded and the Rest of Us Have Claims to Equality*. Oxford: Oxford University Press.

Waldschmidt, A. 1992. 'Against selection of human life: people with disabilities oppose genetic counselling', *Issues in Reproductive and Genetic Engineering*, 5:'155–67.

Ward, L. and Flynn, M. 1994. 'What matters most: disability, research and empowerment', in M. Rioux and M. Bach (eds), *Disability Is Not Measles: New Research Paradigms in Disability*. Ontario: The Roeher Institute, pp. 29–48.

Whyte, S. R. and Ingstad, B. 1995. *Disability and Culture*. Berkeley: University of California Press.

Williams, B. 1962. 'The idea of equality', in P.R. Lasslet and W.G. Runciman (eds), *Philosophy, Politics and Society*. Oxford: Basil Blackwell, pp. 110–31.

Wolfensberger, W. 1972. *Normalisation: The Principle of Normalisation in Human Services*. Toronto: National Institute of Mental Retardation.

World Health Organisation. 1980. *International Classification of Impairments, Disabilities and Handicaps*. Geneva: WHO.

PART 2

Life with a Disability

Introduction

Patrick Devlieger & Renu Addlakha

'Life with a disability' is an area of investigation that appears as one pole of the study of disability. It refers to the possibility of making a distinction between self and other, the progression of life in time, and its situation in space. For research that investigates lives, it is important to understand the particularities of lives characterised by disability, and the progression of such lives. In addition, an understanding of what constitutes a life, sometimes understood as the self, appears to be crucial when approaching both its essence and its constructed nature.

An understanding of a life invariably also refers to its mirror pole, namely, society or culture. Talking or writing about lives, another's or one's own, implies referral to the social, cultural, historical and other contexts in which lives are lived. The consequence is that the study of lives includes commentary on the context in which they are situated. The emphasis of the study of lives then becomes a starting point from which interactions, processes and positioning become important. Through the story of life and its analysis, a rare understanding of the shaping of lives becomes available. Depending on the disciplinary background, this is sometimes referred to as an insider's perspective, the subjective dimension, or, more generally, the construction of the meaning of a life. The articles in this part of the Reader aim to illustrate these interests in the particular case of lives characterised by disability.

In the human sciences, there is a long history of studying lives. This has led to both disciplinary and interdisciplinary approaches. For example, historians have attempted to understand how ordinary lives were lived in the past and how information could be obtained about them, for example, through oral history or the analysis of public records. In the field of anthropology and sociology, life histories are collected to understand more about society and culture. Life-history or biographical methods were accordingly devised. Perhaps one of the best-developed interdisciplinary programmes for the study of lives, known as *life-course studies*, was initiated during the 1980s. It builds on the insight that, complementary to an understanding of the biological basis of a life's development within a life-cycle, the progression of a life can be understood in terms of social, cultural and other dimensions. It involves the impact of family, generations, critical historical events, rituals, and, at a later stage, the intersection of gender, race, ethnic background, age and disability on particular periods or transitions in life.

The five articles chosen for Part 2 are the result of a careful selection process. In that process, the aim was to maximise variety with regard to disciplinary orientation, regions of the world, theoretical concepts, and methods. For some articles, their 'classic' status in the literature also played a pivotal role.

A classic example of the early stage of life-course studies is the article by Bury, 'Chronic Illness as Biographical Disruption'. Disability and chronic illness are disruptive experiences against the background of a normal trajectory. It is remarkable in this article how Bury refers to solutions coming out of one's stock of knowledge and biographical experience. This is quite opposite to a sociological approach that emphasises society's grip on the definition and progression of life, as for example in Deborah Stone's *The Disabled State*, published in 1984.

The study of lives invariably stimulates the bringing out of complexity in knowledge. The issues in generating this knowledge are set against a background of wholeness, as in functional and systems approaches. It is then possible to speak of a person. Another background is the unconscious; a lived life is then a response, a reaction, or an expression of processes. Another framework is that of historical context; the concreteness of a particular life is then situated against the trends and events that define a particular time period. More recently, the impact of power in the shaping of life and its representation has called for a greater reflexivity.

The study of the lives of disabled people has benefited from many of these theoretical and methodological issues. It has served to provide an insider's perspective, a study of the disabled self. This has been accomplished in both the biographical and the autobiographical sense. Robert Bogdan and Steve Taylor (see 'Further Reading') may have initiated one of the classic examples of the use of biography. Their aim was to present an insider's perspective without much theoretical addition or commentary from the authors. They limited the role of the author only to representation, to grasping the richness that could be preserved in description. The development of qualitative research benefited greatly from these experiments.

Writing autobiographically, Robert Murphy accomplishes an understanding of his disabled self. Included in Part 2 is a chapter from his book, *The Body Silent*, about the formation of the disabled self. It refers to specific aspects of American culture and society. Murphy's self is a diminished self, which he refuses to identify solely in negative terms as 'stigma', as is common in the work of Erving Goffman. Rather, he likens it to a ritual situation, following the work of anthropologist Victor Turner, emphasising the essentially undetermined nature of being disabled. For Murphy, being disabled is being suspended in an undefined or 'liminal' status (i.e. on a threshold). One is neither sick nor healthy. It should be said that Murphy's work does not have the great following that Goffman's has; see, for example, Barrett's discussion of the physical expression of social stigma among people with leprosy. While the disability community welcomed the move away from solely negative consequences for the development of the self, Murphy's alternative proved to lack in either further theoretical development or practical application. 'Being suspended' could not be an end stage.

The ethnographic study of lives characterised by disability is usually known as 'life history'. It indicates the way micro-situations point to larger issues in social and cultural, and sometimes global contexts. One early example in the area of mental retardation is a longitudinal study of mental retardation following deinstitutionalisation, conducted by Robert Edgerton (1993). Starting in 1960, Edgerton followed a cohort for over 30 years, focusing especially on how well persons with limited competencies adapted to living in the community. Another notable and more recent study of a single life history is Gelya Frank's. She presents the life of a woman born without arms and legs, in the context of gender and the American cultural context (see 'Further Reading'). We have included an ethnographic study by Renu Addlakha of a single case history. Starting with observations from micro-situations, the focus is on family burdens and adaptive strategies in an Indian cultural context.

The 1990s saw more emphasis on the active improvement of lives. Strategies were devised for developing the self through active engagement in the community and more general power relations. In a context in which it became obvious that disability was not solely an individual matter but also politically and economically produced, a space opened for building a strong self. Empowerment and self-determination became key concepts in the west, to be applied in education and rehabilitation, and supplying the belief that identities can be built.

The 1990s also saw a major resurgence of what became known as the *narrative turn*. Building on phenomenological and post-modern influences, the life story became again a structural device in which place, time, situations and persons could be accounted for, yet in which subjective knowledge could be presented as truth. Sociologists such as Arthur Frank, anthropologists such as Cheryl Mattingly, and literary analysts such as Thomas Couser provided insights into the structuring nature of stories, their necessity for making social situations intelligible, and the widening phenomenon of people finding their own voice, through authorship and authority, in constructing and distributing their own stories.

The passing of disability-rights legislation in many countries, following the Americans with Disabilities Act of 1990, infused the analysis of lives with the terminology of human and civil rights. Disability became understood as a source of discrimination, just as race and gender are. Concurrently, it became the source for the formation of a disability identity and culture.

Coming from the health sciences, the universal concept of 'quality of life' underscored again the authority of the sciences from a perspective of improvement of lives. Perhaps it can be seen as an alternative to stigmatisation of health conditions, which emphasises negative social conditions. Although it is generally assumed that disability leads to poorer quality of life, some research nuances this view by pointing out 'a disability paradox', namely, the acquisition of a relatively good quality of life despite a disability. The study by Taleporos and McCabe (2002), included here, ties in well with these findings. According to these authors, bodily impairment has a negative influence on participants' psychological experiences, feelings and attitudes toward their own bodies. There is, however, evidence suggesting that individuals gradually adjust to their different bodies, and increasingly accept their disabilities over time.

A new approach to studying lives with a disability is in terms of the possibility of creating not only disability identities and disability cultures, but also disability worlds. Such work provides an opening to different sources of knowledge, crossing the boundaries of scientific and artistic work. It includes work by scientists who cross into artistic work, such as Oliver Sacks, of academics who have become disabled, and of disabled writers with links to the academic world. Accepting the possibility of a disability world (or varieties of worlds) leads to new questions regarding disability as a world-creating condition, a transition from one world to another, and on the relations between the little world of disability and the larger social world.

5

Chronic Illness as Biographical Disruption

Michel Bury

INTRODUCTION

The purpose of this paper is to explore a limited range of theoretical and empirical issues thrown up by the study of chronic illness. It focuses on a field study of rheumatoid arthritis carried out by the author between 1976 and 1979 in the north-west of England. The data reported here were gathered by semi-structured interviews with a series of thirty patients being referred, for the first time, to an outpatient rheumatology clinic. These individuals comprised twenty-five women and five men (the disease has a four times higher prevalence among women than among men). The majority of the women were aged between 25 and 54, two being under 24 and six being over 55 years of age. The five men were aged between 45 and 64. Fifteen of the women worked either part-time or full-time; all but one were working-class women, with jobs such as machine operator, school kitchen worker, bakery worker and punch-card operator. All but three respondents were married with families, often including young children.

The selective nature of this series had a purpose. The aim was to concentrate on those with an emerging illness at the earliest possible

Bury, M. 1982. 'Chronic illness as biographical disruption', *Sociology of Health and Illness*, 4 (2): 167–82.

point, to explore the problems of recognition and changes in life situation and relationships occasioned by the development of the illness. I therefore relied on the identification of probable rheumatoid arthritis patients by a consultant rheumatologist, based on referral letters from a general practitioner. In all but one case, a definite diagnosis was subsequently confirmed. The interviews were conducted once at home before attending the clinic, and again after the first two consultations. In addition, observations in the clinic setting were possible, providing informal conversations with respondents and other patients.

CHRONIC ILLNESS AS A DISRUPTIVE EVENT

At the risk of oversimplifying, two traditions have been available to medical sociologists interested in chronic illness. The first stems from the debate over the usefulness or otherwise of Parsons' conceptions of illness and the sick-role. On a negative level, it is maintained that chronic illness appears to deny many of Parsons' assumptions about the patterning of sickness; on a more positive note, it suggests separating and developing deviance and adaptive perspective from his theory (Gerhardt, 1979; Gallagher, 1976). This, it is hoped, will overcome the limitations thought to arise from an overemphasis on acute illness and sick-role behaviour. However, the notion of adapting is often linked to a view of disablement as a relatively stable entity. In fact, the conditions which underpin most forms of disablement involve fluctuating symptoms and uncertain outcome. Taylor (1977) notes that, in the changing spectrum of disablement since the Second World War, chronic illness has come to overshadow the contribution of accident and injury; see also Bury (1979) for a more general discussion of disablement. While residual and permanent disabilities are implicated in conditions such as arthritis, the illness underlying them remains significant. As Mildred Blaxter (1976) has shown, medical definitions are central in disablement, not only from the point of view of doctors' concerns, but also of patients' concerns. While medical definitions may at times be seen as inappropriate in the provision of service and welfare, this does not displace the role of both lay and specialised medical knowledge in explaining experiences or of those behaviours associated with them. My study shows, for example, that a chronically ill person can make adaptations to his lifestyle and still have access to periods of classic sick-role behaviour when such events as surgical intervention or sudden exacerbations of symptoms occur.

The second tradition has been of an interactionist nature. As one would expect, it has concentrated on empirical enquiry, detailing the strategic handling of symptoms and disabilities (Davis, 1964; Wiener, 1975; Strauss, 1975). The insights gained have been important, especially over such matters as the disclosing or disguising of symptoms, but the approach has often been frankly descriptive, with only passing reference to wider theoretical concerns. Strauss (1975), for example, describes the way individuals strategically withdraw from the field of social interaction under the impact of symptoms, but while he argues that this should be seen as understandable, the problematic nature of such behaviour and its deeper implications are left implicit. As Paul Rock (1979) has recently shown, interactionism has been preoccupied with fieldwork rather than explicit theorising. In particular, a willingness to move from descriptive categories of interaction to a wider analysis of cultural and structural forms has been limited.

The perspective to be developed in this article is that of chronic illness as a major kind of disruptive experience or 'critical situation', using Giddens' (1979) term. Giddens makes the point that 'we can learn a good deal about day-to-day situations in routine settings from analysing circumstances in which those settings are radically disturbed' (p. 123). In his discussion, he seems to have in mind disruptions of the social fabric brought about by major events such as war. His reference to Sargant's *Battle for the Mind*, however, suggests that biographically located events such as spirit possession also have the same potential. My contention is that illness, and especially chronic illness, is precisely that kind of experience, where the structures of everyday life and the forms of knowledge which underpin them are disrupted. Chronic illness involves recognition of the worlds of pain and suffering, possibly even of death, which are normally only seen as distant possibilities or the plight of others. In addition, it brings individuals, their families, and wider social networks face to face with the character of their relationships in stark form, disrupting normal rules of reciprocity and mutual support. The growing dependency involved in chronic illness is a major issue here. Further, the expectations and plans that individuals hold for the future need to be re-examined.

Thus, I want to maintain that the development of a chronic illness like rheumatoid arthritis is most usefully regarded as a 'critical situation', a form of biographical disruption, not only as a way of describing what happens, but also to provide a more explicit analytic focus.

For the present, I wish to link three aspects of disruption to the unfolding of a chronic illness. First, there is the disruption of taken-for-granted assumptions and behaviours, the breaching of common-sense boundaries. Dingwall (1976) suggests a 'disruptive' approach to illness in this regard, but goes on to offer a formalistic rather than substantive analysis of its implications. This stage, where one may wonder 'what is going on here', involves attention to bodily states not usually brought into consciousness, and decisions about seeking help. Second, there are more profound disruptions in explanatory systems normally used by people, such that a fundamental rethinking of the person's biography and self-concept is involved. Third, there is the response to disruption involving the mobilisation of resources to face an altered situation.

ONSET AND THE PROBLEM OF RECOGNITION

It is now a sociological commonplace that lay perceptions of symptoms (and the decision to seek help) do not necessarily coincide with those held by professionals (Wadsworth, Butterfield and Blaney 1971; Maclean, 1975). No one in the study group recognised the first signs as indicating rheumatoid arthritis. In the first instance, impairments (a swollen finger, early morning stiffness) were merely regarded as a nuisance, and were seen as a result of, for example, exertion while decorating at home. They were not, even in retrospect, seen as a warning. The only kind of explanation called for was of a 'proximal' kind. That is, common sense partially furnished the answer, particularly in terms of the immediate external environment. This orientation towards the external environment comes close to the views regarding the source of ill health discussed by Herzlich (1973). But the externalising and localising of the sources of discomfort became more problematic as the illness unfolded.

One of the most important features of chronic illness is its insidious onset. Non-communicable diseases do not 'break out'. They 'creep up'. Davis (1963) indicates how the transition from trivial symptoms to a developing and persisting disability has an impact on those concerned. It involves initiation into a new social arena where common-sense guidelines are no longer sufficient. Maclean and Cockshutt (1979) and Cowie (1976), in their studies of heart attacks, indicate how social and biographical factors influence this initiation. Even in the case of heart attacks, people report finding themselves in a critical situation of great uncertainty, where they may have little or no idea of what is happening to them.

The main feature in this instance, somewhat in contrast with that in other studies, is that the emergence of rheumatoid arthritis is an experience unlikely to involve others until a relatively late stage. The role of significant others in recognition is limited, and it is possible for some, though not all, patients to hide their symptoms or disguise their effects for long periods. I came to realise, in the course of interviewing, that even having been referred to a specialist clinic (often some months after onset), some were still hiding their illness from their families. Indeed, two women used the interview situation to help reveal to their spouses the seriousness of their condition. Clearly, where the symptoms of a condition coincide with those widely distributed in a population (in this case aches and pains), the processes of recognition and of legitimating the illness are particularly problematic.

As the symptoms persisted, the probability of some kind of arthritis or rheumatism suggested itself, or was suggested by others. For the younger women, it came as a profound shock to realise that arthritis could begin at their age. Their experience contrasted sharply with the common cultural paradigm of the disease. A reaction of disbelief mixed with anxiety is thus common among those with an emerging illness of this kind. There is rarely anything in the individual's biography which provides an immediate basis for recognition of the symptoms as an illness. Many of the women had been physically active, both in the house and at work, and in sports and leisure activities. The stereotype of arthritis is so sharply contrasted with this that it seems impossible to move from one status to the other. As one woman put it:

> Well, at first I thought I'd broken, chipped, the bone in the finger, with it being a knuckle. I thought, I bet I've banged it, really, because I do bang my hands a lot sometimes, and I thought I'd chipped it, and I thought, 'Oh, it'll go off.' It was months, really, before I got round to going to the

> doctor, because we got married in the July and I didn't go and see the doctor before the end of August, beginning of September. I just thought it was one of those things that would clear up. It never dawned on me it would end up like this.

The significance of age requires underlining. The image of arthritis as a disease of the elderly is common. On the one hand, it makes the possibility of a straightforward process of recognition remote. Arthritis was seen, initially, by those I interviewed, as a 'wear and tear' disease, a result of becoming old, with inevitable disabling consequences, particularly expressed as a fear of 'seizing-up' and becoming crippled. Individuals, even in their forties and fifties, did not think of arthritis as occurring in the way experienced, and this was even more true of the women in their twenties. The emergence of the condition seemed to imply a 'premature ageing' for the individual (Singer, 1974). As such, it marked a biographical shift from a perceived normal trajectory through relatively predictable chronological steps, to one that was fundamentally abnormal and inwardly damaging. The relationship of 'internal reality' to 'external reality' was upset.

Common-sense assumptions lose their grip, yet alternative explanations do not readily present themselves. The individual is unsure about whether and how to disclose the illness, both to significant others and to outsiders such as general practitioners. But for those who decide to consult, a logic is set in motion, although the course of referral is rarely a smooth one. A general practitioner may well have difficulty in diagnosing early rheumatoid arthritis and send a woman home with a strapped-up wrist, in a 'wait and see' exercise. In one case, a man was simply given pain-killers, and he decided to consult a chiropodist for his painful feet. Often, however, the development of more systemic symptoms and growing disabilities made one insist on pursuing referral. Finally, sometimes after considerable delay, referral to a rheumatology outpatient clinic occurred.

This marked the end of the initial stage. The referral was often treated with relief, suggesting as it did that the individual was 'going to get sorted out.' The relief was, however, more than simply that of coping with functional problems and growing pain and discomfort. It was also a sign that the individual was justified in presenting his or her symptoms and that their behaviour in general was warranted. The prospect of official recognition and treatment therefore had a range of expectations attached to it.

EMERGING DISABILITY AND THE PROBLEM OF UNCERTAINTY

The place of uncertainty in the experience of illness, especially chronic illness, is widely recognised (Davis, 1960; Wiener, 1975). This involves both uncertain knowledge about the impact and course of the condition, and appropriate behaviour in the face of its effects. In the case of rheumatoid arthritis, the emergence of obvious signs of disability, as I have indicated, can become overriding. In some instances, respondents were simply 'taken over' by the disease. One man, a manual worker in his forties, developed such severe stiffness and pain, especially on waking, that he could not shave or dress himself. While the tolerance of others in such a situation will be tested, the individual can elicit it, or try to insist on the legitimacy of his actions. But this legitimacy raises a new set of problems, involving a re-evaluation of the relationship between the now-visible disease and selfhood. It is in this context that medical knowledge takes on particular importance.

Access to medical knowledge, at least in the case of physical illness, offers an opportunity to conceptualise the disease as separate from the individual's self. This separation of disease from human contingencies has, in a variety of ways, come in for criticism. In recent years, the idea that disease is itself 'reification' has been taken up by sociologists. In itself it is not a new idea, dating back at least to Virchow in nineteenth-century Germany (Faber, 1923) in his opposition to any kind of nosology based on disease categories. Recently, Taussig (1980) and others have sought to give this approach a sociological revival, drawing on the sociology of knowledge and theories of alienation (e.g. Berger and Luckmann, 1967). But, as Fabrega and Manning (1972) have shown, the separation of disease from self is a powerful cultural resource. The objectivity of disease provides, through medical science, a socially legitimate basis, both for deviant behaviour and clinical intervention. Assertions that scientific objectivity acts as an ideological force frequently fail to address this question of legitimacy. To be able to hold the disease 'at a distance' assists the claim that one is a victim of external forces. To do anything less is to accept fully the burden of responsibility.

However, the point of the argument about reification, at least in chronic illness, is that a strict separation of disease and self (for that matter, disease and social relationships in general) is precarious. The experience of the patients in this study underlined the uneasy balance which is struck between seeing the condition as an outside force and yet feeling its invasion of all aspects of life. Thus, patients approached the specialist with mixed feelings. On the one hand, they wanted definite knowledge of their physical state and its causes, and yet felt, realistically, that there was a limited amount which the doctors could do in effecting a cure. They expected their drugs to be changed or 'sorted out', but often added that the main issue was still going to be learning to live with their condition. Medical intervention was, therefore, regarded at the same time as both important and limited.

On being told that they definitely had rheumatoid arthritis, reactions combined fear and relief. Some said that, as they had known it beforehand, the consultation simply confirmed the worst; others were beset with anxiety and fear, especially about the future. The image of rheumatoid arthritis as a crippling disease is strong, and despite attempts by staff to reassure patients that only a small proportion of sufferers become severely disabled, many saw a future of growing dependency and invalidity. Not only this, but individuals also face the limits of medical knowledge and treatment regimens. Realisation slowly dawns that the latter, involving periods of rest and activity, are difficult to follow and often less than effective. Doctors unwittingly reinforce this by telling patients that no cause of rheumatoid arthritis is known. Thus, while the diagnosis of the disease provides something firm to relate to, and to explain to others, the actual nature of the disease remains elusive and the treatments empirical. One woman said:

> The doctor told me to rest as much as I could. Well, I think if you do too much resting you stiffen up, don't you? I don't really understand what it's all about, to be quite honest ... you know, because one doctor tells you one thing and one tells you another.... One tells you to use your fingers like this and the other tells you to rest your hands. So you don't know where you're up to, do you?

The realisation that medical knowledge is incomplete, and that treatment is based on practical trial and error, throws individuals back on their own stock of knowledge and biographical experience. The search for a more comprehensive level of explanation, a more certain basis of coping with the illness is often a long and profound one. Comaroff and Maguire (1981), following Durkheim's views on the role of science, indicate the need to *complete* the knowledge gained from specialist sources, a need to tie in formal knowledge with the person's total biography.

Interpretative sociology has often made play on a strict separation of the languages of cause and meaning. Many writers assert that there is what amounts to a conceptual gulf between acts of nature and human intention. Crick (1976) has recently argued this position in developing a 'semantic anthropology'. Coulter (1973) argues it in separating the worlds of 'cells and tissues from acts and conduct', and Goffman (1975) says that our culture divides natural events from 'guided doings'. As I have indicated, conceptualising disease relies strongly on this cultural motif, but it seems to me that Giddens (1979) is also right to assert that in lay thought cause and meaning frequently coincide.

In searching for the meaning of events, and answers to questions like 'Why me?' and 'Why now?', incidents from the past are set against presumed knowledge of the disease's causation. Patients in this study assumed that a predisposition to rheumatoid arthritis must be inherited or 'carried in the blood'. The interviews often turned on questions about familial transmission, both in terms of whether the condition might have been inherited and whether it might be passed to offspring. Moral concerns and science-based knowledge overlap. While a few individuals firmly believed that family members had passed on the disease directly, others sought to implicate emotional upset or other serious events in its emergence and onset. One woman patient and her sister (who also had arthritis) decided that emotional shocks were of such importance that their remaining brother needed protecting from upsetting events, in order to forestall the onset of disease.

In discussing more specific events linked to the onset of her illness, another woman, a part-time dinner lady, recounted being called to her seven-year-old son's aid on arriving at the school for work. He had collapsed in the playground. She said:

> I went to the cloakroom and found him in a terrible state. Nobody seemed to be doing anything, so I carried him home myself. I'm not very big and it nearly killed me. In the end, the ambulance came and rushed him off

> to hospital. Appendicitis. He had an emergency operation, and was on a drip for two days. He recovered, but it was such a shock. I often put my trouble down to that time. I'm not saying it caused it. Only, that's when things started happening.

The woman in this interview wanted to express a number of things simultaneously. In the first place, she saw the possibility of a causal or triggering effect of 'shocks to the system'. Similar views were expressed by most respondents in this study. But this woman was conveying more than simple views about causation. First, the meaning of the event of rheumatoid arthritis itself was seen in terms of an analogous shock to her life. Her social situation had been difficult enough before onset, and it was as if the final blow had been delivered. The arthritis appeared as a grossly unfair act, cheating her out of the few hopes she retained for the future. Whilst she 'managed' or 'coped' with the disease, kept it at bay as much as possible, it continually intruded into her sense of self-confidence, upsetting an already precarious balance. Second and as the quotation above shows, she was also hard pressed to mobilise resources around her. She stated that she had a husband who worked long hours in a manual job for low wages, and a marriage which, at the best of times, was not supportive. The illness thus meant not only a disruption of structures of explanation and meaning, but also of relationships and material and practical affairs. And it is to these that I now want to turn in a little more detail.

CHRONIC ILLNESS AND THE MOBILISATION OF RESOURCES

I have tried to show that attempts to impose meaning on threatening and seemingly arbitrary events, such as the appearance of rheumatoid arthritis, involve an examination of the constellation of familial and biographical experiences. In addition, the individual is inevitably drawn into rearranging his or her wider personal and community involvements. The presence or absence of a supportive social network may make a significant difference in the course of disablement, as Smith (1979) has shown. The specification of such networks and their use in routine health-service settings is already being attempted (Capildeo et al., 1976). The maintenance of neighbourliness and friendship, particularly in the ability to reciprocate favours or help offered, is central. The availability of a good friend, especially for many of the female patients in the study being reported here, emerged as a key element in the picture.

The disruption of friendship and community involvement arises not only because of functional limitations, such as restrictions in mobility and the problems of fatigue, but also because of the embarrassment which such disabilities create. Maintaining normal activities, like being able to sit in one position for a long period of time at a cinema, or maintaining normal appearances in a social gathering at a club or pub, have to become deliberately conscious activities, and thus frustrating and tiring. In the end, the effort simply does not seem worth it. The world of everyday life, that was once taken for granted, becomes a burden of conscious and deliberate action. The simplest outing becomes a major occasion for planning, an expedition. Thus, the handicaps of social isolation and dependency which flow from these disruptions in social intercourse are not simply derived from the ability or inability to carry out tasks and activities. Individuals begin to restrict their terrain to local and familiar territory, where they are least likely to be exposed to the gaze and questions of acquaintances and strangers (Goffman, 1968; Barker and Bury, 1978). As a male respondent put it:

> Now the only place I go now is down to the local club. Everybody knows me sort of thing. They might say it's a shame for him, but nobody bothers me, they accept me as I am. But if I go anywhere else, say, if I was to go to another club or another pub somewhere where I am not known as a regular and I see somebody who I haven't seen for years, they try to avoid you. They, people, are embarrassed. People say 'Bloody hell, is that...? Dear me, what's the matter with him?' And they try not to catch your eye, if you will. People tend to stay away from you. I don't know, they just don't want to be involved. You tend to do the same then.

As I mentioned earlier, Strauss (1975) has pointed out that withdrawal from social relationships and growing social isolation are major features of chronic illness. In the early stages of a disease, one of the most difficult places to maintain normal relationships and mobilise resources, especially among younger sufferers, is at work. Two women with jobs which involved the continuous use of their hands exemplified the problems. One felt that her workmates had little sympathy, and that she could demand no special consideration. As was common among the study group, she was reluctant to do so anyway, in case she drew unwelcome attention to herself and her work. She was under pressure to keep pace with the speed of work, and she constantly worried about the loss of her job. Again, the situation is best expressed in the words of the woman herself:

> We're getting all new work now from the fire stations, street reports and that. They take ages. Some of the girls just seem to whistle through them, but it takes me nearly all day to do them. She [her supervisor] wouldn't be too pleased. I know that for a fact. She'd say, 'Oh, it's not worth your while working here,' and all that. That's the type of thing you usually get if they know you're going to be off ever so often. So I don't say anything, and if I'm off I'm just ill. The doctor doesn't even put down what is wrong with me. I invent something and he puts it on the sick note, and then I say what is actually wrong with me.... At the moment I'm treated as an equal, which I am. I do the same amount of work as them. I get more or less the same money, so I think, 'Well, at least I'm keeping my part up.'

The attempt to normalise in the face of disruption is revealed here. Departing from behaviour which is deemed appropriate carries its own specific disadvantages, and thus is avoided as far as possible. Much depends on the degree of flexibility which both formal institutions and informal relationships are prepared to allow. In this case, such latitude appeared to the sufferer to be minimal.

A wider set of provisions were available to the other woman. Her employers were sympathetic and helpful. However, she too suffered strains as a result of her illness, though this time more directly from the informal pressure of her workmates who, she stated, were reluctant to redistribute the workload in her favour. Even though she felt that they were generally sympathetic, her frequent absences meant that the limits of tolerance had been reached. As one telephonist among a group, there was little room for manoeuvre, especially as the work required continual manual dexterity, a situation which became increasingly difficult as the disabling effects of the disease developed. Even though union/management arrangements gave her the right to be absent for both regular hospital visits and when her disabilities and symptoms were at their worst, such explicit acceptance could not circumvent the relationship problems at work itself. The form in which work tasks were organised reduced the opportunities for adopting a strategy to disguise her difficulties and thus reduce her handicap.

Occupation and social class are, of course, closely related, although their relationship in illness is a complex matter. The importance of social class for my discussion lies in the variable distribution of resources in society, and thus the ability of individuals from different social strata to compensate for the effects of disability and offset economic and other handicaps. However, the picture is not always straightforward. In the study, two men, a manual worker to whom I've already referred, and a small businessman, suffered the onset of severe systemic illness. In the short term, the self-employed man suffered relatively greater hardship, as his business was threatened and, unlike the manual worker, he could not rely on state benefits. In the long term, however, the manual worker faced greater difficulties. The administrative definitions of disability bring about their own consequences, as Blaxter (1976) has shown.

For the first six months, the manual worker actually found himself financially as well off being 'off sick' as he did when in work. This came as something of a surprise in the early days, but on passing the six-months point, his long-term disability benefits came into force and he found himself facing permanent hardship. The businessman was able, slowly, to rearrange his work practices and significantly reduce his own hours of work. The manual worker finally struggled back to work after a year's absence, only to find that the tasks, involving re-roofing of factories and warehouses, were impossible, even with considerable support from his workmates. This brought about a new crisis, and at the point of a third interview with him he expressed great bitterness at having worked so hard all his life with little to show for it in times of adversity. Again, the 'unfairness' at having been singled out was hard to bear. Not surprisingly, the pain and discomfort of his arthritis combined with these worries to produce a great deal of unhappiness and depression. Throughout the period of persisting disability and growing handicaps, his contact with his general practitioner had been minimal. From time to time he gave his doctor a routine progress report. Of his feelings and practical hardships he said nothing.

DISCUSSION AND CONCLUDING REMARKS

In describing the experience of the onset and development of rheumatoid arthritis, I have tried to suggest a perspective which conceptualises chronic illness as a particular kind of disruptive experience. This disruption throws into relief the cognitive and material resources available to individuals. It displays the key forms which explanations of pain and suffering in illness take in modern society, the continuity and discontinuity of professional and lay modes of thought, and the sources of variability in experience arising from the influence of structural constraints over the ability to adapt.

Under normal conditions, the relationship between self and others is a precarious enterprise, characterised as it is in contemporary settings by high degrees of self-reflection, individualism and the manipulation of appearances (Berger, Berger and Kellner, 1974). This precariousness is held in check by a wide range of 'cognitive packages' available to individuals and groups, each of which is more or less successful in structuring and maintaining meaning. Insofar as it is possible to identify dominant motifs, those which resonate strongly with scientific and technical imperatives are likely to be the most influential. Not surprisingly, therefore, medical knowledge and medical practice have become central features in modern society. As Foucault (1973) puts it, 'In this [European] culture, medical thought is fully engaged in the philosophical status of man.'

However, knowledge and practice are not necessarily perceived in the same light. Treatments are often empirical in character, and patients may feel let down by the limits of medical intervention and technology, or indeed by a realisation of the limits of medical knowledge itself. But my study provides no ground for assuming that these problems indicate any generalised disillusionment with medicine as a system of knowledge and explanation.

Indeed, the reverse may be the case; criticism is directed at poor communication by doctors, or inappropriate treatment and advice, contrasting with the high expectations held of medicine. From this point of view, the 'medicalisation of life' thesis, while carrying obvious face validity, remains sociologically naive. It is to be expected that areas of experience on the 'margins' of everyday life (Berger and Berger, 1976) require elaborate symbolic expression (in my case, the occurrence of pain, suffering and other features of chronic illness as a whole), and attract attention from those institutions which codify knowledge of the body and mind in the practical management of personal troubles and affliction, specifically, of course, those of medicine and, to a lesser extent, the agencies of social welfare. The assessment of medicine's role as a symbolic system, in facilitating as well as constraining understanding and action in such situations, is jeopardised by the continuance of a one-sided portrayal of medicine's negative influences. The deep involvement of medicine in reorganising the disruptive experiences of chronic illness, in reordering its arbitrary and threatening characteristics, inevitably involves issues of social control. That medical sociology should seek to explore this is important, but to suggest, as some writers do, that the experience of pain, illness, and even death can be faced without recourse to such codes is patently false (see, for example, the recent arguments of Illich, 1975; Kennedy, 1981; and Sontag, 1979).

Medical conceptions of chronic organic disease and its causation are not regarded as illegitimate 'reifications' from a lay point of view. They provide an objective fixed point on a terrain of uncertainty. The problem, however, is that such knowledge itself often turns out to be ambiguous and limited. Thus, rheumatoid arthritis appears as a definite entity, yet its implications for the future are uncertain. Such knowledge is incomplete; it has to be supplemented by, and set against, a body of knowledge and meaning drawn from the individual's own biography. The search for the cause of the illness, which I have described, is at one and the same time a search for its meaning. The separation of cause and meaning has an important but limited place in lay thought. The identification of medical thought with disease and lay thought with illness, in medical sociology, seems to me oversimplified (Eisenberg, 1977; Cassell, 1975). A more careful treatment of the continuity and discontinuity between lay and specialised modes of thought is called for. I wish to suggest that medicine be treated as a cultural system, as both an important resource to people in times of distress and pain, and as a constraint in their search for the deeper meaning of experience. I further wish to suggest a dual view of medicine, or rather, a view of the duality of medicine, one which, following Giddens (1979), has a 'respect for the authenticity of belief' (whether doctors' or patients'), while offering the possibility of a 'critical evaluation of the justification of belief and the involvement of beliefs in the distribution of power'.

Important though the place of medicine is in facilitating and constraining the adaptation of individuals (and those with whom they live and work) to the presence of chronic illness, this is clearly not the only, or necessarily the most important, issue. I have also tried to show that disruptions in biography are, at one and the same time, disruptions of social relationships and of the ability to mobilise material resources. To be sure, medical knowledge and lay knowledge about disease and illness enter these fields, but it is clear that the warrantability of a person's changed behaviour, because of chronic illness, is determined by many other factors. We know relatively little about the 'limits of tolerance' within families and workplaces, and how they vary between different social groups and settings. The disruption of reciprocity, the problems in legitimating changed behaviour, and the overall effects of stigma associated with chronic illness all affect the individual's ability to mobilise resources to advantage. Conversely, the variability in resources between different social groups affects the processes mentioned here. As Illsley (1980) has recently pointed out, the processes involved in the interaction between wider social structures and the experiences of ill-health, within specific cultural and familial contexts, are still poorly understood. The perspectives of biographical disruption and the interplay of lay and professional modes of thought are offered here as a contribution to tackling that problem.

References

Barker, J. and Bury, M.R. 1978. 'Mobility and the elderly: a community challenge', in V. Carver and P. Uddiard (eds), *An Ageing Population*. Sevenoaks: Hodder and Stoughton.

Berger, P. and Berger, B. 1976. *Sociology: A Biographical Approach*. Harmondsworth: Penguin.

Berger, P. and Luckmann, T. 1967. *The Social Construction of Reality*. London: Allen Lane.

Berger, P., Berger, B. and Kellner, H. 1974. *The Homeless Mind*. Harmondsworth: Penguin.

Blaxter, M. 1976. *The Meaning of Disability*. London: Heinemann.

Bury, M.R. 1979. 'Disablement in society: towards an integrated perspective', *International Journal of Rehabilitation Research*, 2 (1): 33–40.

Capildeo, R., Court, C. and Rose, F.C. 1976. 'Social network diagram, *British Medical Journal*, 1: 43–44. Reprinted in V. Carver and P. Uddiard. 1978. (eds) *An Ageing Population*. Sevenoaks: Hodder and Stoughton.

Cassell, E.J. 1975. 'Preliminary explorations of thinking in medicine', *Ethics in Science and Medicine*, 2: 1–12.

Comaroff, J. and Maguire, P. 1981. 'Ambiguity and the search for meaning: childhood leukaemia in the modern clinical context', *Social Science and Medicine*, 1 (5B): 115–23.

Coulter, G. 1973. *Approaches to Insanity*. London: Martin Robertson.

Cowie, B. 1976. 'The cardiac patient's perception of his heart attack', *Social Science and Medicine*, 10: 87–96.

Crick, M. 1976. *Explorations in Language and Meaning: Towards a Semantic Anthropology*. London: Malaby Press.

Davis, F. 1960. 'Uncertainty in medical prognosis: clinical and functional', *American Journal of Sociology*, 66: 41–47.

Davis, F. 1963. *Passage through Crisis: Polio Victims and their Families*. Indianapolis: Bobbs Merrill.

———. 1964. 'Deviance disavowal: the management of strained interaction by the visibly handicapped', in H. Becker (ed.), *The Other Side*. New York: Free Press.

Dingwall, R. 1976. *Aspects of Illness*. London: Martin Robertson.

Eisenberg, L. 1977. 'Disease and illness', *Culture, Medicine and Psychiatry*, 1: 9–23.

Faber, K. 1923. *Nosography in Modern Internal Medicine*. New York: P.B. Hoeber.

Fabrega, H. and Manning, P. 1972. 'Disease, illness and deviant careers', in R.A. Scott and J.D. Douglas (eds), *Theoretical Perspectives on Deviance*. New York: Basic Books.

Foucault, M. 1973. *The Birth of the Clinic*. London: Tavistock.

Gallagher, E. 1976. 'Lines of reconstruction and extension in the Parsonian sociology of illness', *Social Science and Medicine*, 10 (5): 207–18.

Gerhardt, U. 1979. 'The Parsonian paradigm and the identity of medical sociology', *Sociological Review*, 27: 229–51.

Giddens, A. 1979. *Central Problems in Social Theory*. London: Macmillan.

Goffman, E. 1968. *Stigma: Notes on the Management of Spoiled Identity*. Harmondsworth: Penguin.

———. 1975. *Frame Analysis*. Harmondsworth: Penguin.

Herzlich, C. 1973. *Health and Illness: A Social-Psychological Analysis*. European Monographs in Social Psychology, vol. 5. London: Academic Press.

Illich, I. 1975. *Medical Nemesis*. London: Calder and Boyars.

Illsley, R. 1980. *Professional or Public Health?* London: Nuffield Provincial Hospitals Trust.

Kennedy, I. 1981. *The Unmasking of Medicine*. London: Allen and Unwin.

Maclean, U. 1975. 'Patient delay: some observations on medical claims to certainty', *Lancet*, 5 July: 23.

Maclean, U. and Cockshutt, A. 1979. 'How women cope with their menfolk's heart attacks', *New Society*, 26 July: 183–85.

Rock, P. 1979. *The Making of Symbolic Interactionism*. London: Macmillan.

Singer, E. 1974. 'Premature social ageing: the social and psychological consequences of a chronic illness', *Social Science and Medicine*, 18: 143–51.

Smith, R.T. 1979. 'Rehabilitation of the disabled: the role of social networks in the recovery process', *International Rehabilitation Medicine*, I (2): 63–72. See also, R.T.

Smith and L. Midanik. 'The effects of social resources on recovery and perceived sense of control among the disabled', *Sociology of Health and Illness*, 2: 48–63.

Sontag, S. 1979. *Illness as Metaphor*. London: Allen Lane.

Strauss, A.L. 1975. *Chronic Illness and the Quality of Life*. St Louis: Mosby.

Taussig, M. 1980. 'Reification and the consciousness of the patient', *Social Science and Medicine*, 14B: 3–13.

Taylor, D. 1977. *Physical Impairment: Social Handicap*. London: Office of Health Economics.

Wadsworth, M., Butterfield, W.J.H. and Blaney, R. 1971. *Health and Sickness: The Choice of Treatment*, London: Tavistock.

Weiner, C. 1975. 'The burden of rheumatoid arthritis: tolerating the uncertainty', *Social Science and Medicine*, 9: 97–104.

6

The Damaged Self

Robert F. Murphy

From the time my tumour was first diagnosed through my entry into wheelchair life, I had an increasing apprehension that I had lost much more than the full use of my legs. I had also lost a part of my self. It was not just that people acted differently toward me, which they did, but rather that I felt differently toward myself. I had changed in my own mind, in my self-image, and in the basic conditions of my existence. It left me feeling alone and isolated, despite strong support from family and friends; moreover, it was a change for the worse, a diminution of everything I used to be. This was particularly frightening for somebody who had clawed his way up from poverty to a position of respect. I had become a person of substance, and that substance was oozing away. It threatened everything that Yolanda and I had put together over the years. In middle age, the ground beneath me had convulsed. And I had no idea why and how this had happened.

I cannot remember ever before thinking about physical disability, except as something that happened to other, less fortunate people. It certainly had no relevance to me. A disabled person could enter my field of vision, but my mind would fail to register him—a kind of selective blindness quite common among people of our culture. During a year that I spent in the Sahel and Sudan zones of Nigeria and Niger, a region of endemic

Murphy, R.F. 1990. *The Body Silent.* New York: W.W. Norton, pp. 85–104.

leprosy and missing hands, feet and noses, the plight of those people was as alien to me as were their language, culture and circumstances. Because of this gulf, I had no empathy for them, and just enough sympathy to drop coins into cups extended from the ends of stumps. A few pennies were all that it took to buy the dubious grace of almsgiving. It was a bargain, a gesture that did not assert my oneness with them, but rather my separation from them.

With the onset of my own impairment, I became almost morbidly sensitive to the social position and treatment of the disabled, and I began to notice nuances of behaviour that would have gone over my head in times past. One of my earliest observations was that social relations between the disabled and the able-bodied are tense, awkward and problematic. This is something that every handicapped person knows, but it surprised me at the time. For example, when I was in the hospital, a young woman visitor entered my room with a look of total consternation on her face. She exclaimed that she had just seen an awful sight, a girl who was missing half of her skull. I knew the girl as a very sweet, but quite retarded, teenaged patient who used to drop in on me a few times a day; we always had the same conversation. I asked my guest why the sight bothered her so much, but she couldn't tell me. She in turn asked why it didn't trouble me. After a moment's thought, I replied that I was one of 'them', a notion that she rejected vehemently. But why did my visitor, a poised and intelligent person, react in this way? It aroused my curiosity.

There is something quite significant in this small encounter, for it had elements of what Erving Goffman called 'one of the primal scenes of sociology'. Borrowing the Freudian metaphor of the primal scene (a child's traumatic witnessing of the mother and father in sexual intercourse), Goffman used the phrase to mean any social confrontation of people in which there is some great flaw, such as when one of the parties has no nose. This robs the encounter of firm cultural guidelines, traumatising it and leaving the people involved wholly uncertain about what to expect from each other. It has the potential for social calamity.

The intensely problematic character of relations between those with damaged bodies and the more-or-less unmarked cannot be shrugged off simply as a result of the latter's ineptitude, bias, stupidity, and so forth, although they do play a part. Even the best-intentioned able-bodied people have difficulty anticipating the reactions of the disabled, for interpretations are warped by the impairment. To complicate matters, the disabled also enter the social arena with a skewed perspective. Not only are their bodies altered, but their ways of thinking about themselves and about the persons and objects of the external world have become profoundly transformed. They have experienced a revolution of consciousness. They have undergone a metamorphosis.

Nobody has ever asked me what it is like to be a paraplegic—and now a quadriplegic—for this would violate all the rules of middle-class etiquette. A few have asked me what caused my condition, and, after hearing the answer, have looked as though they wished they hadn't. After all, tumours can happen to anybody—even to them. Polite manners may protect us from most such intrusions, but it is remarkable that physicians seldom ask either. They like 'hard facts', obtainable through modern technology or old-fashioned jabbing with a pin and asking whether you feel it. These tests supposedly provide good, 'objective' measures of neurological damage, but, like sociological questionnaires, they reduce experience to neat distinctions of black or white, and ignore the broad range of ideation and emotion that always accompanies disability. The full subjective states of the patient are of little concern in the medical model of disability, which holds that the problem arises wholly from some anatomic or physiological disorder, and is correctible by standard modes of therapy—drugs, surgery, radiation, or whatever. What goes on inside the patient's head is another department, and if there are signs of serious psychological malaise, he is packed off to the proper specialist.

The medical people have had little curiosity about what I think about my condition, although they do know its sensory symptoms: a constant tingling in my hands, forearms and feet, and a steady, low threshold of pain in my legs. The discomfort is similar to the soreness and burning sensation experienced with torn or severely strained muscles, and has much to do with the fact that the musculature of my trunk and legs is always in spasm, despite a generous daily dosage of muscle relaxants. The curious thing about this condition is that a knife could be run through my leg now and I wouldn't feel it. Aside from the tingle and the ache, my legs are otherwise numb and bereft of sensation. For the past four years, I have not tried to move them, for the tumour has long since passed the point at which therapy could maintain function. They don't even twitch anymore.

For a while, I occasionally tried to will the legs to move, but each futile attempt was psychologically devastating, leaving me feeling broken and helpless. I soon stopped trying. The average non-disabled person could be driven to the edge of breakdown if his legs were pinioned and rendered totally immobile for long periods, and an accident victim in a body cast finds his only comfort in the fact that his situation is temporary. I was saved from this, however, because the slow process of paralysis of my limbs was paralleled by a progressive atrophy of the need and impulse for physical activity. I was losing the will to move.

My upper-body functions have suffered some impairment ever since the tumour became symptomatic, although the lower body has deteriorated at a much faster rate. In addition to the diminished lung capacity and, consequently, more rapid and shallow breathing, the musculature of the arms and hands has progressively weakened, their range of movement has become steadily more narrow, my fingers have stiffened, and my hands have become increasingly numb and insensitive to touch and temperature. In common with other paralytics, I have to be careful with hot water or hot dishes and pots, for I can burn myself without knowing it. To complicate the hand problems, the fingers of quadriplegics curl inward toward the palms, a process that by the spring of 1986 has made my left hand almost useless.

Beyond these physical symptoms, I have been overtaken by a profound and deepening sense of tiredness—a total, draining weariness that I must resist every waking minute. It starts in the morning when I struggle to awaken, fighting my way out of the comfort and forgetfulness of sleep into self-awareness and renewed disability. Facing the world everyday is an ordeal for everybody; it is no accident that strokes and heart attacks peak in the period 8 a.m. to 9 a.m. It is much worse to confront the day with a serious deficit. The wish to turn my back to the world continues through the daily ablutions, which grow longer and more tedious every year; it now takes me a quarter-hour to shave. I am fully able to face life by 10 a.m., but by 4 or 5 p.m., I start to flag. Between these hours, I teach, talk to students and attend meetings, after which I go home and lie down for a couple of hours. I also conserve strength by spending only two, or at most three, days a week at the university. Like most professors,

I don't pass the other days in idleness. I read student exams, reports and doctoral dissertations; I keep up on books and journals in my field; and I do research and writing. But the professorial life allows me to work at home at my own tempo, sometimes while lying in bed. In no other line of work, I tell my graduate students, could such a wreck be 100 percent employed. It has to be described as an easy job!

But there is another aspect of my fatigue that cannot be eased by rest. This is a sense of tiredness and ennui with practically everything and everybody, a desire to withdraw from the world, to crawl into a hole and pull the lid over my head. The average person will recognise this wish, for everybody, at some time or other, feels that things have become too much to handle. Then he or she wishes for surcease, for even temporary remission. How tempting to tell all and sundry—family, work and society—to go to hell and leave one alone. Who hasn't said this, even if only under his breath? When an ordinary citizen is overcome by these feelings everyday and all day, however, his family and friends will urge him to seek professional help, for these are the sure symptoms of depression. In contrast, persons who are deeply impaired harbour these urges chronically, sometimes because they are depressed, but more often because they must each day face an inimical world, using the limited resources of a damaged body.

Many give in to the impulse to withdraw, retreating into a little universe sustained by monthly Social Security disability checks, a life circumscribed by the four walls of an apartment and linked to outside society by a television set. Constantina Safilios-Rothschild, a sociologist, has noted that disability may provide a pretext for withdrawal from work for some older workers dissatisfied and weary with their jobs, a kind of 'secondary gain' bought at great price. But this is not the source of the isolation; it's just a way of making the best of a bad thing. Many other disabled people go forth to battle the world everyday, but even they must wage a constant rearguard action against the backward pull. This is a powerful centripetal force, for it is commonly exacerbated by an altered sense of selfhood, one that has been savaged by the partial destruction of the body. Disability is not simply a physical affair for us; it is our ontology, a condition of our being in the world.

Of all the psychological syndromes associated with disability, the most pervasive, and the most destructive, is a radical loss of self-esteem. This sense of damage to the self, the acquisition of what Erving Goffman called a 'stigma' or 'spoiled identity', grew upon me during my first months in a wheelchair, and it hit me hardest when I returned to the university in the fall of 1977. By then, I could no longer hold on to the myth that I was using a wheelchair during convalescence. I had to face the unpalatable fact that I was wedded permanently to it; it had become an indispensable extension of my body. Strangely, I also felt this as a major blow to my pride.

The damage to my ego showed most painfully in an odd and wholly irrational sense of embarrassment and lowered self-worth when I was with people on my social periphery. Most of my colleagues in the anthropology department were old friends, some even from our undergraduate years, and they generally were warm and supportive. But people from other departments and the administration were another matter. During my first semester back at the university, I attended a few lunch meetings at the Faculty Club, but I began to notice that these were strained occasions. People whom I knew did not look my way. And persons with whom I had a nodding acquaintance did not nod; they, too, were busily looking off in another direction. Others gave my wheelchair a wide berth, as if it were surrounded by a penumbra of contamination. These were not happy encounters.

My social isolation became acute during stand-up gatherings, such as receptions and cocktail parties. I discovered that I was now three-and-a-half feet tall, and that most social interaction was taking place two feet above me. When speaking to a standing person, I have to crane my neck back and look upward, a position that stretches my larynx and further weakens my diminished vocal strength. Conversation in such settings has become an effort. Moreover, it was commonplace that I would be virtually ignored in a crowd for long periods broken by short bursts of patronisation. There was no escape from these intermittent attentions, for it is very difficult to manoeuvre a wheelchair through a crowd. My low stature and relative immobility thus made me the defenceless recipient of overtures, rather than their instigator. This is a common plaint of the motor-disabled: They have limited choice in socialising, and often must wait for the others to come to them. As a consequence, I now attend only small, sit-down gatherings.

Not having yet read the literature on the sociology of disability, I did not immediately recognise the pattern of avoidance. Perhaps this was for the best, as my initial hurt and puzzlement ultimately led me to research the subject. In the meantime, I stopped going to the Faculty Club and curtailed my contacts with the university-at-large. This is not hard to do at Columbia University, as each department lies within a 'Maginot Line', everybody is very busy, and the general social atmosphere runs from tepid to cool. None of this is surprising, for it is also the dominant ethos of New York City. On the positive side, this same general mood allows me to work in peace. They leave you alone at Columbia, and I wanted more than ever to be left alone.

Withdrawal only compounds the disabled person's subjective feelings of damage and lowered worth, sentiments that become manifest as shame and guilt. I once suggested to a housebound elderly woman that she should use a walker for going outside. 'I would never do that,' she replied. 'I'd be ashamed to be seen.' 'It's not your fault that you have arthritis,' I argued, adding that I used a walker and I wasn't ashamed. This was untrue, of course, and I knew it. But why should anyone feel shame about his disability? Even more mysterious, why should anyone feel a sense of guilt? In what way could I be responsible for my physical state? It could not be attributed to smoking or drinking, the favourite whipping boys of amateur diagnosticians, and it wasn't the result of an accident, with its possibilities for lifestyle culpability, the accusation that one bought it by living dangerously. No, I didn't do a damned thing to earn my tumour, nor was there any way that I could have prevented it. But such feelings are endemic among the disabled. One young woman, who had been born without lower limbs, told me that she had felt guilt for this since childhood, as had her parents (from whom she probably acquired the guilt). Indeed, a mutuality of guilt is the very life-stuff of the paralytic's family, just as it is, on a smaller scale, central to the cohesion—and turmoil—of all modern families.

Guilt and shame are not in fact as separate as they are often represented to be. In simple form, both are said to involve an assault on the ego: guilt is the attack of the superego, or conscience, and shame arises from the opprobrium of others. Of the two, I believe that shame is the more potent. The sociologist George Herbert Mead wrote that an individual's concept of his or her self is a reflection or, more accurately, a refraction, as in a fun-house mirror, of the way he or she is treated by others; and if a person is treated with ridicule, contempt or aversion, then his own ego is diminished, and his dignity and humanity are called into question. Shaming is an especially potent means of social control in small-scale societies, where everybody is known and behaviour is highly visible, but it is less effective in complex societies like our own, where we can compartmentalise our lives and exist in relative anonymity. But a wheelchair cannot be hidden; it is brutally visible. And to the extent that the wheelchair's occupant is treated with aversion, even disdain, his sense of worth suffers. Damage to the body, then, causes diminution of the self, which is further magnified by debasement by others.

Shame and guilt are one, in that both lower self-esteem and undercut the façade of dignity we present to the world. Moreover, in our culture, they tend to stimulate each other. The usual formula is that a wrongful act leads to a guilty conscience; if the guilt becomes publicly known, then shame must be added to the sequence, followed by punishment. There is then a causal chain that goes from wrongful act to guilt to shame to punishment. A fascinating aspect of disability is that it diametrically and completely reverses this progression, while preserving every step. The sequence of the person damaged in body goes from punishment (the impairment) to shame to guilt and, finally, to the crime. This is not a real crime, but a self-delusion that lurks in our fears and fantasies, in the haunting, never-articulated question: 'What did I do to deserve this?'

In this topsy-turvy world of reversed causality, the punishment—for this is how crippling is unconsciously apprehended—begets the crime. All of this happens despite the fact that the individual may be in no way to blame for his condition; real responsibility is irrelevant. This transmutation of body impairment into guilt is a neat inversion of the Freudian Oedipal drama. According to the psychoanalytic interpretation of the myth, Oedipus unknowingly kills his father and marries his own mother, for which crime the Fates pursue him to Colonus, where he blinds himself. Blinding is seen as a symbolic form of castration, which is, in turn, the fitting punishment for incest. According to Freud, in male socialisation, it is the threat of castration by the father, even if only a fantasised threat, that forces the child to relinquish and repress the guilt-ridden wish to possess the mother. It should be noted, however, that in the myth the father did not blind Oedipus; Oedipus did it to himself. What is usually forgotten in discussions of the Greek tragedy is that the father, after hearing from a soothsayer that his son would one day slay him, crippled young Oedipus. In fact, the name Oedipus can be translated as 'Swollen Foot' or, loosely, 'Gimpy'.

That crippling can be just as proper a punishment for incest as blinding finds ethnographic support. In my own fieldwork, I recorded a Mundurucu myth in which a man who committed incest with his surrogate mother was physically deformed by her husband, a god, and later blinded. And among West African Moslems there is a widespread religious cult centred on a female succubus named Dogwa. (In Morocco, this cult figure is called Aisha Kandisha.) Dogwa is both nurturing and sexually seductive to her devotees; she is both mother and lover. In the former role, she can bring wealth to her followers, but in the latter, she jealously takes swift retaliation against infidelity. Appropriately, the punishment is crippling or blinding. It is worth noting that no father figure is involved here. Instead, there is the ambivalent mother, the giver and nurturer of life, and its potential destroyer. Incest, or even the unconscious wish for it, is a dangerous game, and I would hazard the guess that the unconscious, diffuse sense of guilt that so often bedevils the disabled arises in the first place from the chimerical notion that the crippling is a punishment for this repressed, elusive and forbidden desire. There may be no such thing as Original Sin, but original guilt lurks in the dark recesses of the minds of all humans. These ashes of our first love are the basic stuff of the indefinable, unarticulated and haunting sense that the visitation of paralysis is a form of atonement, a Draconian penance.

Paralytic disability constitutes emasculation of a more direct and total nature. For the male, the weakening and atrophy of the body threaten all the cultural values of masculinity: strength, activeness, speed, virility, stamina and fortitude. Many disabled men, and women, try to compensate for their deficiencies by becoming involved in athletics. Paraplegics play wheelchair basketball, engage in racing, enter marathons, and do weightlifting and many other active things. Those too old or too impaired for physical displays may instead show their competence by becoming 'super-crips'. Just as 'super-moms' supposedly go off to work every morning, cook Cordon Bleu dinners at night, play with the kids, and then become red-hot lovers after the children are put to bed, the super-crip works harder than other people, travels extensively, goes to everything, and takes part in anything that comes along. This is how he shows the world that he is like everybody else, only better.

Becoming a super-crip, or super-mom, often depends less on the personal qualities of the individual than on very fortunate circumstances. In my own case, I was well established in my profession at the time of my disability, so my activity was just a matter of persistence. The real super-crips are those who do everything after they become impaired, like one woman who, after partial remission from totally paralytic multiple sclerosis, went on to finish college and then obtain a Ph.D. She refused to let the disease rob her of a future. There are many such people, but, like super-moms, they are still a minority. The vast majority, as we will see, are unable to conquer the formidable physical and social obstacles that confront them, and they live in the penumbra of society, condemned to lives as outsiders.

Afflictions of the spinal cord have a further devastating effect upon masculinity, aside from paralysis, for they commonly produce some degree of impotence or sexual malfunction. Depending on the extent of damage to the cord, the numbed genital area sends no signals to the brain, nor do the libidinal centres of the brain get messages through to the genitalia and the physiological processes that produce erections. This can result in total and permanent impotence, sporadic impotence, or difficulty in sustaining an erection until orgasm. There are some paraplegic men, on the other hand, who can maintain an erection but are unable to achieve orgasm, even after steady intercourse of a half-hour to an hour. The effects of this on the male psyche are profound. We usually think of 'castration anxiety' as an Oedipal thing, but there is a sort of symbolic castration in impotence that creates a kind of existential anxiety among all men. It is no accident that impotence is a major problem in those lands where masculine values are strongest, nor is it fortuitous that the new sexual freedom in America, with its emphasis on female gratification and male performance, has yielded a bumper crop of impotent men. After all, being a man does not mean just having a penis; it means having a sexually useful one. Anything less is indeed a kind of castration, although I am using this lurid Freudian term primarily as a metaphor for loss of both sexual and social power.

Most forms of paraplegia and quadriplegia cause male impotence and female inability to achieve orgasm. But paralytic women need not be aroused or experience orgasmic pleasure to engage in genital sex, and many indulge regularly in intercourse and even bear children, although by Caesarean section. Human sexuality, Freud tells us, is polymorphously perverse, meaning that the entire body is erogenous, and the joys of sex varied. Paraplegic women claim to derive psychological gratification from the sex act itself, as well as from the stimulation of other parts of their bodies and the knowledge that they are still able to give pleasure to others. They may derive less physical gratification from sex than before becoming disabled, but they are still active participants. Males have far more circumscribed anatomical limits. Other than having a surgical implant that produces a simulated erection, the man can no longer engage in genital sex. He either becomes celibate or practices oral sex, or any of the many other variations in sexual expression devised by our innovative species. Whichever alternative he takes, his standing as a man has been compromised far more than has been the woman's status. He has been effectively emasculated.

Even in those cases in which the paraplegic male retains potency, his stance during the sex act changes. Most must lie still on their backs during intercourse, and it is the woman who must do the mounting and thrusting. In modern America, this is an acceptable alternative position, but in some cultures it would be considered a violation of male dominance: men are on top in society and they should be on top in sex, and that's the end of the matter. And even in the relatively liberated United States of the 1980s, the male usually takes the more active role and the position on top. But the paraplegic male, whether engaging in genital or oral sex, always takes a passive role. Most paralytic men accept this limitation, for they discover that the wells of passion are in the brain, not between the legs, and that pleasure is possible even without orgasm. One man, who had enjoyed an intensely erotic relationship with his wife before an auto accident made him paraplegic and impotent, reported that they simply continued oral sex. The wife derives complete orgasmic satisfaction and the husband achieves deep psychological pleasure, which he describes as a 'mental orgasm'. The sex lives of most paralysed men, however, remain symbolic of a more general passivity and dependency that touches every aspect of their existence and is the antithesis of the male values of direction, activity, initiative and control.

The sexual problems of the disabled are aggravated by a widespread view that they are either malignantly sexual, like libidinous dwarfs, or, more commonly, that they are completely asexual, an attribute frequently ascribed to the elderly as well. These erroneous notions, which I suspect arise from the sexual anxieties of their holders, fail to recognise that a large majority of disabled people have the same urges as the able-bodied, and are just as competent in expressing them. Spinal cord injuries raise special problems, but motor-disabled people with cerebral palsy, the after-effects of polio, and many other conditions, often can lead almost normal sex lives. That asexuality is also attributed sometimes to the blind underlines the utter irrationality of the belief.

Given the prevalence of such ignorance, I was pleased to read in 1985 that educational television was airing a film on sex among the disabled, and I made it a point to watch it. At the beginning of the film, there appeared on the screen a warning that there would be nude scenes, leading me to the happy expectation that a paraplegic or quadriplegic would be shown making love. Not so, for the only nudes were a couple of very healthy-looking young women. And, in deliberate counterpoint, most of the disabled people shown were grossly disfigured. It was a modern-day version of *Beauty and the Beast*, a film that served to perpetuate, not combat, a prejudice. The producers meant well, but they merely illustrated the depth of the problem. This episode reminded me that when one young woman began research among paraplegics, a female friend asked her, 'But you wouldn't go to bed with one of them, would you?' These are indeed primal scenes.

One of Sigmund Freud's enduring contributions to our age was his rejection of classical philosophy's disembodiment of the mind. Instead, Freud started with a theory of instincts that located much of human motivation and thought in the needs of the body, especially the sexual drive. This was not a simple, single-direction, mechanical determinism, however, for Freud's theories held that causality is a two-way street. The human mind also uses its symbolic capacity to reach out and encompass the body, making it just as much a part of the mind as the mind is of the body. The body, particularly the more explicitly erogenous zones, becomes incorporated into human thought, into the very structure of the personality, and the sexual symbolism of pleasure and desire is used by the mind in moulding one's orientation to the world. Sex thus invades thought, but is also intensified and transformed by thought. And so it is that the loss of the use of one's legs, or any other vital function, is an infringement on the integrity of the mind, an assault on character, a vitiation of power.

The unity of mind and body is also an important element of phenomenological philosophy. This school, which arose in the early twentieth century from the writings of Edmund Husserl, sidesteps the old philosophical question, 'How do we know the world (or reality, or truth),' and says that the world is whatever we make it out to be; it is created within the stream of conscious experience. And the way we experience and understand reality is in good part shaped by the language categories through which we sort out what we take to be real, and by the cultural symbolism through which we find significance and meaning in the mess of sense impressions continually bombarding us. Reality, then, isn't a hard-and-fast thing, the same for everybody, but a consensual matter, a social construct that must be reaffirmed and recreated in all our interactions with other people. It would follow from this relativistic view of the human grasp of the world that people of different cultures inhabit somewhat different realities, as do people of the same culture but of radically different circumstances—people, for example, who can't walk.

In his 1962 book *The Phenomenology of Perception*, the French philosopher Maurice Merleau-Ponty states that the starting point for our apprehension and construction of the world is the body. This goes beyond the obvious fact that our sense organs are parts of the body, for he stresses that the landscape of the body is, explicitly or implicitly, the means and the perspective by which we place ourselves in environments and experience their dimensions. As Simone de Beauvoir says, the body is not a thing, an entity separate from the mind and from the rest of the world in which it is situated. The body is also a set of relationships that link the outer world and the mind into a system. Merleau-Ponty illustrates this by reference to the phenomenon of the 'phantom limb', the amputee's illusion that he still possesses the missing arm or leg. He writes, 'What it is in us which refuses mutilation and disablement is an *I* [Merleau-Ponty's emphasis], committed to a certain physical and inter-human world, who continues to tend towards his world despite handicaps and amputations and who, to this extent, does not recognise them *de jure* [openly and avowedly].' The amputee is missing more than a limb: He is also missing one of his conceptual links to the world, an anchor of his very existence.

Gelya Frank, an anthropologist, has written a life history of a woman born without her four limbs, documenting the laborious process by which she became 'embodied', grew to accept her condition, and developed self-love. Frank sees her as a kind of Venus de Milo whose beauty is curiously enhanced, like the statue's, by her lack of limbs. Embodiment is a problem for those born with deficiencies, but at least they can be socialised to their limitations from infancy. On the other hand, most paraplegics and quadriplegics come to their lot through 'the slings and arrows of outrageous fortune' and have a different problem; they have to become re-embodied to their impairments. And if the loss of function is grave enough, they may even have to become disembodied.

My own sense of disembodiment is somewhat akin to that of Christina, the 'disembodied lady' discussed by Oliver Sacks in his book *The Man Who Mistook His Wife for a Hat.* Because of an allergic reaction to an antibiotic drug, Christina lost all sense of her body—a failure of her faculty of proprioception, the delicate, subliminal feedback mechanism that tells the brain about the position, tension and general feeling of the body and its parts. It is this 'sixth sense' that allows for coordination of movement; without it, talking, walking, even standing, are virtually impossible. In similar fashion, I no longer know where my feet are, and without the low-level pain I still feel, I would hardly know I had legs. Indeed, one of the early symptoms of my malady was a tendency to lose my balance when I would take off my pants in the dark, something that happened to me often in my drinking days. Christina's troubles differ from those of the paralytic, however, for her loss has been more complete. Besides, she became disembodied while still capable of movement, and she compensated by using her eyes to coordinate her physical actions. Quadriplegics, too, must watch what they are doing, and I have spilled drinks held in my hand because my wrist had turned and my brain didn't register it. But by the time the paralytic's failure of proprioception is as complete as Christina's, the limb is no longer movable, and the condition is moot.

I have also become rather emotionally detached from my body, often referring to one of my limbs as *the* leg or *the* arm. People who help me on a regular basis have also fallen into this pattern, saying, for example,

'I'll hold the arms and you grab the legs,' as if this depersonalisation would compensate for what otherwise would be an intolerable violation of my personal space. The paralytic becomes accustomed to being lifted, rolled, pushed, pulled and twisted, and he survives this treatment by putting emotional distance between himself and his body. Others join in this effort, and I well remember that after I came to from neurosurgery in 1976, there was a sign pinned to my sheet that read DO NOT LIFT BY ARMS. I weakly suggested to the nurse that they print another sign, saying THIS SIDE UP.

As my condition has deteriorated, I have come increasingly to look upon my body as a faulty life-support system, the only function of which is to sustain my head. It is all a bit like *Donovan's Brain*, an old science-fiction movie in which a quite nefarious brain is kept alive in a jar with mysterious wires and tubes attached to it. Murphy's brain is similarly sitting on a body that has no movement or tactile sense below the arms and shoulders, and that functions mainly to oxygenate the blood, receive nourishment, and eliminate wastes. In none of these capacities does it do a very good job. My solution to this dilemma is radical dissociation from the body, a kind of etherealisation of identity. Perhaps one reason for my success in this adaptation is that I never did take much pride in my body. I am of medium height, rather scrawny, and militantly non-athletic. I was never much to look at, but that didn't bother me greatly. From boyhood onward, I cultivated my wits instead. It is a very different matter for an athletically inclined boy or a girl on the threshold of dating and courtship.

Those who have lost use of some parts of their bodies learn to cultivate the others. The blind develop acute sensitivity to sounds, and quadriplegics, who cannot handle heavy telephone directories, have a remarkable knack for remembering phone numbers. But of a more fundamental order, the quadriplegic's body can no longer speak a 'silent language' in the expression of emotions or concepts too elusive for ordinary speech, for the delicate feedback loops between thought and movement have been broken. Proximity, gesture and body-set have been muted, and the body's ability to articulate thought has been stilled. It is perhaps for this reason that writing has become almost an addiction for me, for in it thought and mind become a system, united in conjunction with the movements of my hands and the responses of the machine. Of even more profound impact on existential states, the thinking activity of the brain cannot be dissolved into motion, and the mind can no longer be lost in an internal dialogue with physical movement. This leaves one adrift in a lonely monologue, an inner soliloquy without rest or surcease, and often without subject matter. Consciousness is overtaken and devoured in contemplation, meditation, ratiocination and reflection without end, relieved only by one's remaining movements, and sleep.

My thoughts and sense of being alive have been driven back into my brain, where I now reside. More than ever before, it is the base from which I reach out and grasp the world. Many paralytics say that they no longer feel attached to their bodies, which is another way of expressing the shattering of Merleau-Ponty's mind-body system. But it also has a few positive aspects. Just as an anthropologist gets a better perspective on his own culture through long and deep study of a radically different one, my extended sojourn in disability has given me, like it or not, a measure of estrangement far beyond the field of any trip. I now stand somewhat apart from American culture, making me in many ways a stranger. And with this estrangement has come a greater urge to penetrate the veneer of cultural differences and reach an understanding of the underlying unity of all human experience.

My own disembodied thoughts are crude when compared with those of many people. A blind Milton painted sweeping landscapes of the heavens in *Paradise Lost*, and Beethoven crafted the Ninth Symphony despite, or perhaps because of, being deaf. And today, one of the world's leading cosmologists, a Cambridge physicist named Stephen Hawking, travels through quarks and black holes in a journey across space and time to the birth of the universe. These are voyages of the mind, for Hawking has an advanced case of amyotrophic lateral sclerosis (familiarly known as Lou Gehrig's disease), which has left him with only slight movement in one hand and an inability to speak above a whisper. There are not many Miltons, Beethovens and Hawkings, however, and their example may be small comfort to a twenty-year-old quadriplegic who has made the mistake of diving into shallow water. For most disabled people, the loss of synchrony between mind and body has little compensation.

Many years ago, long before I became disabled, I was talking to a black anthropologist, a friend from our days as fellow graduate students, and the subject turned to race. In the course of our conversation, my friend said, 'I always think of myself as being black, just as you always think of yourself as white.' I protested this, saying that, even though I did think of myself as white when talking to a black person, my skin colour was not in the forefront of my conscious mind at other times. My friend didn't believe me. But I was neither mistaken nor misleading in my observation, for I grew up in and still lived in a white world. Whiteness was taken for granted; it was standard, part of the usual order of things. I lived in white neighbourhoods; I sailed on a white warship (except for the officers' stewards, who were black); I went to white schools (P.S. 114 in Rockaway Beach never had a black student during my eight years there); and I work in a profession that is still ninety-five percent white. Why think of my whiteness when most of my contacts are with white people? The comedian Martin Mull once did a television programme entitled 'The History of White People in America', a howlingly funny title because its redundancy fractures logic. White is normal; it's what ethnolinguists call an 'unmarked category', a word that is dominant within its class and against which other words of that class are contrasted. Why, I would no more have thought of myself as white than I would have thought of myself as walking on two legs.

Before my disability, I was a standard White, Anglo-Saxon, Agnostic Male (WASAM?), a member of the dominant part of the society. My roots in tattered-lace-curtain Irish Catholicism made me uneasy in academia, but I never gave much thought to the other components of my identity. My black friend was forced by the reality of white society always to think of himself as black. It was his first line of defence against a hostile environment. His was an embattled identity. And in exactly the same way, from the time I first took to the wheelchair up to the present, the fact that I am physically handicapped has been in the background of my conscious thoughts. Busy though I might be with other matters and problems, it lingers as a shadow in a corner of my mind, waiting, ready to come out at any moment to fill my meditations. It is a Presence. I, too, had acquired an embattled identity, a sense of who and what I was that was no longer dominated by my past social attributes, but rather by my physical defects.

7

Body Image and Physical Disability: Personal Perspectives

George Taleporos & Marita P. McCabe

INTRODUCTION

Body image in people with physical disability is an important area of investigation which has received little attention in the research literature. Because of the significant role that body image may play in the lives of people with physical disabilities, this topic warrants empirical investigation. This paper presents qualitative data on the body images of seven adults with physical disability.

Teal and Athelstan (1975, p. 266) defined body image as a psychological experience focused on feelings and attitudes toward one's own body. Smith (1984) provided an elaboration of these feelings and attitudes by claiming that body image includes both conscious and unconscious feelings, and that these may relate to the size, function, appearance and potential of one's body. Slade's (1994, p. 302) definition of body image as a loose mental representation of body shape, size and form which is influenced by a variety of historical, cultural, social, individual and biological factors which operate over varying time spans, recognises

Taleporos, G. and McCabe, M.P. 2002. 'Body image and physical disability: Personal perspectives', *Social Science and Medicine*, 54: 971–80.

the impact of environmental factors. Informed by these definitions, body image is defined in the current study as the combination of an individual's psychological experiences, feelings and attitudes that relate to the form, function, appearance and desirability of one's own body, which is influenced by individual and environmental factors.

Body image in people with physical disability is examined here from a psychosocial perspective that is informed by the social model of disability. Psychosocial theory provides a useful framework for understanding the body-image concerns of people with physical disability. It includes concepts such as 'stigma' and 'otherness', and also integrates the problem of exclusionary social ideals and social norms. The social model of disability 'challenges the traditional view of disability as a medical tragedy, and replaces it with a view of disability as a social oppression, arguing that disability is socially constructed, not biologically determined' (Shakespeare, Gillespie-Sells and Davies, 1996, p. 3). The social model of disability infers that individuals with identical physical impairments are likely to vary in their feelings and attitudes towards their own body because of social factors such as education, social support, and real or perceived social attitudes. Researching body image from this perspective involves investigating the individual's experiences of the social world, as well as learning about the social cues that they have received and the social attitudes to which they have been exposed.

Stigma Theory and the Concept of Otherness

Goffman (1963, p. 12) provided one of the earliest and most notable psychosocial perspectives on physical disability. Goffman built his theoretical discussion around the concept of stigma, which he defined as 'an attribute that is deeply discrediting'. He distinguished between three different types of stigma. The first type he described as abominations of the body; within this category are physical disabilities or disfigurements. The second type is blemishes of individual character, such as mental disorder. He labelled a final category tribal stigma, which covers racial, cultural and religious minorities. In explaining the process of stigmatisation, Goffman wrote:

> While the stranger is present before us, evidence can arise of his possessing an attribute that makes him different from us … of a less desirable kind

.... He is thus reduced in our minds from a whole and usual person to a tainted, discounted one (Goffman, 1963, p. 12).

Thus, according to stigma theory, when a person with a physical disability meets a stranger, the stranger immediately becomes aware of the person's 'discrediting attribute', i.e. the physical impairment. The impairment results in 'stigma', and the stranger makes many other attributions about the person based on this one attribute. These attributions may include that the person with the physical disability is unattractive, impotent, asexual, receiving welfare payments, or of lower intelligence. The person may be immediately discounted as a possible lover or friend. Hence, the disability becomes an all-permeating, overwhelming classification that obscures all other personal characteristics, skills and abilities (Dovey and Graffam, 1994; Lawrence, 1991; Stone, 1995).

Factors such as visibility and obtrusiveness of a stigma are important mediators of the interaction between the stigmatised and the 'normal world' (Goffman, 1963). These concepts are especially relevant to the experience of people with disabilities and their body image, as there are substantial differences among this group in relation to these dimensions. The experience of an individual with a highly visible and obtrusive physical difference is likely to have a greater adverse impact on body image than the experience of an individual whose difference is milder. According to Goffman (1963), the latter individual is less confronting to the normal, less likely to cause embarrassment, and more likely to be capable of initiating behaviours or techniques to disguise the disability or, in Goffman's words, to 'pass' as a 'normal'.

For the researcher or clinician seeking to understand the psychosocial impact of physical disability on body image, Goffman's theory is very useful. It asserts that anomalous attributes are salient, and result in a negative evaluation and perception of the person with the physical disability. Throughout one's lifespan, but more critically during childhood and early adolescence, body image is affected by environmental factors and social attitudes. If an individual has lived in an environment of acceptance, then acceptance by others should lead to the acceptance of oneself (Smith, 1984). It is therefore likely that those people whose bodies are devalued by society may devalue themselves, and these feelings may impact negatively on their body image.

Mayers (1978) also pointed out that it is very difficult for a disabled individual to have a positive body image, because many disabled individuals have received cues from the environment that lead them to believe that they are ugly. Mayers reinforces this notion with an anecdote about a person with a disability, who said that learning to look at herself in a full-length mirror and working toward seeing herself as attractive and not as the ugly creature that she had been trained to believe she was, represented the first step in developing a sexual life.

Goffman's proposition that people with visible physical disabilities are the bearers of stigma appears to have been readily accepted by psychosocial researchers. Researchers studying the effect of stigmatisation commonly use disabled people to form a 'stigmatised' or experimental group, and use able-bodied people to form a 'non-stigmatised' or control group (Stephens and Clark, 1987; Walker, Harriman and Costello, 1980; Ungar, 1979). The findings of these studies have also provided support for Goffman's theory.

In a study of 121 able-bodied children at a summer camp, interpersonal liking had a negative relationship with physical disability and a positive relationship with physical attractiveness (Kleck and De Jong, 1983). Furthermore, physically disabled children were viewed as less attractive (Kleck and De Jong, 1983). With regard to adults, a study of personal space revealed that able-bodied people create less physical distance from other able-bodied people than from people with visible physical disabilities, indicating that people stigmatise others on the basis of a visible disability (Stephens and Clark, 1987). It should also be noted that some studies have reported that people with physical disabilities are evaluated more favourably than people without physical disabilities (Carver et al., 1976, 1977).

Other authors have responded to, and extended upon, Goffman's work, particularly his position that people with disabilities are stigmatised and 'cut off' from the rest of society (Badame, 1981; Blumberg, 1975; Daniels, 1978; Gerschick and Miller, 1994; Hahn, 1981; Wendell, 1996). The concept of 'Otherness' is psychologically important, as it relates to a person's feeling of disconnectedness from the rest of society, a feeling that is likely to affect people with disabilities and their body image (Daniels, 1978). Wendell (1996) wrote that people with disabilities arouse fear in able-bodied people, and it is for this reason that they are made 'Other'. Wendell explains the essential processes involved:

> When we make people 'Other', we group them together as the objects of our experience, instead of regarding them as subjects of experience with whom we might identify, and we see them primarily as symbolic of something else—usually, but not always, something we reject and fear and project onto them. To the non-disabled, people with disabilities and people with dangerous and incurable illnesses symbolise, among other things, imperfection, failure to control the body, and everyone's vulnerability to weakness, pain and death. (Wendell, 1996, p. 60)

Murphy (1995, p. 143) mentions projection, too, saying that disabled people are made particularly threatening through 'psychological mechanisms of projection and identification, by which people impute their feelings, plans and motives to others and, in turn, incorporate those of others as their own'. Gliedman and Roth (1980) provided a detailed discussion of the concept of 'Other' as a living symbol of failure, frailty and emasculation, a counterpoint to normality, a figure whose very humanity is questionable. Daniels (1978) believes that the body of literature supports the application of the concept of 'Other' to people with disabilities.

Social Norms, Values, Ideals and Physical Disability

Social norms and values regarding the ideal body are likely to have an important influence on the body images of people with disabilities. Murphy (1995, p. 143) argued that 'the disabled, individually and as a group, contravene all the values of youth, virility, activity and physical beauty that Americans cherish.' Murphy drew on his personal experience of living with quadriplegia to reflect on the position of physical disability in American society. He believed that disabled people are resented by the able-bodied. They are seen by them as ugly and repulsive, and are perceived as subverters of social values and ideals. According to Murphy (1995), these values and ideals include strength, independence, virility and health, values which are promoted and affirmed constantly in the media, while the disabled body is hidden, or presented as something to be avoided, corrected and pitied. Lawrence (1991) highlighted the difficulties that people with physical disabilities face in forming a positive body image in a world obsessed with physical fitness and body-beautiful images:

> Individuals want to be outstanding in all developmental tasks, serviceable and attractive. Material success, sporting attainment and intellectual

> achievement are signs of personal worth. For physically handicapped people, such appearance and achievement-oriented norms are not good reference points for self-conception because physically handicapped individuals are lacking these socially admired qualities. (Lawrence, 1991, p. 140)

Therefore, people with physically disabilities may experience shame, self-hatred and a negative body image as a consequence of not 'measuring up' to a cultural ideal that has been accepted and internalised. They may wish for bodies that they cannot have; they may reject physical ideals as narrow and oppressive; or they may fluctuate between these points of view (Wendell, 1996). 'In any case, they must struggle harder than non-disabled people for a self-image that is both realistic and positive, and this is made more difficult by other people's reactions to them' (Wendell, 1996, p. 91). In a society that idealises the body, the use of the social norm as an anchoring point for self-concept formation is likely to have a negative impact on people with physical disabilities (Lawrence, 1991). Furthermore, people who cannot come close enough to the ideal may feel like devalued people because of their devalued bodies (Hannaford, 1985). Emotional tension which is painful and unpleasant may become difficult to reduce or eliminate, leading the individual to feel inadequate, inferior and socially unacceptable (Lawrence, 1991). The emotional turmoil described by Lawrence (1991) may cause people with physical disabilities to develop an impaired body-image and low body-esteem. Mackelprang (1993) observed that atrophied limbs, spasticity, urine bags, and the need for physical assistance could all contribute to low sexual self-image. Rousso's (1982, p. 84) observations about the struggles of people with cerebral palsy further illustrate the body-image concerns that result from physical disability:

> People with cerebral palsy often struggle with their body image; they question their desirability and attractiveness, given the visible physical features of their disability. For them, such characteristics as being uncoordinated, having involuntary movements, grimacing, and speaking in an uneven, unmelodious voice, may be in startling contrast to the traditional definitions of desirability and beauty. As a result, their own gestures and mannerisms may be a source of self-disgust.

Quantitative Findings on Physical Disability and Body Image

Generally, quantitative studies support the theoretical and qualitative work that suggests that physical disability has a negative impact on body image. For example, Cromer and others (1990) found that adolescents with disabilities had poorer scores on a body- and self-image subscale than able-bodied adolescents. Another study surveyed body image in over 3,000 adolescents and young adults, and also found that participants with chronic conditions scored lower on body image than their able-bodied peers (Wolman et al., 1994). The large sample size in the above study provides confidence in the results and in the conclusion that physical disability impacts negatively upon body image. However, this research was conducted on young people, and the findings may not apply to an older population. Furthermore, the differences between individuals with visible and non-visible disabilities were not examined.

A study of 47 adult males with spinal-cord injury also highlighted the negative impact of physical disability on body image (Romeo, Wanlass and Arenas, 1993). Using the Derogatis Sexual Functioning Inventory (DSFI), the study revealed that participants scored lowest on body image compared to the other DSFI scales. Furthermore, the mean score on body image was significantly lower than that of the non-disabled DSFI normative group. The authors concluded that body perception and satisfaction with one's bodily capabilities are usually negatively impacted by spinal-cord injury. This study complements the work of Wolman and others (1994) by suggesting that a negative relationship between physical disability and body esteem is likely to exist. Similar findings were obtained in a study of females with spinal-cord injury (Kettl et al., 1991). Twenty-seven women completed a questionnaire investigating their perception of their sexuality, body image and sexual behaviour after injury. The largest change was in the perceived attractiveness of their bodies, with participants rating their bodies as being only half as attractive after their injury. This study could be criticised for its use of retrospective recall. However, a negative change in perceived attractiveness is still indicative of physical disability impacting negatively on body esteem.

Although the above studies appear to provide strong evidence suggesting that physical disability has a negative impact on body image, some studies on body image and physical disability have shown conflicting findings.

Samonds and Cammermeyer (1989) evaluated the body image of 20 males who had been diagnosed with MS for an average of 21 years, and found that their scores on body satisfaction or dissatisfaction were similar to the scores of college-aged men on whom the scales (Body-Cathexis scale and the Self-Cathexis scale) were originally tested. It is possible that the absence of a matched control group and the small number of participants that took part in the study could have produced erroneous results and conclusions. An earlier study also found no difference in body esteem between people with and without a visible physical disability (Gruver and Nelson, 1978).

Summary of the Literature and the Purpose of the Current Study

Overall, psychosocial theory and empirical research both indicate that people with physical disability are likely to have difficulties in establishing a positive body image. Theoretically, negative social attitudes, incongruent social ideals, and the processes of stigmatisation and Otherness may all contribute to the negative body image that has been reported in the research (Cromer et al., 1990; Kettl et al., 1991; Romeo, Wanlass and Arenas, 1993; Wolman et al., 1994).

The current study is motivated by a need to understand the interplay between social factors and the lived experiences of people with physical disability as they relate to body image. Through semi-structured interviews, the intended outcome of this study is to illustrate, through their own words, how people with physical disabilities experience and respond to social attitudes towards physical difference, and how this affects their body image.

METHOD

Theoretical Orientation and Personal Anticipations

In line with the recommendations of Elliott, Fischer and Rennie (1999), it is recognised here that a number of factors have affected this research, primarily the first author's life experiences with a congenital physical disability. Over recent years, through personal struggles and through intimate discussions with his physically disabled friends and colleagues, the first author has developed a number of assumptions and hypotheses about body image, physical disability and society. These include that body image is a problematic issue for people with disabilities, and that social attitudes towards physical differences are largely unfavourable. Furthermore, as a disability activist and a proponent of the social model of disability, the first author regards social forces as having a central role in shaping the experience of physical disability. The second author has spent much of her career researching body image, and has concluded that body image is an important issue for both able-bodied and disabled people. As an able-bodied person, her 15 years of research into the personal lives of people with disability have helped her to overcome the myths and stereotypes that are perpetuated about people with disabilities.

The Participants

The strategy for participant recruitment involved a publicity campaign that was focused on Monash University, the Muscular Dystrophy Association (MDA), wheelchair sporting groups, and the first author's disability-activist peers in Melbourne, Australia. Advertisements were posted at the MDA, at the Disability Liaison Office of Monash University, and in the Monash University Disability Support newsletter, which has a circulation of 400 readers.

The criteria that were established for inclusion in the sample were: (a) to be over 18 years of age; (b) to have a physical disability that severely impairs mobility (mobility was seen to be severely impaired when the person was unable to walk independently); and (c) the absence of an intellectual disability. Attempts were made to create a balanced sample in terms of age, gender and sexual orientation. For example, when the initial three interviews obtained were of three heterosexual women, participants who fell into this category were no longer accepted into the sample. The majority of the participants were active in the disability-rights movement and all but one participant had some post-secondary education.

The participants were aged between 22 and 50 years, and lived in Melbourne, Australia. There were three males and four females: one identified as a gay male, another as lesbian and the remaining participants as heterosexual, although two of these women also said they were bi-curious. The range of disabilities represented were: two spinal-injured quadriplegics, one spinal-injured paraplegic, two participants with neuromuscular diseases, one with cerebral palsy, and one with a brittle-bone disease. The majority had a working-class Anglo-Celtic background and identified as disability activists. Each participant is described below. Because of the personal nature of this research, participants were assigned pseudonyms, and identifiable details were omitted to protect their privacy.

Katie is aged 33. She has severely impaired mobility and uses a motorised wheelchair as a result of a neuromuscular condition called spinal muscular atrophy. Katie is currently in a live-in relationship with a male, and she describes her sexual orientation as 'heterosexual but bi-curious'.

Sue is a 39-year-old single woman with muscular dystrophy. The symptoms, such as difficulty running, began in childhood. She uses a motorised wheelchair and describes herself as 'heterosexual but bi-curious'.

Dave is a 22-year-old male who lives with his family. He is quadriplegic following a recent accident, and uses a manual wheelchair. His injury is incomplete, as he has some movement and feeling below the injury. Dave is in a relationship with a woman he met soon after his injury.

Harry is a 48-year-old male with quadriplegia, who uses a motorised wheelchair since a motor vehicle accident five years ago. He has been exclusively homosexual throughout his life.

Steven is a 50-year-old male paraplegic. He was injured in his twenties. He is a disability activist, a wheelchair-sports athlete, a husband and a grandfather.

Phoebe is a 26-year old who has a small stature and fragile bones (osteogenesis imperfecta). Although she has lived her life primarily as a heterosexual, she describes her sexuality as 'person-specific', and is currently in a relationship with a woman.

Monique is a 31-year-old heterosexual single woman with cerebral palsy. Monique uses a motorised wheelchair, although she is able to walk with the aid of walking sticks.

Procedure

Data were gathered through in-depth interviews that were conducted by the first author. Each participant was asked to choose a pseudonym at the beginning of the interview; one participant wanted to use her real name. The interviews took place in a private location chosen by the participants, and were approximately 2 hours in duration. (Please note that the body-image interview was part of a larger interview that also covered sexuality and gender identity.) The duration of the interview was dependent on the interest and openness displayed by the participant. Each interview was recorded on audiotape and then transcribed. It focused on two open-ended questions. First, the participants were asked about their feelings towards their bodies. Second, they were asked to describe how they saw themselves, i.e., whether they saw themselves as sexy, or if they felt that their disability made them feel unattractive. To increase disclosure, the interviewer used encouraging questions and prompts.

RESULTS AND DISCUSSION

The information provided by the participants is organised and discussed around themes that emerged from the data. These themes were developed after a close study of the data by the two authors, who reached consensus on three major themes: the internalisation of negative social attitudes, bodily acceptance over time, and mediating factors in the experience of an altered body. In order to minimise bias, the data were only edited for the sake of clarity and brevity, and, in the most part, are presented here in full.

The Internalisation of Negative Social Altitudes

The influence of negative social attitudes and the internalisation of these social attitudes by people with disabilities was a strong theme that emerged. The following story, as stated by Phoebe, provides a real-life example of the social attitudes towards the disabled body. For some, disability is perceived as the antithesis of attractiveness.

Phoebe: I was waiting for the train one day, and this guy came up to me and said, 'I'm really sorry that you're in that thing,' referring to my wheelchair, of course. And I said, 'Why is that?' He said, 'You know, you're really not bad looking, you're really quite pretty. It's such a shame that you're actually in that thing. It's such a turn off.' And I was just blown away. I didn't quite know what to say.... This happened again, and I said something that was quite fulfilling.

For people like me with physical disabilities, our disability is likely to be our most obvious external characteristic. Thus, these negative social attitudes towards disability, as described by Phoebe, are unlikely to foster the development of a healthy body image, especially when they are vocalised by strangers. Katie's story reveals a very difficult struggle with her body image, and it demonstrates the influence of social attitudes. She begins by discussing some of the things that she likes about her body.

Katie: There are positive things that I see about my body. I like the way my hair looks, and I like my fingernails when they're done up and I've polished them, and I like the way I put on makeup.... I've got the greatest set of nipples on earth, 'cause they're really sensitive and they give me a lot of pleasure, and I feel the same way about my clit[oris] .... I feel sexy when I'm wearing really sexually provocative clothing. But that's different from feeling like I look sexy. I still pick fault with every aspect of my body. There are minor things that I like but basically, if I could do a body swap, I'd do one in an instant.

Katie makes an important distinction between 'feeling sexy' and 'feeling like she looks sexy'. The former appears to relate to her confidence in herself as a sexual person and as a person who is sexually interested, active and responsive. The latter relates to her feelings about how other people perceive her body. She goes on to clarify this distinction.

Katie: The funny thing is, I feel really negative around body image, but I feel really positive stuff around sexuality.... This is such a contradiction—to feel so negatively about your body, and yet so positive about your sexuality.

Katie believes that her negative feelings about her body are the result of negative feedback from her environment. She explains how rejection by potential sex partners has led her to conclude that she is unattractive.

Katie: At first I thought I was unattractive because I was fat, but now everyone's saying that I'm too bloody skinny, so it can't be that I'm fat. So what conclusion have I got, when I'm a size ten and I still have guys rejecting me? What conclusion can I come up with other than that they see the disability before they see me? On the phone, I can describe myself as sexy, but when they get here they obviously see something else. So it's pretty hard to separate what other people see and not take that on board and see it for myself. I think that society creates an image of beauty, and if you don't conform to it, you get put down so much that you eventually believe the story that they're telling you. So how do you reprogramme the computer in your head that's been programmed to say you're ugly? I'd give just about anything to do that.

For Katie, the negative attitudes are internalised to such an extent that she seeks out ways to modify her body through radical surgery.

Katie: What I want to do is have an apronectomy [the cutting away of loose skin]. I'm on two waiting lists. I want my bum, thighs, stomach, and the skin under my arms done, and what I would love them to do is breast implants as well, and I want a nice tight little bum.... Feminists jump on women about cutting up their bodies to fit the body-beautiful image, and as much as I'm a feminist, when it comes to cosmetic surgery, I'm the first to say: I want it, I want it!

Bodily Acceptance over Time

Sue and Phoebe also experience negative feelings towards their bodies. However, what emerges from their stories is a sense of increasing acceptance of their body.

Sue: My body image has gone through an evolution since my diagnosis. My body image and sexual image have probably improved as I've become more disabled. Before I was diagnosed, I hardly even thought about my body. When you're 18, every female is young, sexy and attractive, and every man runs after you. After I was diagnosed, I thought I wouldn't be attractive anymore. I still thought I was sexual, but I didn't think I'd be able to express it anymore. I thought that having muscular dystrophy would put men off and they'd think that I wasn't attractive because I can't walk very well. I was very angry at my body—I felt betrayed. Although I knew I was a sexual being, I thought I wouldn't be seen as that. I was fighting myself: knowing that I was [sexual] and fighting my belief that somehow I wasn't [sexual] because people outside did not view me as a sexual creature anymore. There was a huge internal conflict. It's been fifteen years, and I've had very positive feedback and experiences from supportive partners. I'm still not entirely happy with my body. And I'm self-conscious about my posture, and various things, but I feel that I don't have to be perfect anymore. I used to think that I was deficient as a disabled woman, but as I've matured I've realised that nobody's perfect.

Sue's experience demonstrates the impact of a progressive disability on a person's body image. The onset of muscular dystrophy made her conscious of her body. She believed that others would not find her attractive because of her disability, and this resulted in anger towards her own body. However, she has adjusted to her disabled body and attributes this to positive feedback from supportive partners. This demonstrates the importance of feedback from significant others on the development of body image. Below, Sue talks more about her current feelings towards her body, conveying both negative and positive feelings, but on the whole a sense of acceptance.

Sue: Basically, I'm quite happy with my body image, except my posture … my standing posture, that is. I'm getting a roll of fat around my waist, which I don't like either, but that's just because I'm a woman. I feel pretty comfortable with my body, probably even better than some of my able-bodied friends, who have worse feelings about their bodies than I do.… I'd run around naked in front of anybody. I have a pretty healthy body image.

A similar experience of adjustment and acceptance is expressed by Phoebe.

Phoebe: I'm now at a point where I think I've got to learn to love this body, 'cause it isn't gonna get any better. I think I've got particular things about me that are attractive, and they tend to become a focus. There are times when I think, I'm too fat, I need to lose weight, but then I think: 'Who cares? There's someone who loves me just the way I am.' Why should I change it, who would I be doing it for? Image is a big thing for me, in that I try to make sure that I look reasonable and that I'm very presentable. My hair is a big thing, and I like to make sure that it's the way I like it. And the whole makeup thing. When I'm asked, what I'd like to change about my body, I kind of think 'Where would I begin?' People ask me, 'Don't you wish you were taller?'… I kind of like being short now. [If I were tall] there'd be lots of things getting in the way. Like, would I straighten my arms, would I straighten my legs, would I rod my back? There's all sorts of things I could do. But then I think: I'm in proportion, I can dress in a way that I look normal, as much as I hate that word.

Phoebe appears to have forged a positive body image by focussing on the positive aspects of her body and accepting those features that she finds less attractive. For both Phoebe and Sue, acceptance of less positive features appears to be enhanced by their recognition that 'nobody is perfect', that is, even able-bodied people never achieve physical perfection. This was also evident in the interview with Monique.

Monique: I feel my body is not where I want it to be. I'm not deformed or anything. I'm like a Michelangelo [laughs]. I've got a scoliosis back, my bum sticks out. My feet are swollen and go purple.... I'm not very happy with it, but I just deal with what I've got. I call myself a piece of art—a Picasso. It's just like with anyone; they're not happy with the way they look.

Steve had similar experiences to those of Phoebe and Sue. Steve's story is of a slow and steady improvement in his body image since an accident led to spinal injury over 25 years ago.

Steve: I feel quite lucky with the nature of my disability. It hasn't really affected the way my body looks, apart from atrophied legs and hips. I'm not in any way negative about my body image, I'm quite happy about it. For a long while, I couldn't get to grips with it. I didn't wear shorts for 20 years. Then I came out and got my legs brown, and now I'm quite happy with them. I couldn't care less. I'm quite comfortable with my body image.

Steve explains how his negative body image was symptomatic of early adjustment processes after his accident.

Steve: I think my bad body image was a symptom of a whole lot of things out of place. Initially, I was still sort of denying my disability, trying to be someone I wasn't. I was trying to pretend I was a non-disabled guy. When I finally came to terms with it, I thought: 'I've got a disability, so what? So I'm glad to have skinny legs. That's fine.' Prior to that, it was denial stuff. I was in the same boat as everyone else. I was thinking this disabled thing is going to be terrible, and that became a self-fulfilling prophecy. I made it as bad as I thought it was going to be. It was one of those things. I don't know how I came to terms with it. But I'm incredibly comfortable with it these days. I don't feel any sense of loss all these years later. I was injured when I was 21. I just turned 50. I don't feel any sense of loss. My sense of gain has been far greater than my sense of loss. Body image is fine. I'm an athlete now and quite strong, and all that masculine crap is still there and it doesn't really concern me. I do what I do. My body is fine. I have fun with my body.

It is clear that Steve has overcome his negative feelings towards his body after a long process of adjustment to, and acceptance of, physical disability. Like Sue, the initial period after the onset of disability was difficult, and he had a negative body image. Like both Sue and Phoebe, he focuses on his positive attributes. Steve has developed a positive body image, which is reinforced by his sport and his identification as an athlete.

Mediating Factors in the Experience of an Altered Body

Harry and Dave were both recently injured. While they both had difficulties working through their negative feelings towards a changed body, there are some obvious differences which shed light on some likely mediating factors in body acceptance in people with spinal-cord injury. Harry, who had his accident only five years ago, appears to be facing the struggles that Steve and Sue faced when they first became disabled. For Harry, a negative body image is something that he continues to struggle with.

Harry: When I'm out in a group of people, I'm very conscious of my differences, although I disguise it very well. I am very conscious that I'm in a wheelchair, and that my body is not the best.... Well, first of all, I am forty-eight and the body is not what it was pre-accident. I come across very confidently, very assertively, very articulately, but underneath I am very insecure and not comfortable with my body. I mean, it's five years. I've lived 43 years able-bodied, and five years is not a very long time. However, I camouflage that very well, because no one except my closest friends would really know how I really felt. I'm different and I'm aware of my difference being what it is. And I see people who I find very attractive, and I'm conscious that my chances of scoring with them are non-existent.... I am conscious of my differences, and I don't have the confidence to go up to other people.

A combination of increasing age and physical disability cause Harry to have negative feelings towards his body. He responds by refusing to shut himself off from others, and portraying a confident nature that masks his feelings of physical inadequacy. For Dave, there is frustration at not being able to sculpt his body the way he could pre-accident, but this appears to be more of an annoyance than a serious concern. Interestingly, like Sue, affirmations from his partner and others support a positive body image.

Dave: It [body image] annoys me a lot. Beforehand, I used to go to the gym about four or five times a week, and I was pretty conscious of the way I looked. By the same token, I can still wear a tank top and look alright, 'cause my body's not too bad. I'm lucky in some respects, because my body hasn't changed a lot. I mean, your legs get a bit smaller. My partner and other people still say, 'You're lookin' pretty good.'... It [the accident] hasn't really changed the way I look. I'm just sitting down, not standing up....

A comparison of Dave's and Harry's experiences indicates that factors other than disability affect body image. In these cases, while both participants had recent injuries resulting in quadriplegia, Dave expresses a more positive body image. This may be due to his relative youth, his participation in sports, and because he entered a long-term relationship soon after his accident.

CONCLUSION

In accordance with earlier studies (Cromer et al., 1990; Wolman et al., 1994; Romeo et al., 1993; Kettl et al., 1991) and with the observations of earlier authors (Lawrence, 1991; Mackelprang, 1993; Mayers, 1978; Rousso, 1982), the current study showed that, for each participant, living with a physical disability had clearly impacted upon their psychological experiences, feelings and attitudes towards their own bodies. At some point in their lives, body image had been a serious struggle for each individual, as negative social attitudes towards physical difference were internalised. Feelings of physical inadequacy and unattractiveness permeate these stories. The participants also indicated that these negative feelings were the result of feedback from the environment, as suggested by Smith (1984) and Mayers (1978). It appears that positive feedback from partners and others can help a person with a disability to achieve a positive body image, even when it does not duplicate the image of beauty that is upheld in our society.

The process of stigmatisation, as described by Goffman (1963), can explain the negative attitudes that are reported here, as well as the difficulties expressed by participants in attracting sexual partners. The different experiences of participants with varying degrees of visible impairment also support Goffman's (1963) proposition that people with more salient differences will be more severely stigmatised. For example, Katie, Harry and Phoebe describe more negative feedback compared to Dave and Steve, who had less obvious physical differences. Murphy's (1995) theory that people with disabilities are subverters of social values and ideals can also explain the rejection that the participants, particularly Katie and Harry, have described. There is also evidence for Wendell's (1996) concept of Otherness in the participants' reports of the way some able-bodied people treated them. Katie's experiences with men provide an obvious example.

This study also suggests that a negative body image could be expected in the initial period after the onset of disability. However, after some time has passed, the individual would be expected to adjust to the disability and begin to accept his or her body. This appears more likely to occur if the individual focused on some aspect of personal achievement, such as sports, family, career or education. Furthermore, an important factor in the development of a positive body image in people with physical disability may involve focusing on the positive aspects of their body and perceiving the impairment as just one sign of physical imperfection, with which we all struggle. The accuracy of this hypothesis requires further investigation.

Overall, the current study provided an insight into the social interaction between able-bodied people and people with physical disabilities from the disabled person's perspective. This is a complex interaction that is mediated by, among other things, the nature of the person's disability and the degree to which their body deviates from the social ideal. This interaction, and the resulting feedback, has a powerful impact on the person's body image, which itself appears to be mediated by other factors, particularly, the amount of time since the onset of disability, the degree of social support, and the amount of positive feedback that the individual has already received. Previous experiences of positive feedback may buffer negative feedback, possibly because a positive body image has already been established, or because the individual can draw on their memories of positive experiences that occurred in the past.

A selection bias and the size of the current sample limit the generalisability of these findings. It is likely that the few individuals who elected to participate in the current investigation are significantly more confident, and possibly more concerned with their body image, than other people with physical disabilities. Future studies need to be conducted with larger and more randomised samples to determine the applicability of the current findings to a more representative sample of respondents.

References

Badame, R.S. 1981. 'Social skills: The process of learning to take risks', in D.G. Bullard and S.E. Knight (eds), *Sexuality and Physical Disability: Personal Perspectives*. St Louis: C.V. Mosby, pp. 242–47.

Blumberg, M.L. 1975. 'Psychodynamics of the young handicapped person', *American Journal of Psychotherapy*, 29 (4): 466–76.

Carver, C.S. et al. 1976. 'Ambivalence and evaluative response amplification', *Bulletin of the Psychonomic Society*, 13 (1): 50–52.

———. 1977. 'Favourable evaluation of stigmatised others', *Personality and Social Psychology Bulletin*, 3: 232–35.

Cromer, B.A. et al. 1990. 'Knowledge, attitudes and behaviour related to sexuality in adolescents with chronic disability', *Developmental Medicine and Child Neurology*, 32: 602–10.

Daniels, S.M. 1978. 'Correlates of attitudes toward the sexuality of the disabled person in selected health professionals', *Sexuality and Disability*, 1 (2): 112–26.

Dovey, K. and Graffam, J. 1994. *The Experience of Disability: Social Construction and Imposed Limitation*. Geelong: Deakin University Press.

Elliott, R., Fischer, C. and Rennie, D. 1999. 'Evolving guidelines for publication of qualitative research in psychology and related fields', *The British Journal of Clinical Psychology*, 38: 215–29.

Gerschick, T.J. and Miller, A.S. 1994. 'Gender identities at the crossroads of masculinity and physical disability', *Masculinities*, 2 (1): 34–55.

Gliedman, J. and Roth, W. 1980. *The Unexpected Minority: Handicapped Children in America*. New York: Harcourt Brace Javanovitch.

Goffman, E. 1963. *Stigma: Notes on the Management of Spoiled Identity*. Englewood Cliffs: Prentice-Hall.

Gruver, G. and Nelson, M. 1978. 'Self-esteem and body-image concept in paraplegics', *Rehabilitation Counseling Bulletin*, 22 (2): 108–13.

Hahn, H. 1981. 'The social component of sexuality and disability: Some problems and proposals', *Sexuality and Disability*, 4 (4): 220–33.

Hannaford, S. 1985. *Living Outside Inside: A Disabled Woman's Experience*. Berkeley: Canterbury Press.

Kettl, P. et al. 1991. 'Female sexuality after spinal-cord injury', *Sexuality and Disability*, 9 (4): 287–95.

Kleck, R. and De Jong, W. 1983. 'Physical disability, physical attractiveness, and social outcomes in children's small groups', *Rehabilitation Psychology*, 28 (2): 79–91.

Lawrence, B. 1991. 'Self-concept formation and physical handicap: Some educational implications for integration', *Disability, Handicap and Society*, 6 (2): 139–46.

Mackelprang, R.W. 1993. 'A holistic social-work approach to providing sexuality education and counseling for persons with severe disabilities', *Journal of Social Work and Human Sexuality*, 8 (2): 63–87.

Mayers, K.S. 1978. 'Sexual and social concerns of the disabled: A group-counselling approach', *Sexuality and Disability*, 1 (2): 100–11.

Murphy, R. 1995. 'Encounters: The Body Silent in America', in B. Ingstad and S. Reynolds Whyte (eds), *Disability and Culture*. Berkeley: University of California Press.

Romeo, A.J., Wanlass, R. and Arenas, S. 1993. 'A profile of psychosexual functioning in males following spinal-cord injury', *Sexuality and Disability*, 11 (4): 269–76.

Rousso, H. 1982. 'Special considerations in counselling clients with cerebral palsy', *Sexuality and Disability*, 5 (2): 78–88.

Samonds, R.J. and Cammermeyer, M. 1989. 'Perceptions of body image in subjects with multiple sclerosis: a pilot study', *Journal of Neuroscience Nursing*, 21 (3): 190–94.

Shakespeare, T., Gillespie-Sells, K. and Davies, D. 1996. *The Sexual Politics of Disability: Untold Desires*. London: Cassell.

Slade, P.D. 1994. 'What is body image?', *Behaviour Research and Therapy*, 32: 497–502.

Smith, R. 1984. 'Identity crisis', *Nursing Mirror*, 158: i–vi.

Stephens, K.K. and Clark, D.W. 1987. 'A pilot study on the effect of visible physical stigma on personal space', *Journal of Applied Rehabilitation Counselling*, 18 (3): 52–54.

Stone, S.D. 1995. 'The myth of bodily perfection', *Disability and Society*, 10 (4): 413–24.

Teal, J.C. and Athelstan, G.T. 1975. 'Sexuality and spinal-cord injury: Some psychosocial considerations', *Archives of Physical Medicine and Rehabilitation*, 56: 264–68.

Ungar, S. 1979. 'The effects of effort and stigma on helping', *Journal of Social Psychology*, 107 (1): 23–28.

Walker, M., Harriman, S. and Costello, S. 1980. 'The influence of appearance on compliance with a request', *Journal of Social Psychology*, 112 (1): 159–60.

Wendell, S. 1996. *The Rejected Body: Feminist Philosophical Reflections on Disability*. New York: Routledge.

Wolman, C. et al. 1994. 'Emotional well-being among adolescents with and without chronic conditions', *Journal of Adolescent Health*, 15 (3): 199–204.

8

Self-Mortification and the Stigma of Leprosy in Northern India

Ronald F. Barrett

The burden is worse than the bacteria. You see, the infection is easily treated, easily cured with [multi-drug therapy]. But even when the leprosy has been totally eliminated, many people will treat you as someone who is cursed for all time. That is the major problem.

The statement above was made by Ramchandra, a middle-aged man from Benares, interviewed as part of a 22-month ethnographic study of social discrimination among people with Hansen's Disease (HD), also known as leprosy, in northern India. Ramchandra's statement echoed a common assertion among Indian HD workers that the social stigma of leprosy is far worse than the disease itself. Contrary to many popular beliefs, HD is a mildly contagious condition that can be readily treated with antibiotics in most cases (Bryceson and Pfalzgraff, 1990). In the minority of more prolonged and difficult cases, simple precautions and careful observation are all that are needed to prevent the onset of permanent disabilities (Srinivasan, 1994). In contrast to these clinical realities, however, Indians with HD are often permanently ascribed to the most untouchable categories of humanity (Frist, 2000). Moreover,

Barrett, Ronald F. 2005. 'Self mortification and the stigma of leprosy in Northern India', *Medical Anthropology Quarterly*, 19 (2): 216–30.

this untouchability often persists long after they have been 'cured' of the disease, creating lifelong prospects of divorce, eviction, loss of employment and ostracism from family and social networks (Kopparty, Karup and Sivaram, 1995).

The extreme discrepancies between the clinical and social realities of HD in India underscore a common distinction in medical anthropology between the pathophysiology of disease and the human experience of illness as suffering (Kleinman, 1988).[1] As such, it is tempting to segregate the bacteria of Hansen's Disease from the social burden of leprosy. Yet, although this distinction may be useful for initial criticism, further examination reveals that, like many other discredited medical conditions, the physical and social stigmata of HD are too interconnected to be adequately disentangled. As such, leprosy is best approached as an illness of discrimination *inclusive* of its physical condition.

In this article, I examine the biocultural dynamics of social discrimination and physical disfigurement among people with HD in the Benares district of Uttar Pradesh, northern India. Drawing on the illness narratives and observations of people living in colony and street settings, I trace three destructive processes by which their social stigmata became physically expressed: (1) concealment leading to undertreatment; (2) dissociation and self-neglect; and (3) self-mutilation under conditions of extreme poverty. These processes represent self-mortification in every sense of the word—shaming, necrosis, and the subjection of the flesh by discipline or denial. As such, these people came to embody, quite literally, the local prejudices that exacerbated their condition in the first place. Although deeply experienced by a few, the marks of leprosy are situated in a perpetuating cycle that extends well beyond the patient communities themselves.

THE BACTERIA AND THE BURDEN

There is both a sharp contrast and intimate connection between the clinical and social realities of leprosy in India. *Mycobacterium leprae* is among the least contagious of human pathogens. It is estimated that the bacterium

[1] Kleinman's (1988) case studies illustrate that, while distinctive, illness and disease need not be exclusive categories.

produces symptoms in less than 10 percent of the human population, and only after prolonged exposure and a five-year incubation period (Bryceson and Pfalzgraff, 1990). Although evidence suggests a hereditary component to this susceptibility, in most cases spouses and children of those infected never contract the disease (Mira et al., 2004; Sehgal, 1994). *M. leprae* fares even worse outside its human hosts. Indeed, it grows so poorly under most conditions, natural or artificial, that its exact mode of transmission has yet to be proven (Sasaki et al., 2001).[2]

In contrast to the bacterium, the social mark of leprosy in India is highly contagious. Consistent with Goffman's so-called courtesy stigma (1963), friends and relatives of people with HD risk severe social and economic losses for their affiliations. Consequently, many Indian families would rather banish their diagnosed relatives to a distant town or city than risk discrimination against the entire household (Kopparty, Karup and Sivaram, 1995). With very poor chances of employment and little, if any, support from home, these exiles have few options for survival. Typically, they must find subsidised living in an isolated colony, or else live on the streets and beg in areas frequented by tourists and pilgrims. Both of these subsistence modes contribute, in turn, to the stereotypes from which their discrimination originated. Among those susceptible to *M. leprae* infection, the disease is usually treatable with a combination of three antibiotics, commonly referred to as multi-drug therapy (MDT). In most cases, this regimen can render a patient noninfectious in 30 days, and noninfected in six to nine months (Ponnighaus, 1995).[3] Yet, for people like Ramchandra, the social stigma of leprosy can last a lifetime, regardless of whether they have been biomedically cured of the disease.

[2] The highest bacterial titres can be found in nasal secretions, and a number of transmission modes have been hypothesised (see Naafs et al., 2001): water (Matsuoka et al., 1999) or an anaerobic soil intermediary (Chakrabarty and Dastidar, 2001). However, the model cannot be proven until the organism can be feasibly grown under laboratory conditions. To date, the only naturally infected nonhuman host for leprosy is the armadillo, an animal that does not reproduce easily under captive conditions (Bruce et al., 2000).

[3] A minority of those infected are particularly susceptible to the mycobacterium. Known as lepromatous, or LL, these cases often require a longer and more involved course of treatment over three to five years (Bryceson and Pfalzgraff, 1990).

I followed 72 such cases in three groups, over periods ranging from two to four years.[4] Although a few were able to mitigate their untouchability in urban public spaces, no one had gone so far as to permanently reunite with their original households during that time. Later in this article, I present case studies that demonstrate how the intense and intractable nature of this social burden contributes to the spread of the bacteria through the avoidance of leprosy treatment workers and clinics.

Some of the most prevalent myths about HD concern its associated deformities and disabilities. Contrary to many popular beliefs, HD does not cause limbs to rot off. Although a small percentage of cases experience internal loss of cartilage and bone at the face and digits, the vast majority of physical deformities result from accumulated trauma. Typically, the selective infection of peripheral nerves results in limb anaesthesia, diminishing people's ability to rely on touch and pain to prevent injuries to their hands and feet, and to make the constant micro-adjustments necessary to prevent pressure ulcers. The resultant injuries and ulcers accumulate and, along with secondary infections, lead to progressive amputations not unlike those found among people with diabetes (Brand and Yancey, 1997; Bryceson and Pfalzgraff, 1990; Jopling, 1988). Even in cases of permanent neuropathy, physical deformities and disabilities can be prevented through basic measures like custom footwear and training in injury prevention. But that which is basic is not always easy. Because of the ever-present threat of injury to anaesthetic limbs, people with HD neuropathies must be hyperaware of their bodies in relation to their surrounding environments (Brand and Yancey, 1997). Without constant visual inspection of an insensate hand, a cigarette or hot stove could result in a third-degree burn in less than a minute. More insidiously, without regular attention to footwear, or scheduled readjustments while sleeping, a pressure ulcer could work its way to the bone in a matter of weeks. Although straightforward, such preventative measures are challenging to

[4] These 72 cases resided in three different living and treatment areas: (1) Dashashvamedha (N = 17); (2) Kusht Seva Ashram (N = 31); and (3) Asapur (N = 24). I first came to know the Dashashvamedha group in the winter of 1996–97. Although highly transient, I was able to follow up with most of them, and work with the two other groups, during my main fieldwork in 1999–2000, and again during a follow-up visit in the spring of 2001.

maintain under the best of conditions. They become formidable under the conditions of extreme poverty and demoralisation that is common among people who are publicly branded as 'lepers' in India.[5] The social and physical disabilities of HD are not only mutually engendering, they actually impede efforts to prevent one another.

LEPROSY ON THE GANGES

Benares (also known as Varanasi or Kashi) is one of the oldest and largest centres of pilgrimage in India, revered by Hindus, Muslims, Buddhists and Jains, who come by the millions to visit its myriad temples and shrines and bathe along a three-mile stretch of *ghats* (steps) leading to the holy Ganges river (called Ganga in India). Like the Ganges itself, the sanctity of Benares is closely linked to its capacity for absorbing the ritual pollution and sins of any and all who reside within its sacred spaces (Barrett, 2002). Its many pilgrims bring a steady flow of donations, and the city's numerous ashrams, settlements and squatter camps are ready possibilities for transient living. As such, Benares is a major destination for a variety of indigent and socially discredited populations, people with HD among them.

Part of my ethnographic fieldwork focused on the lives and illness narratives of two HD-diagnosed communities in the greater Benares area: the long-term residents of a leprosy treatment facility within an isolated religious retreat, or ashram; and an indigent squatter community beside the river. These two communities represented only a small subset of the nearly half million registered cases in India (WHO, 2000) at the time of my research, many of whom would not have been discredited because they were treated without ever being publicly identified. Yet these marginalised groups are especially relevant in that they have come to characterise the most common stereotypes of people with leprosy whom everyone seeks to avoid: the colony resident and the street-dwelling beggar.

The treatment centre of the Kusht Seva Ashram (KSA) is situated in a village-plus-truck stop, just across the river from Benares. The KSA clinic is one of the most popular leprosy treatment centres in northern India,

[5] Understandably, the term leper is considered highly derogatory by activists within the international HD community (Gussow and Tracy, 1968).

visited by thousands of patients every year. It is sponsored by a heterodox religious sect known as the Aghori, and staffed by Ayurvedic physicians who provide free services and low-cost herbal medicines that are manufactured in the ashram. Although it mainly serves an outpatient population, KSA has separate facilities for up to 40 residential patients.

When I conducted interviews at KSA in the late winter of 1999, 31 HD-diagnosed adults (26 males, 5 females) resided within the walls of the ashram. Although all were ostensibly inpatients, their average length of stay was 5.2 years, with nearly a third residing longer than their recommended three years of treatment. These extended stays had more to do with social than medical needs, such that the KSA effectively functioned as a religiously sanctioned leprosy colony.

The second community consisted of outpatients served by an NGO-sponsored street clinic. Through clinic contacts, I interviewed 17 of approximately 25 people who were then living in squatter camps around Dashashvamedha Ghat, the area beside the river frequented by the majority of pilgrims when they first arrive in the city. Although all of these people had been cured of the *M. leprae* infection, residual deformities marked them as *korhia* (lepers) for life.[6]

The indigent community of Dashashvamedha made their living off the alms of pilgrims, who would drop small coins and handfuls of rice into outstretched hands and waiting bowls in order to cast off a bit of sin before bathing in the Ganges. As such, begging provided a service not unlike that of the many ritual specialists in this area, who take on the karma of others in exchange for basic resources (see Parry, 1986; Raheja, 1988). For this reason, I have argued that they are the true Mahabrahmins of the ghats (Barrett, 2002). Yet, unlike the many high-status pundits and priests of Benares, the absolving role of its beggars only reinforced their social and economic poverty.

The KSA and Dashashvamedha groups were mainly comprised of people from Bhojpuri-speaking rural areas of eastern Uttar Pradesh and western Bihar. Most were tenant farmers, unskilled labourers, and housewives from poor and landless families, a situation consistent with

[6] In this part of northern India, the term *korhia* is considered so inauspicious that some people will spit after saying it, lest the word itself contaminate them.

the long-time association of leprosy and poverty in India (Buckingham, 2002). All but one identified with a Hindu religious tradition.

The significant demographic differences between the Dashashvamedha and KSA populations occurred along the lines of gender and education. The 2:1 ratio of men to women in Dashashvamedha was consistent with the sex distribution of HD in India (Kumar et al., 2001; Noordeen, 1994), an ongoing puzzle that may well be explained by the diminished autonomy of women with respect to medical decisions and access to essential health resources (Beals, 1976; Bloom, Wypij and Das Gupta, 2001), as well as possible gender differences in manual labour practices (Barrett, 1997).[7] With regard to the even lower representation of women at KSA however, gender inequalities were closely linked to issues of childcare, for the ashram did not allow children to live on its grounds.

Table 8.1
Kusht Seva Ashram (KSA) and Dashashvamedha (DAS) individuals by years of formal education (X^2 = 5.42; DF = 1)

Education	0	1	2	3	4	5	6	7	8	9	10	11	12	Total
KSA	19	0	1	0	0	2	1	1	1	1	2	2	1	31
DAS	16	0	0	0	0	0	0	0	0	0	0	1	0	17

The members of the Dashashvamedha group were significantly less educated than those of the KSA (Table 8.1). Except for a single outlier, none of the former had even a year of formal education. The KSA community had a bimodal distribution of some education and none whatsoever. Such data strongly suggest that some combination of knowledge and class had influenced the different life trajectories of these two groups in the latter stages of their illness.

Whatever combinations of gender and class may have channeled these people into colonies versus squatter camps, both shared common themes

[7] Although it is well documented that Indian women have worse access to health-care resources than men, one would expect a higher proportion of physical deformities among those women who eventually obtained treatment. On the contrary, however, men have an even higher ratio (4 : 1) of physical deformities than women. Extending the hypotheses posed in Note 2 above, and based on some preliminary observations, I suggest that the way in which men engage in manual labour subjects them to higher rates of physical trauma and, therefore, a greater frequency of high-titre infections. This phenomenon is very much in need of further research.

of social discrimination that exacerbated the progress of their disease at its early stages and excluded them from their home communities when their condition could no longer be concealed. The following case studies illustrate these themes and the particular ways that they physically expressed themselves.

DISAVOWAL AND UNDERTREATMENT

Sita was an energetic and outspoken woman in her early forties who belonged to a community of goldsmiths in a small town about 70 kilometers from Benares. She was illiterate beyond the ability to sign her own name, and cynically laughed at the slim chance that she or any other woman from her community would have a formal education. She had been living at the Kusht Seva Ashram for 22 years, and repeatedly spoke about the loneliness she felt from the years of separation from her natal family.

Sita was 14 when she first noticed a gray patch on her upper arm. This caused great concern in her family, because any skin blemishes or spots would have adversely affected her chances for marriage. Although she could still conceal the patch beneath her sari, there was no telling whether the condition would spread. The senior males of Sita's family decided to send her to a doctor of 'English medicine', who diagnosed the HD and prescribed a course of dapsone.[8] She was then sequestered at home while the family hastily arranged her marriage. Her condition kept secret, Sita was married within a month and ceased taking any medications lest it be discovered.

Sita's condition remained unchanged until the birth of her first child, a daughter, four years later. She then began having numbness along her left arm and leg and contractions in her toes. Her condition no longer concealable, Sita feigned surprise when she was diagnosed a second time. To avoid being recognised at a regional leprosy clinic, her affines accompanied her on long trips for treatment in the adjacent state of

[8] Dapsone was the leading treatment for *M. leprae* infection until the early 1980s. Unfortunately, the organism began showing resistance to this sulfa drug within a decade of its introduction in 1943. Today, dapsone is considered to be merely bacteriostatic against *M. leprae*.

Bihar. Sita's daughter died of undisclosed causes at six months of age, and her husband died the following year. With no male children, and no one to advocate for her within the family, Sita's already marginal status declined even further. With strong pressure from her mother-in-law, Sita took up residence at KSA. To this date, both her natal and affinal families publicly maintain that she is living the pious life of a widow in an ashram somewhere in Benares.

Sita's story illustrates the tragic consequences of denial and concealment in the progression and spread of a discredited disease. Given the social consequences, it is understandable that people would go to great lengths to conceal their condition. Unfortunately, such strategies usually result in delays between initial symptoms and diagnosis, and in adherence to medication regimens (Kopparty, Karup and Sivaram, 1995; Mull et al., 1989). This problem is compounded by the segregation of HD treatment services in India (Arole et al., 2002).[9] Under these conditions, the most public sign of early-stage HD is for someone to be seen near a leprosy treatment worker or clinic. To prevent such associations, people often travel great distances to non-local clinics or avoid treatment altogether (Arole et al., 2002; Dharmshaktu, 1992).

The majority of HD-diagnosed people from Dashashvamedha and the KSA—59 percent and 61 percent, respectively—reported delays between initial symptoms and their first visit to a licensed professional healer. Most of these delays were described in the context of concealment strategies, as in Sita's history, or some form of denial (e.g. 'I did not want to know'). Others reported that not only were they ignorant of early signs of HD, but their health providers were as well. The latter issue reflects discrimination of another sort, for the segregation of leprosy treatment services also results in a segregation of clinical knowledge.

In his reformulation of deviance as stigma, Goffman (1963) includes a taxonomy of strategies for disavowing the social mark: (1) sheltering—segregation within protective social environments; (2) passing—concealing or camouflaging the mark; and (3) covering—minimising tensions during social interactions. Yet it is clear that these disavowal strategies provide only limited benefits to the discredited, and might very well reinforce

[9] The solution of reintegrating leprosy treatment into primary-care services can also be problematic. For a critical perspective, see Justice (1986).

the stigma of a given condition over time (Goffman, 1963; Jones, Scott and Markus, 1984). This is even more the case when the stigmatised condition is an infectious disease and the disavowal results in delayed testing or incomplete adherence to treatment (Alonzo and Reynolds, 1995; Rubel and Garro, 1992).[10]

Such dynamics forge a direct link between social stigma and the epidemiology of Hansen's Disease in India. Unfortunately, however, this link has yet to be adequately measured. In accordance with World Bank guidelines, statistics for India's National Leprosy Elimination Programme are based solely on the passive detection of registered cases in WHO-approved treatment centres (Ponnighaus, 1995). Among such centres that I have observed in the Benares district, registered cases are assumed to have sought treatment elsewhere and are dropped from the books when patients fail to return after six months. Many among the KSA and Dashashvamedha had discontinued official MDT programs, and all had since sought treatment through non-official sources. As such, none of these people existed in national or WHO statistics. The concealment of leprosy is not only pervasive but institutional as well.

DISSOCIATION AND SELF-NEGLECT

Sadness and resignation were pervasive emotions among the residents of the KSA. Laxman was no exception in this regard. At 25 years of age, he had a ninth-grade education and an acre of land, which would have made him an attractive marriage prospect in many parts of rural Bihar, were it not for contracted fingers and the wounds on his toes and feet. Ten years ago, he began having difficulty holding onto farm implements and repeatedly injured himself while working in the fields. Initially misdiagnosed, his condition worsened until he started MDT six months later. Unlike Sita, however, Laxman was never able to conceal his condition, because soon after diagnosis, his neighbours saw him being visited by a local leprosy treatment worker. It took little time for word to spread among prospective in-laws, and Laxman's family gave up trying

[10] See Nichter (2002) for a counterexample in which health providers relabel tuberculosis within a less stigmatising ethnomedical category in order to improve health-seeking and adherence to treatment.

to get him married after two abortive attempts. Laxman related these latter events as if they marked the end of his life.

Laxman continued MDT on a sporadic basis, and I suspected that he was eventually cured. Yet, although he was tolerated in his family and village, no one spoke with him and he kept to himself. In accordance with ritual pollution taboos, he ate his meals from separate pots and *thalis* (plates), and sat alone during village celebrations. Laxman stated that, 'In our society, people hate anyone with this disease.' He insisted, however, that the problem did not lie with his village, but rather with himself.

I was struck, not only by the content of Laxman's story, but also the manner in which he related it. Laxman kept his hands to his sides throughout most of the interview. He related his loss of manual dexterity and subsequent injuries without making a single gesture. This gesture-free narrative was repeated by nearly all of the KSA residents with whom I spoke. They kept their affected limbs beneath garments whenever possible, and assumed positions and postures that minimised whatever was left exposed. It seemed that, even within the isolated confines of the ashram, disavowal persisted as a deeply ingrained habit.

In addition to these habits, the KSA residents also expressed linguistic dispossession from their affected limbs. During the course of their illness narratives, all dropped the possessive pronoun when narrating the succession of injuries to, and problems with, their hands and feet. Thus, when recalling a cut or burn in regional Bhojpuri, *hamare hath* (my hand) simply became *hath* ([the] hand). In standard Hindi, it was *Doctor ne payr ka elaj kiya* (The doctor treated [the] foot) instead of *mera payr* (my foot). A few even went so far as to say *yah anguli* (this finger) or *yah panja* (this toe), without any look or gesture toward the digit. It was as if the appendages that remained had already been amputated, or those that were amputated had left no signs of previous attachment. These habits of word and gesture were particularly disconcerting, given that many KSA residents continued to suffer from limb anaesthesia, necessitating constant visual inspection and a hyperawareness of affected limbs to prevent further injuries. Although they may have been all too aware of their situation on the whole, these data indicate that the residents of KSA were actively dissociating themselves from their physical disabilities on a moment-by-moment basis. If so, this behaviour would have significant consequences for the further progression of their physical condition, even in the absence of infection.

With this background, it is interesting to note that leprologists from Hansen's Disease Centre in Carville, Louisiana, in the U.S., relate anecdotal observations of disdain and neglect of affected limbs among some of their patients (personal communication, Leo J. Yoder, 1998). Although situated in very different cultural contexts, many Carville patients describe themes of isolation and shame very similar to those of the KSA residents (Gussow, 1989). While conducting life-history interviews in Carville in 1997, two patients presented their narratives to me free of gestures and personal pronouns for disabled limbs (personal communication).

Murphy (1990) describes a similar process of dissociation during the progression of his paralysis and cancer. He examines the 'silencing' of his body, beginning with loss of proprioception and ending with emotional detachment. He refers to his limbs as 'the arm' or 'the leg', his body as a 'faulty life-support system', and his remaining self as 'Donovan's Brain'. Murphy and others examine issues of stigmatisation among people with paralysis, characterising them in terms of liminality due to the loss of social roles associated with sexuality and physical independence (Murphy et al., 1988). Within the same time frame, Murphy ignores parts of his own body to the point that he becomes nearly septic from bone-deep pressure ulcers (1990).

For stigmatised neurological conditions with anaesthesia, the loss of physical sensation combined with the loss of social identity creates a strong potential for bodily neglect, thereby perpetuating feedback between the physical pathology and the social pathology of its discrimination. Moreover, the internalisation of stigma is likely to be deeper when such conditions are acquired in adulthood, given that disability prejudices are often learned early through socially ascribed prototypes of health and beauty (Ablon, 1995; Jones, Scott and Markus, 1984). Thus, when confronting the physical parts by which they once identified themselves, parts that have since become misshapen and senseless, it is not surprising that some of these people would dissociate themselves from that which they have long known to be alien, and which marked their alienation from the world around them—a disembodiment of leprosy.

POVERTY AND SELF-MUTILATION

Ram Dev insisted that I cut him. He wanted me to expand the two-inch wound on the ball of his foot with a scalpel. In biomedical terms, it was a Stage 4 ulcer: a crater formed by weeks of constant pressure that had gradually extended down to the bone. Because of his neuropathies, Ram Dev never felt the wound, nor would he have felt the scalpel if I had agreed to his request. The healing of such wounds sometimes requires the removal of dead tissue, which can usually be achieved though vigorous cleaning and a proper dressing. Such was the case for Ram Dev on this particular day, but he would have none of it.

I had been volunteering as nurse at a biweekly street clinic for people with HD near the main bathing ghat at Dashashvamedha. There, I encountered Ram Dev and several other patients who regularly sought the removal of healthy tissue and enlargement of the wounds in their hands and feet. They explained that the additional cutting dispelled the 'bad blood' that was causing their condition. Although none would admit it themselves, statements made about one another suggested that this explanatory model of bloodletting was strongly motivated by the desire to enhance physical deformities for begging. Along similar lines, a few initially resisted taking MDT on the grounds that the medicines might cause their fingers to grow back. After all, these people were marked for life, and deformities were often their primary means of survival.

The mutilation was a gradual process, one that took place in the day-to-day struggle for meagre resources. People would request additional bandages. In combination with exposed deformities, the bandages would be thought to conceal something much worse in the horrors of the pilgrim's imagination. Those with additional bandages might earn slightly more on a given day. Those with bloody bandages might do better, exposed wounds even more, the larger the better, and so on. With fierce competition for alms on the ghats, medical debridement provided a legitimate means to gain a slight advantage under the worst of circumstances. It did not happen all at once. It did not happen every day. But from time to time, some people would trade a bit of flesh for a bit more rice and money.

To fully appreciate these actions, one must understand the desperate conditions under which they occurred. The Dashashvamedha poor were crowded into makeshift shelters of loose brick covered with plastic sheets or corrugated tin. They had no access to clean water or sanitation, and were chronically undernourished. It was therefore hardly surprising that HD was the least of their medical problems. Rather, it was diseases of poverty such as tuberculosis, parasitic infections, diarrhoea, and sexually transmitted diseases that presented the greatest health challenges. Among the women, the stigma of leprosy was compounded by gender inequalities and a lack of protection. Many suffered physical and sexual abuse, and were forced into prostitution under the worst possible conditions. Although none of the children had ever been diagnosed, they carried the mark of their parents, and spent most of their days scavenging through garbage and begging. Unfortunately, the children were exceptionally gifted at the latter, and their earning abilities often dissuaded parents from sending them to school. The social mark of leprosy was not only physically harmful, but heritable as well.

In addition to these problems, heroin abuse was endemic among the adult males of Dashashvamedha, Ram Dev included. Benares is a major retail centre for heroin, and a day's supply can be readily obtained with the earnings from a few hours of begging. It is a sad irony that people would seek pain medication for the socioeconomic consequences of a condition noted for the absence of physical sensation, but this is exactly what Ram Dev and many of his friends were doing. Pain was the chief metaphor in their illness histories, in their losses of family, friends and social identity. Pain was also their chief somatic complaint, a generalised discomfort that was present even among those who were not seeking drugs. The association of chronic pain with alienation and loss recurs in studies of people with discredited medical conditions, which have argued that social suffering is internalised and expressed through somatic symptoms that are indistinguishable from those of physical pathology (Good, 1992; Jackson, 1992; Kleinman, 1992). I suggest that the same was true for Ram Dev and other drug-using members of the Dashashvamedha community. For these people, heroin was an attempt to palliate a deeply internalised suffering. It was a means to detach from the past, the poverty, and the somatic experience of self—another disembodiment of leprosy.

With this background, Ram Dev's particular method of self-mortification fits a classic picture of stigma amplification under conditions of extreme poverty and social alienation. Such amplification can be both a means of destruction and of sustenance, for it is in the interests of the discredited to maximise their out-group identity when they have no other opportunities for social integration (Becker, 1963; Pfuhl and Henry, 1993). Relegated to the lowest rung of humanity, the indigent community at Dashashvamedha could do no worse for their social status, and might even make slight improvements to their economic status, by becoming more of what everyone expects them to be. In this manner, Ram Dev fulfilled his community expectations by becoming poor, addicted to drugs, and physically deformed, inscribing on to his body the very models of discrimination that put him on the streets in the first place. Waxler (1981) discusses how people 'learn to become lepers [sic]' by being socialised into the discriminatory models around them. In the case of Ram Dev and others at Dashashvamedha, these models were not only deeply internalised. They were inscribed onto flesh in accordance with the original definition of stigma: a permanent mark, cut or burned on the skin of people so as to publicly brand them as members of a socially discredited group.

CONCLUSION

The 'self'-mortifications described in this article refer not to individual notions of self but rather to the mutually reinforcing cycle of social discrimination and physical disfigurement that destroy people's lives. Strategies of concealment may further the course and spread of HD through late detection and incomplete treatment. Nevertheless, concealment may be the least damaging alternative, given the more severe consequences of social exposure for the lives of extended families. The threshold for neglect of insensitive limbs may be inversely related to people's aversions to those disabilities, especially when these aversions have been internalised among the patients themselves. And, finally, the deliberate pursuit of bodily mutilation is only conceivable as a short-term survival tactic when someone's life has declined beyond any other hope of change. In each of these processes, the social stigma of leprosy furthers its physical stigma, which returns to reinforce individual and collective models of discrimination.

Although not universally discredited, leprosy is the archetype of disease stigma in many parts of the world, as evidenced by the popular saying

'AIDS is the present-day leprosy.'[11] These diseases share more than a common metaphor. HIV/AIDS persists in many countries under similar conditions of structural violence as those of HD in India, such as when economic desperation creates circumstances of pathogen exposure, or the costs of social exposure outweigh the benefits of early testing and treatment (Barrett, 1995; Farmer, 1992; Wojcicki and Malala, 2001). Similarly, the stigma of tuberculosis and the distrust that it creates between patients and providers can impede health-seeking behaviours and adherence to long-term drug regimens (Ruhel and Garro, 1992), both of which are necessary to control the spread of infection and the emergence of multi-drug resistance (Farmer, 1999). For all these 'leprosies', the forces of inequality (read discrimination) are more prevalent than the infections themselves. At the same time, though, such forces are intimately tied to the epidemiology and pathology of their concomitant infections by constraints on the individual choices that would otherwise affect their prevention and treatment.

The biocultural dynamics of stigmatised diseases strongly supports their framing as illnesses of discrimination, inclusive of their pathology, epidemiology, and both the affliction and infliction of human suffering that they entail. This holistic approach not only mandates active engagement between clinical and critical perspectives. It expands the scope of research beyond the locus of the marked patient, to the broader socioeconomic and historical processes from which the mark originates. As such, anthropologists are well positioned to develop a systematic framework for the understanding and prevention of socially discredited diseases.

References

Ablon, Joan. 1995. 'The "Elephant Man" as "Self" and "Other": The psychosocial costs of a misdiagnosis', *Social Science and Medicine*, 40 (11): 1481–89.

Alsonso, A.A. and Reynolds, N.R. 1995. 'Stigma, HIV and AIDS: An exploration and elaboration of a stigma trajectory', *Social Science and Medicine*, 41 (3): 303–15.

Arole, S. et al. 2002. 'Social stigma: A comparative qualitative study of integrated and vertical care approaches to leprosy', *Leprosy Review*, 73 (2): 186–96.

Barrett, Ronald. 1995. 'The sexual economy of women and HIV in Uganda: A critical biocultural analysis', *Southern Anthropologist*, 22 (3): 27–43.

[11] This metaphor is commonly used by Christian service organisations. See http://www.umc.org and http://www.truechristianity.org for examples.

———. 1997. 'Male health and leprosy in northern India: A biocultural perspective'. Paper presented at the 96th Annual Meeting of the American Anthropological Association, Washington, D.C.

———. 2002. 'Aghor Medicine: Pollution, Power and Healing in Benares, Northern India'. Doctoral dissertation. Emory University.

Beals, Alan. 1976. 'Strategies of resort to curers in south India', in Charles Leslie (ed.), *Asian Medical Systems: A Comparative Study*. Berkeley: University of California Press, pp. 184–200.

Becker, Howard S. 1963. *Outsiders: Studies in the Sociology of Deviance*. New York: Macmillan.

Bloom, Shelah S., Wypij, David and Das Gupta, Monica. 2001. 'Dimensions of women's autonomy and the influence on maternal health-care utilisation in a north Indian city', *Demography*, 38 (1): 67–78.

Brand, Paul and Yancey, Phillip. 1997. *The Gift of Pain*. Grand Rapids: Zondervan.

Bruce, Suzanne et al. 2000. 'Armadillo exposure and Hansen's Disease: An epidemiologic survey in southern Texas', *Journal of the American Academy of Dermatology*, 43 (2): 223–28.

Bryceson, Anthony and Pfalzgraff, Roy E. 1990. *Leprosy*. London: Churchill Livingstone.

Buckingham, Jane. 2002. *Leprosy in Colonial South India: Medicine and Confinement*. New York: Palgrave.

Chakrabarty, A.N. and Dastidar, S.G. 2001. 'Is soil an alternative source of leprosy infection?', *Acta Leprologica*, 12 (2): 79–84.

Dharmshaktu, N.S. 1992. 'A project model for attempting integration of leprosy services with general health-care services after the prevalence of the disease is reduced in the endemic districts on multi-drug therapy for over five years', *Indian Journal of Leprosy*, 64 (3): 349–57.

Farmer, Paul. 1992. *AIDS and Accusation: Haiti and the Geography of Blame*. Berkeley: University of California Press.

———. 1999. *Infections and Inequalities*. Berkeley: University of California Press.

Frist, Thomas F. 2000. 'Stigma and societal response to leprosy: Experience of the last half-century', *Indian Journal of Leprosy*, 72 (1): 1–3.

Goffman, Erving. 1963. *Stigma: Notes on the Management of Spoiled Identity*. Englewood Cliffs: Prentice-Hall.

Good, Byron J. 1992. 'The body in pain: The making of a world of chronic pain', in B.J. Good (ed.), *Pain as Human Experience: An Anthropological Perspective*. Berkeley: University of California Press, pp. 29–48.

Gussow, Zachary. 1989. *Leprosy, Racism and Public Health: Social Policy in Chronic Disease Control*. Boulder: Westview.

Gussow, Zachary and Tracy, George S. 1968. 'Status, ideology and adaptation to stigmatised illness: A study of leprosy', *Human Organisation*, 27 (4): 316–25.

Jackson, Jean E. 1992. '"After a While No One Believes You": Real and Unreal Pain', in B.J. Good (ed.), *Pain as Human Experience*. Berkeley: University of California Press, pp. 138–68.

Jones, Edward E., Scott, Robert A. and Markus, Hazel. 1984. *Social Stigma: The Psychology of Marked Relationships*. New York: W. H. Freeman.

Jopling, William H. 1988. *Handbook of Leprosy*. London: William Heinemann.

Justice, Judith. 1986. *Policies, Plans and People: Culture and Health Development in Nepal.* Berkeley: University of California Press.

Kleinman, Arthur. 1988. *The Illness Narratives: Suffering, Healing and the Human Condition*. New York: Basic Books.

———. 1992. 'Pain and resistance: The delegitimation and relegitimation of local worlds', in B.J. Good (ed.), *Pain as Human Experience*. Berkeley: University of California Press, pp. 169–97.

Kopparty, S.N.M., Karup, A.M. and Sivaram, M. 1995. 'Problems and coping strategies of families having patients with or without deformities', *Indian Journal of Leprosy*, 67 (2): 133–51.

Kumar, A. et al. 2001. 'Some epidemiological observations on leprosy in India, *International Journal of Leprosy and Other Mycobacterial Diseases*, 69 (3): 234–40.

Matsuoka, M. et al. 1999. '*Mycobacterium leprae* DNA in daily using water as a possible source of leprosy infection', *Indian Journal of Leprosy*, 71 (1): 61–67.

Mira, Marcelo T. et al. 2004. 'Susceptibility to leprosy is associated with PARK2 and PACRG', *Nature*, 427 (6975): 636–40.

Mull, J. Dennis et al. 1989. 'Culture and compliance among leprosy patients in Pakistan', *Social Science and Medicine*, 29 (7): 199–211.

Murphy, Robert F. 1990. *The Body Silent*. New York: W.W. Norton.

Murphy, Robert F. et al. 1988. 'Physical disability and social liminality: A study in the rituals of adversity', *Social Science and Medicine*, 26 (2): 235–42.

Naafs, B. et al. 2001. 'Factors influencing the development of leprosy: An overview', *International Journal of Leprosy and Other Mycobacterial Diseases*, 69 (1): 26–33.

Nichter, Mimi. 2002. 'The social relations of therapy management', in Mimi Nichter (ed.), *New Horizons in Medical Anthropology: Essays in Honour of Charles Leslie*. New York: Routledge, pp. 81–110.

Noordeen, Shaik Khader. 1994. 'The epidemiology of leprosy', in R.C. Hasting (ed.), *Leprosy*. Edinburgh: Churchill Livingstone, pp. 29–45.

Parry, Jonathan P. 1986. '"*The Gift*", the Indian Gift and "The Indian Gift"', *Man*, 21: 453–73.

Pfuhl, Erdwin H. and Henry, Stuart. 1993. *The Deviance Process*. New York: Aldine de Gruyter.

Ponnighaus, Jorg M. 1995. 'Leprosy: The beginning of an end to a public health problem?', *Dermatological Clinics*, 19 (3): 525–36.

Raheja, Gloria G. 1988. *The Poison in the Gift: Ritual, Prestation and the Dominant Caste in a North Indian Village*. Chicago: University of Chicago Press.

Rubel, Arthur J. and Garro, Linda C. 1992. 'Social and cultural factors in the successful control of tuberculosis', *Public Health Reports*, 107 (6): 626–35.

Sasaki, Shin et al. 2001. '*Mycobacterium leprae* and leprosy: A compendium', *Microbiology and Immunology*, 45 (11): 729–36.

Sehgal, V.N. 1994. 'Leprosy', *Contemporary Tropical Dermatology*, 12 (4): 629–44.

Srinivasan, H. 1994. 'Disability, deformity and rehabilitation', in Robert C. Hasting (ed.), *Leprosy*, pp. 411–47.

Waxler, Nancy. 1981. 'Learning to be a leper: A case study in the social construction of illness', in Elliot G. Mishler (ed.), *Social Contexts of Health, Fitness and Patient Care*. Cambridge: Cambridge University Press, pp. 169–94.

World Health Organization. 2000. 'Leprosy—global situation', *Weekly Epidemiological Record*, 75 (28): 226–31.

Wojcicki, Janet M. and Malala, Josephine. 2001. 'Condom Use, Power and HIV/AIDS Risk: Sex-workers bargain for survival in Hillbrow/Joubert Park/Berea, Johannesburg', *Social Science and Medicine*, 53 (1): 99–121.

9

An Ethnography of Family Burden and Coping Strategies in Chronic Schizophrenia

Renu Addlakha

General hospital psychiatry is premised on a strategic alliance between the institutions of family and hospital. In the context of poor families managing chronic schizophrenia in the home, the services of a general hospital psychiatry unit can preserve patients from total destitution by offering them temporary but periodic refuge, especially during illness exacerbations. It is important to note that in such cases the principal aim of hospitalisation, i.e. the temporary separation of a sick person from society for the purpose of re-socialisation into the norms of health, is relegated to the background. The concern shifts to the procurement of even more basic needs, such as board and lodging. In this sense, the general hospital psychiatry ward may emerge as 'a home away from home'.

Readers will be familiar with the range of psychiatric studies in India that have tried to tap the rehabilitative potential of the family system in the long-term management of chronicity in the community (Kazi, Kavitha and Shariff, 1993; Muralidhar and Shariff, 1981; Muralidhar, Narayana Reddy and Shariff, 1987; Suman et al., 1980). Other studies

Addlakha, Renu. 1999. 'Living with chronic schizophrenia: An ethnographic account of family burden and coping strategies', *Indian Journal of Psychiatry*, 41 (2): 91–95.

have focussed on the family as a therapeutic ally in clinical settings (Prasad, 1981; Sarda Menon and Shankar, 1993; Shariff et al., 1982a and 1982b). Family wards were set up at NIMHANS (Bhatti, Janakiramaiah and Channabasavanna, 1980; Geeta, Channabasavanna and Bhatti, 1980; Narayan, Embar and Reddy, 1972) and at Vellore (Verghese, 1971 and 1988). Another significant development at NIMHANS is the home-care programme for chronic schizophrenic patients. Recovery was found to be faster, and fewer relapses were reported in comparison to hospital care. Follow-up by a trained visiting nurse and continuous counselling ensured a better clinical outcome and social functioning of the patient, in addition to a decrease in family burden (Pai and Nagarajaiah, 1982; Pai and Kapur, 1982). Subsequently, other therapeutic programmes actively engaging the family have been developed which have produced good results (Shankar and Sarda Menon, 1991). While these studies address the patient-hospital-family triad from the providers' perspective, the present paper seeks to reconfigure this theme from the users' perspective.

RESEARCH METHODOLOGY

The data for this study was obtained in the course of fieldwork for a doctorate conducted between 1990 and 1992 in the psychiatry unit of a government hospital in Delhi. The tools employed for data collection were direct observation, and over six informal interviews with the patient and others close to her in the hospital ward, the OPD and at her home. Information was obtained on such broad issues as the perception and experience of the disorder, emic categories of explanation, nature of contact with medical-care systems (both biomedical and alternative), and in addition the day-to-day coping strategies involved in management of chronic psychiatric disability. In this regard, I wish to make special mention of the sheer wealth of information and insight that patients themselves, irrespective of their psychiatric status, may furnish to an empathic listener. Thus, Sita, the subject of this case study, was my chief and most cooperative informant. Content analysis of the descriptive material highlights both the actual modalities and the experienced burden in the management of chronicity.

A HOME AWAY FROM HOME

Sita is a forty-year-old Punjabi woman with a diagnosis of chronic schizophrenia spanning fifteen years. Her illness history is punctuated by several acute exacerbations. A resident of Delhi, she has been hospitalised several times in the psychiatry ward of the major government-owned general hospitals in the city, in addition to a three-month stay at the Shahdara Mental Hospital. The case sheet revealed that she had dropped out of school in the tenth class.

Her elder sister told me that Sita was married about fifteen years ago to a man thirteen years older than her. He too is reported to be psychiatrically disturbed. The couple have three daughters, aged thirteen, nine and five. The other members of her affinal joint-family household are her widowed mother-in-law, two married brothers-in-law, and their families. They reside in the Khari Baoli area of central Delhi.

In addition to the patient, my other informants were her two younger sisters, both married. The elder, Pratibha, is a primary-school teacher living with her husband and two sons in Paschim Vihar, a residential suburb in west Delhi. Sita's other sister, Bimla, is a nurse in a government-owned hospital in Delhi. She too has two children. Sita's eldest daughter, Gita, who was her mother's attendant in the ward, was also very communicative.

My first encounter with Sita was on a hot June afternoon, a day after her admission into the ward. She presented herself at that time as a short, stocky, dark-skinned woman dressed in an old and rather unclean nightgown. Her grey hair was dishevelled, and her clothes were soaking wet. Pratibha, who had accompanied her to the hospital, told me that Sita had started throwing buckets of water over herself ten to fifteen times during the course of a day. She said:

> This is what she has been doing for the past few days. She is also eating a lot, and talking nonsense all the time.

After a few days in the ward on psychotropic medication, Sita was calmer and more amenable to communication. She told me of her own accord:

> I got this illness when I was in the tenth class. I drank too much Coca Cola. My throat began to hurt, and then I got sick. Since then, I have been taking Largactil and Magactil.

This unvarying, albeit incoherent, aetiological explanation of the onset of her suffering was accompanied by such physical complaints as: a sinking feeling in the heart, constipation, and general bodily discomfort. During her stay in the ward, she was obsessed by the idea that she had high blood pressure. Whenever she saw any doctor, she would rush up to him, and implore him to take her blood pressure, saying, 'My pressure has gone up (pressure *badh gaya hai*).'

In the course of a conversation with Pratibha, some of the family's management strategies were delineated. Upon my asking her whether anyone from Sita's conjugal home had come to see her since her current admission into the ward, Pratibha explained in the course of an interview:

Pratibha: When she has an attack, she either comes to my house or to Bimla's. Then we bring her to a hospital.

Renu: But when she is all right, then does she stay at Khari Baoli?
P: Off and on. Last year, she stayed for six months with our brother in Orissa. They look after neither her nor her children at Khari Baoli. We also have to take care of the children.

R: That must be a great burden on you. How do you manage?
P: Yes, it is very difficult. I myself have two sons, and Bimla's husband died a few years ago. Just food, clothing and school fees for one more person makes so much of a difference. But she is our elder sister. If we don't look after her, then who will? Gita stays with me, and the other daughter, Pooja, is in Orissa. Her husband has kept the youngest daughter with him.

R: Is this a permanent arrangement?
P: No, nothing is permanent. Pooja was staying with Bimla before she went to Orissa. If they had been boys instead of girls, then they would have kept them at Khari Baoli. After Anju, the youngest daughter, was born, we got Sita sterilised, because they would never have thought of it themselves.

R: And where does Sita stay when she is not in Khari Baoli?
P: Sometimes here, sometimes there. She was in Orissa for a year. When she stays either with me or my sister, our brother sends some money for

her every month. It has been going on like this for many years. There is also the hospital. Invariably, she becomes ill once a year. Then she has to be hospitalised for a month or so.

In addition to providing sustenance to Sita, especially during periods of relapse, her siblings (and by extension their conjugal families) are also engaged in the more arduous and long-term task of bringing up her children. Their responsibilities include the provision of basic needs, such as food, shelter and medical treatment for Sita, and the upkeep of her three daughters. This even involves, on the part of Sita's sisters, reproductive decision-making on her behalf. The hospital emerges as a convenient and necessary resort in this carefully worked-out, ongoing family-based system of management and care.

When I asked Sita how she felt about being looked after by her siblings, especially during her illness, she replied in a quiet tone of voice:

If they were not there, who would look after us? My children and I would die. Our *bhabhi* [brother's wife] always fights about me. When I was in Orissa, I lived in the servant quarters. She told my brother, 'I won't keep this madwoman in my house.' I cooked my own food on a stove. In Pratibha's house, they too fight when I go there. At least there is no such problem when I am here in the ward. Then, Gita only has to miss school to be with me.

But when I asked her, on the day of her discharge from the ward, where she wanted to go, she said solemnly, 'Khari Baoli.'

Renu: But you say that your husband beats you?
Sita: So let him beat me!

Bimla, who had come to collect her, told me that Sita would stay with her for the time being.

Renu: And after that, where will she go?
Bimla: We will see. Pratibha and I have been thinking of finding her some job as an *ayah* [maid]. She can do that sort of work. When she is all right, she can earn a little money and keep herself occupied. The trouble is that after some time she will fall ill again.

Sita (*interrupting*): He does not allow me to take the medicines. He sits in the temple the whole day, he forgets things, and he beats me.
B: Yes, her husband is also mental.

R: Was he like that at the time of marriage too?

B: Yes. They were both of weak mind. Otherwise, who else would have married her? But her in-laws should look after her as they look after him.

Although most members of Sita's conjugal family, including her husband, do not provide either financial or emotional support, her own children have come to function as her caregivers, especially when she is hospitalised. Gita looked after her mother in the ward with great solicitude. In addition to reporting on her mother's condition to the doctors, she cleaned her utensils, ensured that she kept herself clean, and patiently bore with her frequent outbursts of temper. She did not seem to mind the burden imposed on her by this role reversal with her mother. On the contrary, she told me cheerfully:

She has always been like this. Even when she is not ill, she doesn't do much work. When she is sleeping, or talking with other patients, I try to study, because I have to give a 'compartment' [exam] when school reopens.

A sense of alienation is expressed by Sita's longing for a space of her own. Deprived of a normal home with her husband and children, she often expressed the wish, 'I want to build my own house.' It seems that the closest that she could get to the fulfilment of this wish, in her circumstances, was coming to the ward. Like several other patients, Sita sought refuge in the hospital from her domestic woes. I saw her one day, towards the end of my fieldwork, in the OPD with Pratibha and her youngest daughter. She begged the doctors with tears in her eyes to be admitted into the ward, saying, 'Don't send me home. I am very sick. I have nowhere to go. They are tired of me.' When Pratibha was asked what had happened, she shook her head and said:

I don't know. She came from Khari Baoli and was looking confused. So I brought her here. I too think she needs to be admitted. Can Anju be with her in the ward? Gita has to study for her exams.

The poignancy of the family's plight is revealed by the fact that they had brought the five-year old girl to fulfil the hospital's requirement for ward admission, namely, the presence of an attendant for each patient, provided or paid for by the family.

CONCLUSION

The analysis of this narrative highlights the crucial role of the natal family in the care and management of a chronic, mentally-disturbed woman, and in the rearing of her children. This continuous support, even after her marriage (when a woman in the Indian context is considered to be largely socially and morally the responsibility of her affinal family), is not as uncommon under the given circumstances as it might at first appear. Similarly, pairing the handicapped in the arranged matrimonial system is another management technique employed by families of both the physically and mentally disabled. Although her siblings, despite adverse circumstances in their own lives, provide Sita and her daughters with sustenance and care, the underlying financial strains are evident. This, in turn, creates interpersonal tension. One indicator of this is the patient's frequent relapses. Second, the conscious seeking out of the hospital by both the patient and her family shows a differential appropriation of biomedical space as more welfare than therapeutic.

References

Bhatti, R.S., Janakiramaiah, N. and Channabasavanna, S.M. 1980. 'Family psychiatric ward treatment in India', *Family Process*, 19: 193–200.

Geeta, P.R., Channabasavanna, S.M. and Bhatti, R.S. 1980. 'The study of efficacy of family ward treatment in hysteria in comparison with the open ward and the outpatient treatment', *Indian Journal of Psychiatry*, 22 (4): 317–23.

Kapur, R.L. 1992. 'Family and schizophrenia: Priority areas for intervention research in India', *Indian Journal of Psychiatry*, 34 (1): 3–7.

Kazi, S.A., Kavitha, M.A. and Shariff, I.A. 1993. 'Indicators of social support in the families of mentally ill belonging to scheduled castes', *Indian Journal of Clinical Psychology*, 20 (2): 69–72.

Muralidhar, D. and Shariff, I.A. 1981. 'Obstacles in the way of readjustment of mental patients in the family', *Journal of Rehabilitation in Asia*, 21 (4): 37–41.

Muralidhar, D., Narayana Reddy, G.N. and Shariff, I.A. 1987. 'Rehabilitation potentials in the families of mentally ill', *Journal of Medical and Psychiatric Social Work*, 1 (1): 21–25.

Narayanan, H.S., Embar, P. and Reddy, G.N.N. 1972. 'Review of treatment in family ward', *Indian Journal of Psychiatry*, 14 (2): 123–26.

Pai, S. and Kapur, R.L. 1982. 'Impact of treatment intervention on the relationship between dimensions of clinical psychopathology, social dysfunction and burden on the family of a psychiatric patient', *Psychological Medicine*, 12 (3): 651–59.

Pai, S. and Nagarajaiah. 1982. 'Treatment of schizophrenic patients in their homes through a visiting nurse: Some issues in the nurses' training', *Journal of Nursing Studies*, 19: 167–72.

Prasad, R. 1981. 'Family as a support in crisis situations in clinical settings', *Indian Journal of Social Research*, 22 (3): 279–84.

Sarda Menon, M. and Shankar, R. 1993. 'Family and professionals working together in the management of schizophrenia', in P. Mane and K.Y. Gandevia (eds), *Mental Health in India: Issues and Concerns*. Bombay: Tata Institute of Social Sciences, pp. 261–76.

Shankar, R. and Sarda Menon, M. 1991. 'Family intervention programme in schizophrenia: The SCARF experience', in Unit for Family Studies, Tata Institute of Social Sciences (eds), *Research on Families with Problems in India*, Vol. I. Bombay: Tata Institute of Social Sciences, pp. 28–144.

Shariff, I.A. et al. 1982a. 'Hospital treatment of the mentally ill with periodic family participation: A boon for better rehabilitation', *Journal of Rehabilitation in Asia*, 23 (3): 35–39.

———. 1982b. 'Involvement of the families in the treatment of mentally ill in the hospital', *Indian Journal of Social Research*, 23 (2): 151–54.

Suman, C. et al. 1980. 'Helping the chronic schizophrenics and their families in the community: Initial observations', *Indian Journal of Psychiatry*, 22 (1): 97–102.

Verghese, A. 1971. 'Involvement of families in mental health care', *Journal of Christian Medical Association of India*, 46: 84–87.

———. 1988. 'Family participation in mental health care: The Vellore experiment', *Indian Journal of Psychiatry*, 30 (2): 117–21.

PART 3

Social Life with a Disability: Integration and Social Organisation

Introduction

Renu Addlakha & Osamu Nagase

The fundamental assumption of the social model of disability is that impairment *per se* is not disabling, but it is the limitations imposed by society that give birth to multiple forms of disability. Indeed, given that diversity is the cornerstone of life, it is not individuals who are disabled but society which is disabling. *Disabilism* is the term used to describe an ideology that systematically marginalises and isolates persons with disabilities through a range of social barriers: material, cultural and psychological. Consequently, if social barriers are the root of the oppression faced by persons with disabilities, then the source of positive transformation and empowerment also lies in the social system. That is, society can also be enabling by removing negative attitudes and discriminatory practices that systematically exclude persons with disabilities from spheres of socio-economic life.

The four articles in Part 3 highlight how social institutions and practices impact the lives of persons with disabilities in different cultural contexts. While Fred Davis discusses how persons with visible disabilities and their non-disabled counterparts attempt to attain interpersonal normalisation in a typical North American social milieu, John Hinnant shifts the analytical lens to processes of assimilation that have historically emerged to accommodate the deaf in a part of Bali, Indonesia, predisposed to a hereditary form of deafness. Meenu Bhambani, a physically disabled woman, presents a gender-based analysis of the plight of women with disabilities in contemporary India. Patriarchy has a transcultural resonance reflected in the experiences of, and attitudes to, women with disabilities in different cultural settings. Carol Thomas shows multiple forms of devaluation experienced by women with disabilities in the context of pregnancy and motherhood in contemporary western societies like that of Great Britain.

In his microanalysis of routine social transactions between the visibly disabled and the non-disabled, Davis highlights the manner in which 'deviance is disavowed' when mutual attempts are made to reject societal imputations of negativity. In a society in which disability carries enormous negative connotations, the handicapped person becomes a threat to sociable interaction due to a number of factors. The visible handicap becomes the focal point of interaction. A further source of strain is the attempt of the non-disabled person to disguise his feelings of fear, pity and repugnance in the face of the disability by an outward show of civility and warmth towards the disabled person. Social awkwardness is further exacerbated by the need of the non-disabled to ascertain the extent of the disability and the nature of the limitations without showing undue curiosity by word or deed. In his attempt to normalise the social encounter and reject negative ascriptions of what it means to be a disabled person, the disabled person also struggles to help the other understand him without compromising his dignity or self-respect. A politically correct fiction of equality and normality may be erected by both parties to diminish the discomfort. Furthermore, the disabled participant may explicitly expand the field of interaction to create niches of identification with his non-disabled counterpart in an attempt to diminish the social barriers. Drawing upon commonplace situations of sociability, such as attending a party or business meeting, having a conversation with a fellow traveller, staying at a hotel, or getting to know neighbours, Davis creates an ideal methodological context to demonstrate the many coping strategies used by disabled and non-disabled participants to facilitate the flow of interaction in situations characterised by high levels of embarrassment and discomfort.

In the second article of Part 3, Hinnant shows how culture and society may attenuate the taint of disability through processes of structural integration. Drawing upon fieldwork in Bengkala village in Bali, Indonesia, he shows how deafness in a substantial number of the population, on account of a genetic predisposition, has resulted over time in the creation of a unique deaf community accommodative to hearing people, mediated by a local sign language. The author contends that religious beliefs in reincarnation and ancestor worship create solidarity between deaf and hearing individuals in an already kin-based social system. The deaf participate in religious ceremonies and rituals on a par with their hearing counterparts. Sign language, learnt by both hearing and deaf children, facilitates social integration.

Nevertheless, being deaf has its disadvantages, even in the context of a high level of integration. When exploring deaf persons' perceptions of their disability, the author found that the disability limited employment opportunities, in addition to exposing them to public ridicule. The local term for deaf (*kolok*) is somewhat derogatory, since it implies a lack of mental ability. Deaf women fared particularly badly, because the general segregation of the sexes left them more socially isolated than their male counterparts, who could become members of village organisations and even take up certain types of employment.

Gender emerges as a critical variable mediating the experience of disability for women, irrespective of the socio-cultural context of their lives. Meenu Bhambani highlights the triple burdens of gender, disability and poverty that frame the lives of women with disabilities in developing countries like India. While declining sex ratios, rejection of the girl child, under-nutrition, high school drop-out rates, dowry, and multiple forms of violence affect the lives of all women, their impact is multiplied in the case of women with disabilities, making them a socially altogether invisible category. In her paper, Bhambani traces the negative depiction of women with disabilities in popular Indian mythology and cinema. Since women with disabilities are seen to depart from dominant constructions of femininity as objects of physical beauty and providers of services for the maintenance of home and family, they are considered a perennial liability for the family, objects of pity to be shunned, utterly undesirable and unwanted. They are never considered as capable, efficient persons in their own right. In addition to expanding educational and employment opportunities, the author underscores the need to treat women with disabilities with respect and dignity, as whole persons, without forgetting the disability, but at the same time avoiding comparison with non-disabled women.

Economic prosperity, education and employment opportunities may attenuate some of the more extreme forms of gender discrimination, but they do not necessarily guarantee gender equity. In her article on reproductive experiences of women with disabilities in the north of England, Carol Thomas shows the multiple forms of disabilism suffered by these women in the context of pregnancy, childbirth and motherhood, especially at the hands of healthcare and social-service providers. Indeed, disabled women's reproductive journeys are strewn with ideological, attitudinal and material barriers. The author divides the difficulties faced by them in the reproductive arena into three categories: engagement with the medical-risk discourse, pressure to demonstrate capacity to be good-enough mothers, and experiences of receiving unhelpful offers of assistance from healthcare and social-care providers. A disabled woman's choice to have children is itself fraught with emotional, moral and medical implications: risk to her own health, stringent medical monitoring during pregnancy, fear of giving birth to deformed children, accepting responsibility for possible disability in the child, etc. Disabled women are under additional pressure to perform well as mothers, because of the social perceptions of disabled persons as objects of care rather than as caregivers. They are often considered incapable of fulfilling the role of good mothers even by their relatives, making them more prone to feelings of vulnerability and insecurity. There is always the fear of losing their children to foster care, if they are found lacking. Furthermore, the paternalistic stance of professionals like doctors, nurses and social workers exacerbates the situation. A professional ideology of 'we know best', combined with the fear of asking for help out of fear of being rated incapable, makes many disabled mothers avoid seeking assistance. In the complex interplay of personal anxiety and professional dominance, the right to parenthood of women with disabilities is constantly challenged.

The four articles in this section show that impairment *per se* is not disabling. Indeed, disability is largely a social construction embedded in social institutions and cultural practices. The path to enhancing the status of persons with disabilities lies in the removal of social, economic and psychological barriers that devalue and discriminate against persons with disabilities, while guaranteeing unfettered access to quality healthcare, education, employment and recreation.

10

Deviance Disavowal: The Management of Strained Interaction by the Visibly Handicapped

Fred Davis

A recurring issue in social relations is the refusal of those who are viewed as deviant[1] to concur in the verdict. Or, if in some sense it can be said that they do concur, they usually place a very different interpretation on the fact or allegation than do their judges. In our society, this is especially true of deviance which results from ascription (e.g. the Negro), as against that which partakes to some significant degree of election (e.g. the homosexual). And, while it may be conjectured that ultimately

---

Davis, F. 1961. 'Deviance disavowal: The management of strained interaction by the visibly handicapped', *Social Problems*, 9 (2): 120–32.

[1] Following Lemert, as used here the term deviant (or deviance) (1) refers to a person's deviation from prevalent or valued norms, to which (2) the community-at-large reacts negatively or punitively, which then (3) leads the person to define his situation largely in terms of this reaction. All three conditions must be fulfilled for it to be said that deviancy exists (secondary deviation, in Lemert's definition). In this sense, the Negro, the career woman, the criminal, the communist, the physically handicapped, the mentally ill, the homosexual, to mention but a few, are all deviants, albeit in different ways and with markedly different consequences for their life careers. See Lemert, Edwin M. 1951. *Social Pathology*. New York: McGraw-Hill, pp. 75–77.

neither the Negro nor the homosexual would be cast in a deviant role were it not for society's devaluation of these attributes in the first place, barring such a hypothetical contingency it remains the more persuasive argument in a democracy to be able to claim that the social injury from which one suffers was in no way self-inflicted.

In these pages I wish to discuss another kind of non-self-inflicted social injury, the visible physical handicap. My aim, though, is not to survey and describe the many hardships of the visibly handicapped,[2] but to analyse certain facets of their coping behaviour as it relates to the generalised imputations of deviance they elicit from society, imputations which many of them feel it necessary to resist and reject.

There are, of course, many areas in which such imputations bear heavily upon them: employment, friendship, courtship, sex, travel, recreation, residence and education. But the area I treat here is enmeshed to some extent in all of these, without being as categorically specific as any. I refer to situations of sociability, and more specifically to that genre of everyday intercourse which has the characteristics of being: (1) face-to-face; (2) prolonged enough to permit more than a fleeting glimpse or exchange, but not so prolonged that close familiarity immediately ensues; (3) intimate to the extent that the parties must pay more than perfunctory attention to one another, but not so intimate that the customary social graces can be dispensed with; and (4) ritualised to the extent that all know in general what to expect, but not so ritualised as to preclude spontaneity and the slightly novel turn of events. A party or other social affair, a business introduction, getting to know a person at work, meeting neighbours, dealing with a salesman, conversing with a fellow passenger, staying at a resort hotel—these are but a few of the everyday social situations which fall within this portion of the spectrum of sociability, a range of involvement which can also be thought of as the zone of first impressions.

[2] Comprehensive and excellent reviews are to be found in Baker, R.G. et al. 1953. *Adjustment to Physical Handicap and Illness: A Survey of the Social Psychology of Physique and Disability*. New York: Soc. Sci. Res. Council, Bulletin 55, 2nd edn.; and in Wright, Beatrice A. 1960. *Physical Disability, A Psychological Approach*. New York: Harper.

In interviews I conducted with a small number of very articulate and socially skilled informants who were visibly handicapped,[3] I inquired into their handling of the imputation that they were not 'normal, like everyone else.' This imputation usually expresses itself in a pronounced stickiness of interactional flow, and in the embarrassment of the normal, by which he conveys the all-too-obvious message that he is having more difficulty in relating to the handicapped person[4] than he would to 'just an ordinary man or woman'. Frequently, he will make *faux pas*, slips of the tongue, revealing gestures and inadvertent remarks which overtly betray this attitude and place the handicapped person in an even more delicate situation.[5] The triggering of such a chain of interpersonal incidents is more likely with new persons than with those with whom the handicapped have well-established and continuing relations. Hence, the focus here is on more or less sociable occasions, for it is these in which interactional discomfort is felt most acutely and coping behaviour is brought into relief most sharply.

Because the visibly handicapped do not comprise a distinct minority group or subculture, the imputations of generalised deviance that they elicit from many normals are more nearly genuine interactional emergents than conventionalised sequelae to intergroup stereotyping as, for example, might obtain between a Negro and a white. A sociable encounter between a visibly handicapped person and a normal is usually more subject to

[3] Six were orthopaedically handicapped, three blind, and two facially disfigured. Additional detailed biographical and clinical materials were secured on one blind and four facially disfigured persons, making for a total of sixteen records.

[4] Throughout this paper, whether or not the term 'handicap' or 'handicapped' is joined by the qualifier 'visible', it should be read in this way. Unfortunately, it will not be possible to discuss here that which sociologically distinguishes the situation of the visibly handicapped from that of persons whose physical handicaps are not visible or readily apparent, and how both differ from what is termed the 'sick role'. These are important distinctions, though, whose analysis might illuminate key questions in the study of deviance.

[5] In the sections that follow, the discussion draws heavily on the framework of dramaturgic analysis developed by Erving Goffman. See, especially, Goffman, Erving. November 1956. 'Embarrassment and Social Organisation', *American Journal of Sociology*, 62: 246–71; Goffman, Erving. 1957. 'Alienation from Interaction', *Human Relations*, 10: 47–60; Goffman, Erving. 1959. *Presentation of Self in Everyday Life.* New York: Doubleday.

ambiguity and experimentation in role postures than would be the case were the parties perceived by each other primarily in terms of member-group characteristics. The visibly handicapped person must, with each new acquaintance, explore the *possibilities* of a relationship. As a rule, there is no ready-made symbolic shorthand (e.g. 'a Southerner can't treat a Negro as a social equal,' 'the Irish are anti-Semitic,' 'working-class people think intellectuals are effeminate') for anticipating the quality and degree of acceptance to be accorded him. The exchange must be struck before its dangers and potentialities can be seen, and before appropriate corrective manoeuvres can be fed into the interaction (Strauss, 1959, pp. 31–43).

THE HANDICAP AS THREAT TO SOCIABLE INTERACTION

Before discussing how the visibly handicapped cope with difficult interaction, it is appropriate to first consider the general nature of the threat posed to the interactional situation *per se* as a result of their being perceived routinely (if not necessarily according to some prevalent stereotype) as 'different', 'odd', 'estranged from the common run of humanity', etc.; in short, other than normal. (Achieving ease and naturalness of interaction with normals serves naturally as an important index to the handicapped person of the extent to which his preferred definition of self, i.e. that of someone who is merely different physically but not socially deviant, has been accepted. Symbolically, as long as the interaction remains stiff, strained or otherwise mired in inhibition, he has good reason to believe that he is in effect being denied the status of social normalcy he aspires to, or regards as, his due.) The threat posed by the handicap to sociability is, at minimum, fourfold: its tendency to become an exclusive focal point of the interaction, its potential for inundating expressive boundaries, its discordance with other attributes of the person, and, finally, its ambiguity as a predicator of joint activity. These are not discrete entities in themselves as much as varying contextual emergents which, depending on the particular situation, serve singly or in combination to strain the framework of normative rules and assumptions in which sociability develops. Let us briefly consider each in turn.

A Focal Point of Interaction

The rules of sociable interaction stipulate a certain generality and diffuseness in the attentions that parties are expected to direct to each other. Even if only superficially, one is expected to remain oriented to the whole person, and to avoid the expression of a precipitous or fixed concern with any single attribute of his, however noteworthy or laudable it may be (Wolff, 1950, pp. 45–46). When meeting someone with a visible handicap, a number of perceptual and interpretative responses occur which make adherence to this rule tenuous for many. First, there is the matter of visibility as such. By definition, the visibly handicapped person cannot control his appearance sufficiently so that its striking particularity will not call a certain amount of concentrated attention to itself (White, Wright and Dembo, 1948). Second, the normal, while having his attention so narrowly channelled, is immediately constrained by the requirements of sociability to act as if he were oriented to the totality of the other rather than to that which is uppermost in his awareness, i.e., the handicap. Although the art of sociability may be said to thrive on a certain playful discrepancy between felt and expressed interests, it is perhaps equally true that when these are too discrepant, strain and tension begin to undermine the interaction. (Conversely, when not discrepant enough, flatness and boredom frequently ensue.)[6] Whether the handicap is overtly and tactlessly responded to as such, or, as is more commonly the case, no explicit reference is made to it, the underlying condition of heightened, narrowed awareness causes the interaction to be articulated too exclusively in terms of it. This, as my informants described it, is usually accompanied by one or more of the familiar signs of discomfort and stickiness: the guarded references, the common everyday words suddenly made taboo, the fixed stare elsewhere, the artificial levity, the compulsive loquaciousness, the awkward solemnity.[7]

Second-order interactional elaborations of the underlying impedance are also not uncommon. Thus, for example, the normal may take great pains to disguise his awareness, an exertion that is usually so effortful and transparent that the handicapped person is then enjoined to disguise

[6] In his paper 'Fun in Games: An Analysis of the Dynamics of Social Interaction', Goffman discusses the relationship between spontaneous involvement in interaction and the manner in which 'external attributes'—those which, in a formal sense, are not situationally relevant—are permitted to penetrate the situation's boundaries.

[7] Cf. Goffman on 'other-consciousness' as a type of faulty interaction: Goffman, Erving. 1957. 'Alienation from Interaction', *Human Relations*, 10: 47–60.

his awareness of the normal's disguise. In turn, the normal, sensing the disguise erected in response to his disguise ... and so forth. But unlike the infinitely multiplying reflections of an object located between opposing mirrors, this process cannot sustain itself for long without the pretence of unawareness collapsing, as witness the following report by a young woman:

> I get suspicious when somebody says, 'Let's go for a uh, ah [imitates confused and halting speech] push with me down the hall,' or something like that. This to me is suspicious, because it means that they're aware, really aware, that there's a wheelchair here, and that this is probably uppermost with them.... A lot of people, in trying to show you that they don't care that you're in a chair, will do crazy things. Oh, there's one person I know who constantly kicks my chair, as if to say, 'I don't care that you're in a wheelchair. I don't even know that it's there.' But that is just an indication that he *really* knows it's there.

Inundating Potential

The expressive requirements of sociability are such that rather strict limits obtain with respect to the types and amount of emotional display that are deemed appropriate. Even such fitting expressions as gaiety and laughter can, we know, reach excess and lessen satisfaction with the occasion. For many normals, the problem of sustaining sociable relations with someone who is visibly handicapped is not wholly that of the discrepancy of the inner feeling evoked, e.g. pity, fear, repugnance, avoidance. As with much else in sociability, a mere discrepancy of the actor's inner state with the social expectation need not result in a disturbance of interaction. In this instance, it is specifically the marked dissonance of such emotions with those outward expressions deemed most salient for the occasion (e.g. pleasure, identification, warm interest) that seems to result frequently in an inundation and enfeeblement of the expressive controls of the individual. With some persons, the felt intrusion of this kind of situationally inappropriate emotion is so swift and overwhelming that it approximates a state of shock, leaving them expressively naked, so to speak. A pointed incident is told by a young blind girl:

> One night, when I was going to visit a friend, two of the people from my office put me into a taxi. I could tell that at first the taxi driver didn't

> know I was blind, because for a while there he was quite a conversationalist. Then he asked me what 'these sticks' [a collapsible cane] were for. I told him it was a cane, and then he got so different.... He didn't talk about the same things that he did at first. Before this happened he joked and said, 'Oh, you're a very quiet person. I don't like quiet people, they think too much.' And he probably wouldn't have said that to me had he known I was blind, because he'd be afraid of hurting my feelings. He didn't say anything like that afterwards.

The visibly handicapped are of course aware of this potential for inundating the expressive boundaries of situations, and many take precautions to minimise such occurrences as much as possible. Thus, an interior decorator with a facial deformity would, when admitted to a client's house by the maid, station himself, whenever he could, so that the client's entrance would find him in a distantly direct line of vision from her. This, he stated, gave the client an opportunity to compose herself, as she might not be able to were she to come upon him at short range.

Contradiction of Attributes

Even when the inundating potential is well contained by the parties, and the normal proves fully capable of responding in a more differentiated fashion to the variety of attributes presented by the handicapped person (e.g. his occupational identity, clothes, speech, intelligence, interests, etc.), there is frequently felt to be an unsettling discordance between these and the handicap. Sociable interaction is made more difficult as a result, because many normals can only resolve the seeming incongruence by assimilating or subsuming (often in a patronising or condescending way) the other attributes to that of the handicap, a phenomenon which, in analogous connections, has been well described by Hughes (Hughes, 1958, pp. 102–6). Thus, one informant, a strikingly attractive girl, reports that she frequently elicits from new acquaintances the comment, 'How strange that someone so pretty should be in a wheelchair.' Another informant, a professional worker for a government agency, tells of a fashionable female client who, after having inquired on how long the informant had been in her job, remarked, 'How nice that you have something to do.' Because the art of sociability deigns this kind of reductionism of the person, expressions of this type, even when much less blatant, almost invariably cast a pall on the interaction and embarrass the recovery of smooth social posture. The general threat inherent in the perceived discordance of personal attributes is given pointed expression by still another informant, a paraplegic of upper middle-class background, who comments on the attitude of many persons in his class:

> Now, where this affects them, where this brace and a crutch would affect them, is if they are going someplace or if they are doing something, they feel that, first, you would call attention and, second, you wouldn't believe this but it's true—I'll use the cruellest words I can, no cripple could possibly be in their social stratum.

Ambiguous Predicator

Finally, to the extent to which sociability is furthered by the free and spontaneous initiation of joint activity (e.g. dancing, games, going out to eat; in short, 'doing things') there is frequently considerable ambiguity as regards the ability of the handicapped person to so participate, and as regards the propriety of efforts which seek to ascertain whether he wants to. For the normal who has had limited experience with the handicapped, it is by no means always clear whether, for example, a blind person can be included in a theatre party or a crippled person in a bowling game. Even if not able to engage in the projected activity as such, will he want to come along mainly for the sake of company? How may his preferences be gauged without, on the one hand, appearing to 'make a thing' out of the proposal or, on the other, conveying the impression that his needs and limitations are not being sufficiently considered? Should he refuse, is it genuine or is he merely offering his hosts a polite, though half-hearted, out? And, for each enigma thus posed for the normal, a counter-enigma is posed for the handicapped person. Do they really want him? Are they merely being polite? In spite of the open invitation, will his acceptance and presence lessen somehow their enjoyment of the activity? It is easy to see how a profusion of anticipatory ambiguities of this kind can strain the operative assumptions underlying sociable relations.

PROCESS OF DEVIANCE DISAVOWAL AND NORMALISATION

The above features, then, may be said to comprise the threat that a visible handicap poses to the framework of rules and assumptions that guide sociability. We may now ask how socially adept handicapped persons cope with it so as to either keep it at bay, dissipate it, or lessen its impact upon the interaction. In answering this question, we will not consider those broad personality adjustments of the person (e.g. aggression, denial, compensation, dissociation, etc.) which, at a level once removed, so to speak, can be thought of as adaptive or maladaptive for, among other things, sociability. Nor, at the other extreme, is it possible in the allotted space to review the tremendous variety of specific approaches, ploys and stratagems that the visibly handicapped employ in social situations. Instead, the analysis will attempt to delineate in transactional terms the stages through which a sociable relationship with a normal typically passes, assuming, of course, that the confrontation takes place and that both parties possess sufficient social skill to sustain a more than momentary engagement.

For present purposes, we shall designate these stages as: (1) fictional acceptance; (2) the facilitation of reciprocal role-taking around a normalised projection of self; and (3) the institutionalisation in the relationship of a definition of self that is normal in its moral dimension, however qualified it may be with respect to its situational contexts. As we shall indicate, the unfolding of these stages comprises what may be thought of as a process of deviance disavowal or normalisation,[8] depending on whether one views the process from the vantage point of the 'deviant' actor or his alters.[9]

Fictional Acceptance

In western society, the overture phases of a sociable encounter are to a pronounced degree regulated by highly elastic fictions of equality and

[8] As used here, the term 'normalisation' denotes a process whereby alter, for whatever reason, comes to view as normal and morally acceptable that which initially strikes him as odd, unnatural, 'crazy', deviant, etc., irrespective of whether his perception was in the first instance reasonable, accurate or justifiable. Cf. Schwarz, Charlotte G. August 1957. 'Perspectives on Deviance—Wives' Definitions of their Husbands' Mental Illness', *Psychiatry*, 20: 275–91.

[9] Because of the paper's focus on the visibly handicapped person, in what follows, his interactional work is highlighted to the relative glossing over of that of the normal. Actually, the work of normalisation calls for perhaps as much empathic expenditure as that of deviance disavowal and is, obviously, fully as essential for repairing the interactional breach occasioned by the encounter.

normalcy. In meeting those with whom we are neither close nor familiar, manners dictate that we refrain from remarking on, or otherwise reacting too obviously to, those aspects of their persons which in the privacy of our thoughts betoken important differences between ourselves. In America, at least, these fictions tend to encompass sometimes marked divergencies in social status, as well as a great variety of expressive styles. It is perhaps the extreme flexibility of such fictions in our culture, rather than, as is mistakenly assumed by many foreign observers, their absence, that accounts for the seeming lack of punctiliousness in American manners. The point is nicely illustrated in the following news item:

> Nude Takes a Stroll in Miami
>
> MIAMI, Fla., Nov. 13 (UPI) - A shapely brunette slowed traffic to a snail's pace here yesterday with a 20-minute nude stroll through downtown Miami, ...
>
> 'The first thing I knew something was wrong,' said Biscayne Bay bridge tender E.E. Currey, who was working at his post about one block away, 'was when I saw traffic was going unusually slow.'
>
> Currey said he looked out and called police. They told him to stop the woman, he said.
>
> Currey said he walked out of his little bridge house, approached the woman nervously, and asked, 'Say, girl, are you lost?'
>
> 'Yes,' she replied. 'I'm looking for my hotel.'
>
> Currey offered help and asked, 'Say, did you lose your clothes?'
>
> 'No,' he said the woman replied. 'Why?'
>
> Currey said that he had to step away for a moment to raise the bridge for a ship and the woman walked away....[10]

Unlike earlier societies and some present-day ones, in which a visible handicap automatically relegates the person to a caste-like inferior status, like that of a mendicant, clown or thief, or, more rarely, to an elevated one, like that of an oracle or healer, in our society the visibly handicapped

[10] *San Francisco Chronicle*, 14 November 1960.

are customarily accorded, save by children,[11] the surface acceptance that democratic manners guarantee to nearly all. But, as regards sociability, this proves a mixed blessing for many. Although the polite fictions do afford certain entrée rights, as fictions they can too easily come to serve as substitutes for 'the real thing' in the minds of their perpetrators. The interaction is kept starved at a bare subsistence level of sociability. As with the poor relation at the wedding party, so is the reception given the handicapped person in many social situations: it is sufficient that he is here; he should not expect to dance with the bride.

At this stage of the encounter, the interactional problem confronting the visibly handicapped person is the delicate one of not permitting his identity to be circumscribed by the fiction, while at the same time playing along with it and showing appropriate regard for its social legitimacy. For, as transparent and confining as the fiction is, it frequently is the only basis upon which the contact can develop into something more genuinely sociable. In those instances in which the normal fails or refuses to render even so small a gesture toward normalising the situation, there exists almost no basis for the handicapped person to successfully disavow his deviance.[12] The following occurrence related by a young female informant is an apt, if somewhat extreme, illustration:

[11] The blunt questions and stares of small children are typically of the 'Emperor's Clothes' variety. 'Mister, why is your face like that?' 'Lady, what are you riding around in that for? Can't you walk?' Nearly all of my informants tell of how unnerving such incidents were for them, particularly when other adults were present. Nonetheless, some claimed to value the child's forthrightness a good deal more than they did the genteel hypocrisy of many adults.

[12] On the other side of the coin, there are of course some handicapped persons who are equally given to undermining sociable relations by intentionally flaunting the handicap, so that the fiction becomes extremely difficult to sustain. An equivalent of the 'bad nigger' type described by Strong, such persons are (as in Strong's study) regarded with a mixture of admiration and censure by a number of informants. Admiration, because the cruel stripping away of pretences and forcing of issues is thought morally refreshing, especially since, as the informants themselves recognised, many normals refuse to grant anything more than fictional acceptance, while at the same time imagining themselves ennobled for having made the small sacrifice. Censure, because of the conviction that such behaviour can hardly improve matters in the long

> I was visiting my girl friend's house and I was sitting in the lobby, waiting for her, when this woman comes out of her apartment and starts asking me questions. She just walked right up. I didn't know her from Adam, I never saw her before in my life. 'Gee, what do you have? How long have you been that way? Oh gee, that's terrible.' And so I answered her questions, but I got very annoyed and wanted to say, 'Lady, mind your own business.'

'Breaking Through': Facilitating Normalised Role-Taking

In moving beyond fictional acceptance, what takes place essentially is a redefinitional process in which the handicapped person projects images, attitudes and concepts of self which encourage the normal to identify with him (i.e. 'take his role') in terms other than those associated with imputations of deviance (Mead, 1934). Coincidentally, in broadening the area of minor verbal involvements, this also functions to drain away some of the stifling burden of unspoken awareness that, as we have seen, so taxes ease of interaction. The normal is cued into a larger repertoire of appropriate responses, and even when making what he, perhaps mistakenly, regards as an inappropriate response (for example, catching himself in the use of such words as cripple or blind) the handicapped person can, by his response, relieve him of his embarrassment. One young informant insightfully termed the process 'breaking through':

> The first reaction a normal individual or good-legger has is, 'Oh gee, there's a fellow in a wheelchair,' or 'there's a fellow with a brace.' And they don't say, 'Oh gee, there is so-and-so, he's handsome,' or 'he's intelligent,' or 'he's a boor,' or what have you. And then, as the relationship develops, they don't see the handicap. It doesn't exist any more. And that's the point that you, as a handicapped individual, become sensitive to. You know, after talking with someone for a while, when they don't see the handicap any more. That's when you've broken through.

What this process signifies from a social-psychological standpoint is that, as the handicapped person expands the interactional nexus, he

---

run, and would make acceptance even more difficult for other handicapped persons who later come into contact with a normal who has received such treatment. Cf. Strong, Samuel M. July 1946. 'Negro-White Relations as Reflected in Social Types', *American Journal of Sociology*, 52: 24.

simultaneously disavows the deviancy latent in his status; concurrently, to the degree to which the normal is led to reciprocally assume the redefining (and perhaps unanticipated) self-attitudes proffered by the handicapped person, he comes to normalise (i.e. view as more like himself) those aspects of the other which at first connoted deviance for him. (Sometimes, as we shall see, the normal's normalising is so complete that it is unwittingly applied to situations in which the handicapped person cannot possibly function 'normally' due to sheer physical limitations.) These dynamics might also be termed a process of identification. The term is immaterial, except that, in 'identifying' or 'taking the role of the other', much more is implicated sociologically than a mere subjective congruence of responses. The fashioning of shared perspectives also implies a progressively more binding legitimation of the altered self-representations enacted in the encounter; that is, having once normalised his perception of the handicapped person, it becomes increasingly more compromising—self-discrediting, as it were—for the normal to revert to treating him as a deviant again.

The ways in which the visibly handicapped person can go about disavowing deviance are, as we have stated, many and varied. These range from relatively straightforward conversational offerings in which he alludes in passing to his involvement in a normal round of activities, to such forms of indirection as interjecting taboo or privatised references by way of letting the normal know that he does not take offence at the latter's uneasiness, or regard it as a fixed obstacle toward achieving rapport. In the above quote, for example, the informant speaks of 'good-leggers', an in-group term from his rehabilitation hospital days which, along with 'dirty normals', he sometimes uses with new acquaintances 'because it has a humorous connotation … and lots of times it puts people at their ease.'[13]

Still other approaches to disavowing deviance and bridging fictional acceptance include: an especially attentive and sympathetic stance with

[13] Parallel instances can easily be cited from minority-group relations as, for example, when a Jew in conversation with a non-Jew might introduce a Yiddish phrase by way of suggesting that the other's covert identification of him as a Jew need not inhibit the interaction unduly. In some situations, this serves as a subtle means of declaring, 'O.K., I know what's bothering you. Now I've said it, let's forget about it and move on to something else.'

respect to topics introduced by the normal; showing oneself to be a comic, wit or other kind of gifted participant; and, for some, utilising the normalisation potential inherent in being seen in the company of a highly presentable normal companion (Gowman, 1956). These, and others too numerous to mention, are not of course invariably or equally successful in all cases; neither are such resources equally available to all handicapped persons, nor are the handicapped equally adept at exploiting them. As a class of corrective strategies, however, they have the common aim of overcoming the interactional barrier that lies between narrow fictional acceptance and more spontaneous forms of relatedness.

Inextricably tied in with the matter of approach are considerations of setting, activity and social category of participants, certain constellations of which are generally regarded as favourable for successful deviance disavowal and normalisation, while others are thought unfavourable. Again, the ruling contingencies appear to be the extent to which the situation is seen as containing elements in it which: (1) contextually reduce the threat posed by the visible handicap to the rules and assumptions of the particular sociable occasion; and (2) afford the handicapped person opportunities for 'breaking through' beyond fictional acceptance.

The relevance of one or both of these is apparent in the following social situations and settings about which my informants expressed considerable agreement as regards their preferences, aversions and inner reactions. To begin with, mention might again be made of the interactional rule violations frequently experienced at the hands of small children. Many of the informants were quite open in stating that a small child at a social occasion caused them much uneasiness and cramped their style because they were concerned with how, with other adults present, they would handle some barefaced question from the child. Another category of persons with whom many claimed to have difficulty is the elderly. Here the problem was felt to be the tendency of old people to indulge in patronising sympathy, an attitude which peculiarly resists redefinition because of the fulsome virtue it attributes to itself. In another context, several of the informants laid great stress on the importance of maintaining a calm exterior whenever the physical setting unavoidably exposed them to considerable bodily awkwardness. (At the same time, of course, they spoke of the wisdom of avoiding, whenever possible, such occasions altogether.) Their attitude was that to expressively reflect gracelessness and a loss of control would result in further interactional obstacles toward assimilating the handicapped person to a normal status:

> It makes me uncomfortable to watch anyone struggling, so I try to do what I must as inconspicuously as possible. In new situations or in strange places, even though I may be very anxious, I will maintain a deadly calm. For example, if people have to lift the chair and I'm scared that they are going to do it wrong, I remain perfectly calm and am very direct in the instructions I give.

As a final example, there is the unanimity with which the informants expressed a strong preference for the small, as against the large or semi-public social gathering. Not only do they believe that, as one handicapped person among the non-handicapped, they stand out more at large social gatherings, but also that in the anonymity which numbers further there resides a heightened structural tendency for normals to practice avoidance relations with them. The easy assumption on such occasions is that 'some other good soul' will take responsibility for socialising with the handicapped person. Even in the case of the handicapped person who is forward and quite prepared to take the initiative in talking to others, the organisation and ecology of the large social gathering is usually such as to frustrate his attempts to achieve a natural, non-deviant place for himself in the group. As one young man, a paraplegic, explained:

> The large social gathering presents a special problem. It's a matter of repetition. When you're in a very large group of people whom you don't know, you don't have an opportunity of talking to three, four or five at a time. Maybe you'll talk to one or two usually. After you've gone through a whole basic breakdown in making a relationship with one—after all, it's only a cocktail party—to do it again, and again, and again, it's wearing and it's no good. You don't get the opportunity to really develop something.

Institutionalisation of the Normalised Relationship

In 'breaking through', many of the handicapped are confronted by a delicate paradox, particularly in those of their relationships which continue beyond the immediate occasion. Having disavowed deviance and induced the Other to respond to him as he would to a normal, the problem then becomes one of sustaining the normalised definition in the face of the many small amendments and qualifications that must frequently be made to it. The person confined to a wheelchair, for example, must brief a new acquaintance on what to do and how to help when they come to stairs, doorways, vehicle entrances, etc. Further briefings and rehearsals may be required for social obstructions as well: for example, how to act in an encounter with, to cite some typical situations at random, an overly helpful person, a waitress who communicates to the handicapped person only through his companion, a person who stares in morbid fascination (Gowman, 1956).

Generally, such amendments and special considerations are as much as possible underplayed in the early stages of the relationship because, as in the case of much minority-group protest, the fundamental demand of the handicapped is that they first be granted an irreducibly equal and normal status, it being only then regarded as fitting and safe to admit to certain incidental incapacities, limitations and needs. At some point, however, the latter must be broached if the relationship to the normal is to endure in viable form. But to integrate effectively, a major claim to 'normalcy', with numerous minor waivers of the same claim, is a tricky feat, and one which exposes the relationship to the many situational and psychic hazards of apparent duplicity: the tension of transferring the special arrangements and understandings worked out between the two to situations and settings in which everyone else is 'behaving normally'; the sometimes lurking suspicion of the one that it is only guilt or pity that cements the relationship, of the other that the infirmity is being used exploitatively, and of onlookers that there is something 'neurotic' and 'unhealthy' about it all.[14]

From my informants' descriptions, it appears that this third, 'normal, but …' stage of the relationship, if it endures, is institutionalised mainly in either one of two ways. In the first, the normal normalises his perceptions

[14] The rhetoric of race relations reflects almost identical rationalisations and 'insights', which are meant, among other things, to serve as cautions for would-be transgressors. 'Personally, I have nothing against Negroes (the handicapped), but it would be bad for my reputation if I were seen socialising with them.' 'She acts nice now, but with the first argument she will call you a dirty Jew (good-for-nothing cripple).' 'Regardless of how sympathetic you are toward Negroes (the disabled), the way society feels about them, you'd have to be a masochist to marry one.'

to such an extent as to suppress his effective awareness of many of the areas in which the handicapped person's behaviour unavoidably deviates from the normal standard. In this connection, several of the informants complained that a recurring problem they have with close friends is that the latter frequently overlook the fact of the handicap and the restrictions it imposes on them. The friends thoughtlessly make arrangements and involve them in activities in which they, the handicapped, cannot participate conveniently or comfortably.

The other major direction in which the relationship is sometimes institutionalised is for the normal to surrender some of his normalcy by joining the handicapped person in a marginal, half-alienated, half-tolerant, outsider's orientation to 'the Philistine world of normals.'[15] Gowman nicely describes the tenor and style of this relationship, and its possibilities for sharply disabusing normals of their stereotyped approaches to the handicapped. *Épater le bourgeois* (shock the bourgeois) behaviour is often prominently associated with it, as is a certain strictly in-group license to lampoon and mock the handicap in a way which would be regarded as highly offensive were it to come from an uninitiated normal. Thus, a blind girl relates how a sighted friend sometimes chides her by calling her 'a silly blink'. A paraplegic tells of the old friend who tries to revive his flagging spirits by telling him not to act 'like a helpless cripple'. Unlike that based on over-normalisation, the peculiar strength of this relationship is perhaps its very capacity to give expressive scope to the negative reality of the larger world of which it is inescapably a part, while simultaneously removing itself from a primary identification with it.

IMPLICATIONS

Two, more general, implications seem worth drawing from this analysis.[16]

First, in studies which trace the process wherein an actor who deviates comes to be increasingly defined as a deviant (e.g. the pre-mental patient,

[15] Students of race relations will recognise in this a phenomenon closely akin to 'inverse passing', as when a white becomes closely identified with Negroes and passes into a Negro subculture.

[16] I am indebted to Sheldon Messinger for his valuable comments in these connections.

the pre-alcoholic, the pre-juvenile delinquent), unusual prominence is given to the normalising behaviour of those close to him (spouse, parents, friends, etc.). The picture that emerges is one of these persons assuming nearly the whole burden—by rationalising, denying and overlooking his offensive acts—of attempting to re-establish a socially acceptable relationship with him. He is depicted typically as compulsively wedded to his deviance and incapable or uninterested in making restitutive efforts of his own. In the end, following some critical act of his, normalisation fails *in toto*, and community agencies are called in to relieve the primary group of its unmanageable burden.

There is much about this picture that is doubtlessly true and consonant with the ascertainable facts as we later come to learn of them from family, friends, police, courts and social agencies. We may question, however, whether it is a wholly balanced picture, and whether, given the situational biases of these informational sources, all of the relevant facts have had an equal chance to surface. The perspective developed here suggests that it may be useful to consider whether, and to what extent, the deviator himself is not also engaged, albeit ineffectively, in somehow trying to sustain a normal definition of his person. Were research to indicate that such is the case, we might then ask what it is about his reparative efforts and the situations in which they occur that, as contrasted with the subjects of this study, so often lead to failure and an exacerbation of the troublesome behaviour. (We probably will never know, except inferentially by gross extrapolation, of the possibly many cases in which some such interactive process succeeds in favourably resolving the deviating behaviour.) In other words, as against the simplistic model of a compulsive deviant and a futile normaliser, we would propose one in which it is postulated that both are likely to become engaged in making corrective interactional efforts toward healing the breach. And, when such efforts fail, as they frequently do, it is as important in accounting for the failure to weigh the interactional dynamics and situational contexts of these efforts as it is the nature of the deviant acts and the actor.

Second, we would note that the interactional problems of the visibly handicapped are not so dissimilar from those which all of us confront, if only now and then, and to a lesser degree. We too on occasion find ourselves in situations in which some uncamouflageable attribute of ours jars the activity and the expectations of our company. We too, if we wish to sustain—and, as is typically the case, our company wishes us to sustain—a fitting and valued representation of ourselves, will tacitly begin to explore with them ways of redressing, insulating and separating the discrepant attribute from ourselves (Goffman, 1956). Our predicament, though, is much less charged with awareness, more easily set to rights, than that of the visibly handicapped person and his company. But it is precisely this exaggeration of a common interactional predicament that affords us an added insight into the prerequisites and unwitting assumptions of sociable behaviour in general. Put differently, it can be said that our understanding of a mechanism is often crude and incomplete until it breaks down and we try to repair it. Breakdown and repair of interaction is what many of the visibly handicapped experience constantly in their lives. In studying this with them we are also studying much about ourselves of which we were heretofore unaware.

References

Baker, R.G. et al. 1953. *Adjustment to Physical Handicap and Illness: A Survey of the Social Psychology of Physique and Disability*, Bulletin 55, 2nd edn. New York: Social Science Research Council.

Goffman, Erving. 1956. 'Embarrassment and Social Organisation', *American Journal of Sociology*, 62: 246–71.

———. 1957. 'Alienation from Interaction', *Human Relations*, 10: 47–60.

———. 1959. *Presentation of Self in Everyday Life*. New York: Doubleday.

Gowman, Alan G. 1956. 'Blindness and the role of the companion', *Social Problems*, 4.

Hughes, Everett C. 1958. *Men and their Work*. Glencoe: Free Press.

Lemert, Edwin M. 1951. *Social Pathology*. New York: McGraw-Hill

Mead, George H. 1934. *Mind, Self and Society*. Chicago: University of Chicago Press.

Schwarz, Charlotte G. 1957. 'Perspectives on deviance: Wives' definitions of their husbands' mental illness', *Psychiatry*, 20: 275–91.

Strauss, Anselm. 1959. *Mirrors and Masks*. Glencoe: Free Press.

Strong, Samuel M. 1946. 'Negro-white relations as reflected in social types', *American Journal of Sociology*, 52.

White, R.K., Wright, B.A. and Dembo, T. 1948. 'Studies in adjustment to visible injuries', *Journal of Abnormal and Social Psychology*, 43: 13–28.

Wolff, Kurt H. 1950. (ed.) *The Sociology of Georg Simmel*. Glencoe: Free Press.

Wright, Beatrice A. 1960. *Physical Disability: A Psychological Approach*. New York: Harper.

11

Adaptation to Deafness in a Balinese Community

John T. Hinnant

Communities have recently come to light in various parts of the world in which a fairly substantial deaf population has become integrated into the life of a larger populace. One of the most successful such adaptations occurred on Martha's Vineyard, Massachusetts, in the nineteenth century (Groce, 1985). According to the memory of the oldest living inhabitants, a sign language known both to the deaf and the hearing citizens of the island enabled them to interact with apparent ease. Another such community is Providence Island, Colombia (Washtabaugh, 1980). In this case, also, the presence of a mutually intelligible sign language allowed a degree of interaction between deaf and hearing people. There are additional communities in Latin America, Africa, Nepal and elsewhere in which a local sign language made possible both an interactive deaf community and adaptation to hearing people. Because communities in which successful accommodations to hearing loss are rare, each of these situations allows a special opportunity to understand the means by which hearing and deaf people can live together successfully.

Hinnant, John T. 2000. 'Adaptation to deafness in a Balinese community', in John T. Hinnant, I. Berlin and B. Keats (eds), *Genetics and Hearing Loss.* Dalmar Learning, a part of Cengage Learning Inc., pp. 111–23.

Bengkala, Bali, is another example of a successful accommodation of a deaf population to a community that has developed a unique sign language shared by deaf and hearing residents.

THE VILLAGE OF BENGKALA, BALI

The village of Bengkala is located in the hill country of North Bali. As Friedman has noted, *prasasti* (metal plates inscribed with proclamations from local kings, written in ancient Balinese script) associated with Bengkala are dated 1178 A.D. They promulgate a legal code and set the geographical boundaries for a community that was apparently already flourishing and very much in need of regulation by the king of that time. Quite likely, the village antedates the arrival of the Hindu religion on Bali.

Bengkala is a poor village. Because of its altitude, easily accessible ground water is not available for the ubiquitous Balinese wet rice farming. Irrigation water, from Bali's famous Subak aqueduct system (Lansing, 1991), is only available for part of the village. Consequently, a variety of crops, centring on fruit production, are used to partially replace the vital rice crop as a source of food and income.

THE DEAF POPULATION OF BENGKALA

It is not possible to know exactly when the first deaf person was born in the village. Balinese Hindu ancestral beliefs cause a kind of genealogical amnesia (Geertz and Geertz, 1975). Two generations after a person has died, all memory of his name is lost. This makes good sense. In Balinese Hindu belief, each individual is reincarnated, and so a family's ancestors are now its children. There is no need to remember the ancestral names of individuals who are reincarnated. Not surprisingly, the first deaf person whose name appears on our genealogical charts has only been dead for two generations. Even if this person is not the first deaf individual, it is clear that there has been a steady increase, generation by generation, in the number of deaf people in the village. We have identified a total of 62 deaf individuals in the history of Bengkala, of whom 48 are still living. In families where deaf people have married deaf people, there are up to four generations of living deaf individuals present.

DEAF SOCIAL INTEGRATION IN BENGKALA

An understanding of the reasons Bengkala is one of the very few communities worldwide in which deaf people are well integrated into the social life of a community requires an excursion into the nature of Balinese Hindu society and into the organisation of this particular village. Balinese villages are kin-based. Groups of patrilineally related kinsmen live in residential clusters, or house yards (Geertz and Geertz, 1975). In Bengkala, the deaf people live interspersed among their hearing relatives in several of the house yards. Consequently, the deaf grow up among a large number of hearing relatives. Small hearing and deaf children learn the unique sign language of the village together. Hearing children who grow up in this environment seem to learn sign language before they learn to speak. Signing is both part of communications and part of play. For the deaf children, exposure to the sign language occurs at birth. There is no part of their development in which they are deprived of the potential for symbolic communication. The crucial communicative contact between baby and mother is insured. Wherever a deaf baby looks, there is signing.

LIFE CYCLE AND SOCIAL IDENTITY

In discussing the lives of deaf people, it is perhaps best to start at the point which is, for us, the beginning—the birth of the baby. However, in the Balinese Hindu religion, birth is merely one moment in a chain of births, deaths and rebirths. Since babies are considered to be reincarnations of their ancestors, they are therefore sacred. For the first six months of their lives, their feet may not touch the profane earth. They must be carried everywhere by adults.

Reincarnation and Social Identity

When the baby is one month old, its father must go to a trance medium (*balian*) who contacts the ancestral realm to find out its former identity. Usually, the baby is identified as the reincarnation of one of its grandparents, or of a dead relative from the grandparents' generation. On a few occasions, the trip to the trance medium can have genetic consequences. If, later in life, this baby-grown-to-adulthood has chronic misfortune, another trance medium may decide that the first medium was wrong. Instead of being the child of a particular family and the reincarnation of a particular ancestor, the individual in fact turns out to belong to an entirely different kin group. To remedy this situation, the individual must go through an identity change ritual, which involves a *wayang kulit* (leather puppet) performance.

In Balinese conception, our world is a place of little importance. The realm of gods, temple spirits and ancestors is the real world, which can only be seen through the screen of the puppet performance (Lansing, 1983). The puppets impersonate divinities, and during the performances they re-enact the lives of the gods portrayed in the great Hindu sagas, the Mahabharata and Ramayana. The puppet master, the *dalang*, is a man of enormous power, for it is he who mediates between this world and the world of the gods by controlling the actions of the puppets and speaking with all of their voices. During the puppet performance, through a particular puppet, the dalang will indicate the new name and kinship affiliation of the distressed individual.

I have enough faith in western empiricism to believe that the genetic material of the individual belongs to the first, culturally mistaken identity. During the process of preparing a comprehensive genealogy of Bengkala, I came across cases of individuals and their descendants being shifted entirely away from their biological parentage, and placed in the genealogies of other clans. For purposes of genetic analysis, we relocated them in their original kin groups. This instance is an example of the generally slippery nature of kinship systems, which are actually culturally determined and therefore variable. It also illustrates the fluid nature of personal identity in Bali.

The First Years of Life and Deafness

The general pattern of Balinese social maturation also applies to the deaf people. For six months, they are considered to be divinities whose feet must never touch the earth. Occasionally, during this six-month period of very intense interaction with adults, it becomes apparent that a baby cannot hear. The infant is then subjected to sharp noises to see if it reacts. If the baby's parents are deaf, there is already the general expectation that the child will be deaf. Only in cases of hearing parents giving birth to deaf children is there any surprise.

There have been a number of situations in which a deaf baby is born to hearing parents who are heterozygotes for the recessive gene causing deafness in this community. The deaf members of the community, once they learn of such a child, visit and ensure that it learns to sign. Usually, the parents are already familiar with sign language and are able to teach the baby. However, in 1998, a deaf baby was born to hearing parents who did not know the sign language. They were put in the awkward position of having to learn to sign as adults.

Maturation, Voluntary Groups and Deaf Social Networks

As deaf children mature, they will join organisations that are peculiar to Balinese society. These organisations are called *sekeha*, and are voluntary groups that form around certain activities. When the activities are completed, the sekeha disband. There are sekeha for planting and harvesting rice. There are sekeha for a range of other agricultural tasks. There are even sekeha for making music and drinking palm wine. The financial goal of the sekeha in Bengkala is to save money to buy pigs for pork distribution at the festival of Galungan every six Balinese months. Additionally, for the deaf, the sekeha provide the opportunity to interact with hearing people in work situations that are not necessarily kinship-based.

Deaf Exclusion from Age Grades and the Adat System

There is one area of the life of the village, a form of age-grade organisation, in which deaf people do not participate. The first grade, called *teruna/teruni* (for male/female members), begins when boys and girls are around the age of puberty. The young teruna/teruni form one of the most active groups in the village. They must always be present at temple ceremonies, and must carry out most of the work of preparing the Hindu temples for rituals. They also prepare secular celebrations. This organisation is obviously an important means of socialising young adults.

The promotion out of this age grade occurs at marriage. Young men, who, through marriage, have recently become heads of households, join the *Desa Adat*. This is the council of household heads of the village. In

Balinese villages, there are two systems of law. One is the traditional or Adat system and the other is the Indonesian legal system. Members of the Desa Adat regularly meet to discuss village issues, particularly issues concerning religious practice and the maintenance of the village's temples. Members of the Adat must contribute food and labour to major ceremonies, and they receive a special and highly prized ritual food called *lawar* in return.

Deaf children do not join the teruna/teruni system, and young deaf men do not join the Desa Adat at marriage. Issues that the deaf people wish to present at Adat meetings are voiced by a hearing member on their behalf; decisions reached by the Adat are signed to the deaf people after the meetings. Also, while the deaf do not contribute ingredients for the making of the all-important lawar at temple festivals, they do receive the same portion of the prepared ritual food as do members of the Adat.

Marriage

Throughout the fieldwork, issues centring on marriage, divorce and domestic relations were the dominant topics of discourse. The deaf people marry at a fairly early age, even though finding a spouse is a difficult problem. Generally, deaf people marry one another, although there have been some deaf-hearing marriages. Several of the deaf have had a succession of spouses, both hearing and deaf. Recently, some of the deaf people have begun to marry deaf people from other villages in hopes that children produced by these inter-village unions may not be deaf. Reciprocally, deaf men from other villages in the vicinity (in which there are very few deaf people) have begun visiting Bengkala in hopes of finding a wife.

Adult Life and Subsistence

The deaf people are farmers like the rest of the village community, and they inherit and use land like anyone else in the community. At present, many of the men are also employed as day labourers in the village and in other communities. Several of the women are seamstresses. According to oral history collected from the deaf and hearing members of the community, employment opportunities for the deaf have greatly improved in recent times. In the past, there was little wage labour, and what there was centred on water. As mentioned earlier, the village, with its high altitude, has a chronic water shortage. Deaf men received money (although very little) from village households for carrying water in buckets from the river, which is located in a deep ravine at the edge of the village.

Today, there are two systems of piped-in water. The head of the village has continued the historical association between water and deaf people by placing them in charge of all of the water systems of the village. This involves continual effort and interaction with hearing people to keep the water pipes mended and operating. Deaf people are also in charge of water for temple ceremonies and festivals.

RELIGIOUS PARTICIPATION

There is an additional, all-embracing dimension of Balinese culture: its unique form of the Hindu religion. It is with good reason that Margaret Mead, in the 1940s, wrote of the 'the incredible busyness of the Balinese Hindus' (Bateson and Mead, 1942). On the village level, the Hinduism of Bali is a matter of continual ritual performance. Triggered by significant days in the island's ritual calendar, the more than 20,000 temples of Bali take turns in a continual cycle of elaborate celebration. Much of the effort of ritual preparation falls to women. Offerings, called *banten*, are constructed by women from flowers, banana and palm leaves, fruit, and cooked meat. Men are also involved in preparing *babi guling* (roast suckling pig) and other ritual essentials. Performances involve both sexes. Formal temple ceremonies require the recitation of mantras, which the deaf people do not know; however, they participate in the rest of the temple ceremonies. Women, particularly, are able to perform as well as their hearing friends in the preparation of ritual offerings.

There is a widespread belief in Bali that there are individuals capable of practicing magic, both good and bad. Other individuals, called *leyak*, are thought to be capable of transforming themselves at night into animals, travelling to people's homes, and mystically consuming their bodies over a course of many visits. In addition, there is a belief in *hantus*, the unquiet ghosts of those who have not been properly cremated. The deaf people are especially aware of this realm of beliefs. I have sat with them many evenings, watching individuals sign stories of leyaks that they have seen and other extranormal events they claim to have witnessed. The evil doers are always hearing. This realm of belief seems to be more immediately real for the deaf people than are the mantra-based temple ceremonies.

SIGN LANGUAGE AND DEAFNESS

Indonesia has an official sign language, which is taught in schools for the deaf but is not understood by the citizens of Bengkala. Bengkala sign language developed in the context of this one village and reflects the life of the village. It would be extremely difficult for an outsider to understand the language without having lived in the village with the deaf people.

Although there are many specific signs that can be applied in different contexts, much of the signing involves a complex narration of events (and gossip) using signs created specifically to communicate those events. The narration not only indicates what happens, but by the use of facial expressions and by body language the whole feeling and tone of the event are conveyed in ways more complete than mere speech allows. This narrational quality of the sign language poses a problem for a researcher from outside the village. By the end of each research trip, I have caught up on the narration of events and can usually understand what is being discussed. However, at the beginning of each new research trip, it becomes necessary to learn what has been happening lately and how it is represented in sign narration.

Bengkala sign language has developed independently of writing. In Bali, there are many written languages: Indonesian, three Balinese languages, three Javanese languages, and Sanskrit. However, like many of the older hearing citizens of the village, the deaf people cannot read. Consequently, there is no finger spelling of unfamiliar terms. Also, the deaf do not know the names assigned them by their hearing relatives. Instead, they have an alternate system for identifying one another and their hearing compatriots. They use name signs. The unofficial leader of the deaf community has the privilege of assigning a name sign to each individual, deaf and hearing. The name signs are based either on some distinctive physical trait (a scar, a big nose in my case, and so on) or some aspect of character. These signs are not necessarily flattering or permanent. When some new and appealing aspect of an individual occurs to the deaf leader, he creates a new name sign and puts it into circulation.

Hearing loss is congenital. There is no evidence that the deaf people have ever heard sound. Tests, using a portable audiometer, were conducted with all of the deaf people. There was no evidence from the tests that anyone of any age was able to hear. The deaf, therefore, have no direct contact with spoken language. Their only contact with speech is possibly an indirect one. While the history of the development of the Bengkala sign language is not known, it seems reasonable to assume that hearing people were involved in its development. A question for future analysis is whether the grammatical structure of the sign language has parallels with the structure of spoken Balinese. My best guess at this point is that the sign language, like languages in general, has developed its own unique grammatical structure.

Although the sign language centres on the use of hands, facial expressions and body language, the deaf people are not silent when communicating. For example, an intensifier used to give emphasis involves making a popping sound with the lips. There are also sounds intended to attract the attention of hearing people. Each deaf person has his or her own distinctive attention-getting sound. Also, some deaf individuals emphasise their general signing with a variety of vocalisations, especially during emotionally charged situations.

Although they are unable to hear in the usual sense, it is apparent that the deaf people are extremely sensitive to vibration. This first came to my attention when I was showing them a videotape I had made of them. At the same time, I was rewinding another videotape with a rather noisy rewinding machine. One of the deaf men turned around, puzzled, and seemed to be seeking the source of the sound. I showed him and then asked how he knew about it. He indicated that he felt it in his body. This sensitivity to vibration is particularly important for the involvement of some of the deaf people in a dance performance group.

MARTIAL ARTS AND DANCE

In the 1960s, two hearing men began independently teaching performance skills to a group of deaf men. The first of these hearing men was a gymnast and martial-arts practitioner. Over a lengthy period of time, he taught the complex and difficult sport called *pencak silat* to eight of the deaf men. They, in turn, instructed virtually the entire deaf community. Today, even very small deaf children practice the sport.

The second hearing individual began the process of teaching classical Balinese dance to the same deaf men. In Bali, dance is a vital part of worship. It is believed that the Balinese gods periodically descend on each of the temples of Bali in turn, expecting to be entertained with beautiful clothing, complex offerings, gamelan music, and dance. In any Balinese village, most people, male and female alike, have had some experience attempting classical Balinese dance. The instructor for the deaf dance group used a drum, rather than the usual gamelan orchestra, to provide the musical accompaniment for the dance. The deaf performers received their cues from the base vibration of the drum and the movement of the instructor's hands while drumming. Also, unknown to the audience at performances, the instructor signed instructions to the deaf performers between beats.

History of the Deaf Performance Group

The new-found skills in both silat and dance were put to use when the eight deaf men formed a performance company under the direction of their hearing dance teacher. In the 1960s, this troupe travelled from village to village, putting on performances before police groups (emphasising silat combat) and in village settings (emphasising dance performance). The troupe was well known. People from other villages have told me that they remember, as children, seeing the dancers from Bengkala perform. After being active for several years, the dance troupe disbanded because the hearing director and teacher became involved with commercial activities that demanded all of his time. The troupe was revived in the mid-1990s, after the governor of Bali became interested in the deaf people. He assigned a professional dance teacher to prepare the troupe for public performances. While the original teacher had emphasised classical Balinese dance, the new instructor began lessons in dances of his own invention. He was apparently of the opinion that deafness is a great tragedy and that the deaf people are indeed sad. Several of his dances have them lamenting their deafness. He also taught them to perform using vocalisations. There are Balinese dances in which vocalisations are used, but they are rare. Under this new teacher, a somewhat macabre form of dance has recently emerged.

Both silat and dance skills have given the members of the deaf community a new series of options. Silat is used not only for personal defence and occasional performance, but also is the basis for membership by many of' the deaf men and teenagers in the village guard or *hancip*. Each evening, the hancip members, both hearing and deaf, gather and prepare to spend the evening sitting in the administrative offices at the centre of the village. Occasionally, they go out on patrol, but most of the time is spent exchanging stories and gossip. Sign language is used throughout, because almost always several of the deaf people participate in the rotating membership of the village guard. This interaction provides yet another situation for close communication between deaf and hearing people.

The Contemporary Importance of Performance

The combined silat and dance performances by the deaf people have put Bengkala on the media map. The deaf group has performed for both Balinese and national Indonesian television groups. Newspaper reporters have come to the village and have written about the deaf people. The deaf can see themselves occasionally performing on television. There is a plan for the deaf troupe to perform at the great Festival of Bali, which is held each summer for an international audience. All of this has created a real sense of accomplishment and recognition among the deaf community of Bengkala.

The finely honed skills required by silat and dance performance amply demonstrate that there do not seem to be significant vestibular problems in this deaf community in terms of body control. In some forms of deafness, individuals experience dizziness and other problems when attempting to carry out activities requiring a refined sense of balance. However, when a number of deaf and hearing people in Bengkala were specifically tested by asking them to close their eyes and walk in a straight line, the subjective state of several deaf individuals belied their obvious ability. They reported seeing stars behind their eyelids, dizziness, and a kind of drunken feeling. Many of the deaf people did not react in this manner, and none of the hearing people did so, including the hearing parents (obligate heterozygotes) of deaf individuals.

ATTITUDES ABOUT DEAFNESS

The word *kolok* is used to refer to the deaf. It refers to inability to speak, more than inability to hear. It is a somewhat derogatory word, implying a lack of mental ability. It is generally used by people in the village who have little contact with the deaf people and little or no ability to sign. The kin, affines and neighbours of deaf people generally refer to them by name or relationship, just as they would to anyone else in the community. They attach no stigma to deafness.

When asked about their own attitudes toward deafness, the deaf indicated that they want to hear. They believe their deafness limits their employment options. Several people, especially the teenagers, signed their suspicion that hearing people laugh at them. Also, in a culture where music of many types fills the air, several of the deaf men and boys have lamented their inability to hear it. There is one exception. One young boy signed that he likes being deaf because it makes him special. Given the attention the deaf people have received from the governor of Bali, the Indonesian media, and various visiting geneticists and anthropologists, his observation is reasonable. He intends to marry a deaf woman someday, and wants to have deaf children. In 1998, he found an Indonesian sponsor who has taken him to Denpasar, the capital, where he has begun attending a school for the deaf.

DO THE DEAF HAVE A SEPARATE DEAF CULTURE?

One issue that should be discussed is whether there is a deaf community with a capital 'D' having its own distinctive culture in Bengkala. The evidence is somewhat mixed. On several occasions, deaf people have told me how happy they are to leave behind the hearing members of the village, go out into the gardens, and simply be with one another. There they can sign much more quickly and do not have to worry about explaining the context of their signs to hearing people. There are many gatherings in the gardens for the purpose of feasting, drinking palm wine, sports, and just gossiping about the hearing people. The deaf move about the village in one another's company, and generally know more about one another's activities than they know about the activities of hearing people.

On the other hand, several of the deaf people, particularly women, do not participate in activities with the deaf community. They live at home and seldom appear with other deaf people. Also, when the deaf community throws a party in the gardens, inevitably a few of the particularly able signers among their hearing relatives are invited. Balinese people, hearing and deaf, are profoundly social. Connections among people based on kinship and marriage, along with membership in sekeha groups, temple groups and so on, make it very difficult for any exclusive organisation to exist among either the hearing or the deaf. The deaf people are immersed in the same complex social and cultural world as the hearing. They do not seem to have invented a distinct Deaf Culture that can be differentiated from that of the hearing. However, they have highly distinctive interests and experiences by virtue of deafness itself.

One thing is certain. Communication between the deaf and many hearing members of the community is continuous. There is a saying by the hearing community that the deaf people have no secrets. Since they communicate by signing and are forever signing with their hearing relatives and friends, events in their lives are widely known. Reciprocally, they care about the hearing people, and are extraordinarily keen observers of their behaviour and their foibles.

ONGOING RESEARCH

Since interdisciplinary research on deaf communities is a relatively new endeavour, it is perhaps useful to mention the types of social data that have been collected. To facilitate the genetic research, a comprehensive genealogy, of the entire village of 2,285 living individuals and more than 800 dead people, was constructed. At the same time, a database was created with a record for each individual appearing in the genealogy. Using this information, we were able to connect 12 of the 13 kindreds, originally collected by the two Indonesian physicians who discovered the village, into one comprehensive picture of the deaf families. The construction of accurate genealogies is probably the most useful thing an anthropologist can do for human genetic research. Because systems of kinship and marriage often have unpleasant surprises built into them as far as genetic research is concerned, it is also the job of the anthropologist to acquire a broad understanding of the culture and its impact on kinship and marriage.

In terms of the broader cultural and linguistic aspects of the research, I have so far spent almost two years living in the village with the deaf people, participating in events, and watching what they do on a daily basis. This technique is called 'participant observation' by anthropologists. It seems like no technique at all, but it is probably the most important one we have. In addition to daily observation, specific inquiries were made concerning the traditional history of the village and beliefs about the origin of its citizens. Medical beliefs were examined with a special emphasis on understanding the nature of deafness. The general economic and political life of the village was studied in order to evaluate the role of the deaf people. Extensive autobiographies of almost all of the deaf people were videotaped, and then laboriously translated from sign. Biographies of the deaf people were collected from many of their hearing neighbours and relatives. Nearly 100 hours of videotape and thousands of photographs (many taken by the deaf people themselves) were collected, and will serve as one basis for further analysis of the language and social contexts of the deaf. And, of course, observation of the continual performance of Balinese Hindu rituals, and of those who participate in them, has been a backdrop for all other activities in the village.

CONCLUSION

A full account of the language and lives of the deaf people of Bengkala must await a book-length presentation, which is currently in preparation. As additional communities such as Bengkala are studied in detail, a clearer picture of the factors that differentiate between successful and unsuccessful social adaptations to profound deafness should emerge. Evidence from communities already studied suggests that a sign language known by deaf and hearing alike is vital. Social means for integrating deaf people into the larger community are also essential. In Bengkala, co-residence in kin-based house yards, obligations among kinsmen and affines, *sekeha* voluntary-organisation membership, civic responsibilities for water system maintenance and village guard duties, along with the endless cycle of religious events provide ample social integration of the deaf into the larger community.

References

Bateson, G. and Mead, M. 1942. *Balinese Character, a Photographic Analysis*. New York: The New York Academy of Sciences.

Geertz, H. and Geertz, C. 1975. *Kinship in Bali*. Chicago: University of Chicago Press.

Groce, N.E. 1985. *Everyone Here Spoke Sign Language: Hereditary Deafness on Martha's Vineyard*. Cambridge: Harvard University Press.

Lansing, J.S. 1983. *The Three Worlds of Bali*. New York: Praeger.

———. 1991. *Priests and Programmers: Technologies of Power in the Engineered Landscape of Bali*. Princeton: Princeton University Press.

Washtabaugh, W. 1980. 'The organisation and use of Providence Island sign language', in W.C. Stokoe (ed.), *Sign Language Structure*. Silver Spring: Linstok Press.

12

Societal Responses to Women with Disabilities in India

Meenu Bhambani

A brief review of feminist literature reveals that women's studies in the beginning of the twenty-first century have reached a paradigmatic stage. The global issues pertaining to women have been pursued from political, social, cultural, economic, developmental, ecological and psychological perspectives. But the issues pertaining to women with disabilities have not even been approached, and to even think of paradigms in the context of disabled women is a very distant dream.

It would be a cliché to state that women form the 'marginal component' of society. We suggest that, within this component, there is a subgroup of disabled women which is even more marginalised. What is ironical in the case of this group is that it is virtually ignored, not only by their own able-bodied gender but also by disabled men.

Despite their significant numbers, women and girls with disabilities, especially in the developed countries of the ESCAP region, remain hidden and silent, their concerns unknown and their rights overlooked. Throughout the region, in urban and rural communities alike, they have to face triple discrimination because of their disabilities, gender

Bhambani, Meenu. 2003. 'Societal responses to women with disabilities in India', in Asha Hans and Annie Patri (eds), *Women, Disability and Identity*. New Delhi: Sage Publications.

and economic status. Prejudice prevails even within each of the three categories. Among women, disabled women are seen as inferior, resulting in isolation and marginalisation. They become the poorest of the poor (Mohit, 1996, p. 25). A glaring example of their marginalisation and neglect is that to date there is no reliable data available with regard to the number of disabled women. This is more so in the case of disabled women in the developing countries.

Nisar Ahmed Ganai suggests that one of the causes of female infanticide is deprivation of a malformed or deformed baby from her basic right to life. Even if she is born and survives this attempt on her life, she becomes a victim of passive abuse. Lack of care and affection can result in maternal rejection syndrome or deprivational dwarfism (Ganai, 1994, p. 259).

Undoubtedly, several problems concerning girls and women, both with and without disabilities, are common. Despite an increasing literacy rate, the overall female- male sex ratio has declined. As per NSSO survey reports of 1991, the national sex ratio of females is 86 per 100 males. In some states like Rajasthan, it is 60 women per 100 men. In India, the dropout rate from schools is higher for girls (42.4 per cent) than for boys, which stands at 35.4 per cent. Thus, we find that women are usually at the receiving end of our society. They are left out of all decision-making processes, and their performance is based on three pillars: low status, low pay and low skills. This has resulted in the 'non-status of women's work' (Patel, 1995, p. 49).

It has often been pointed out that being a woman means being poorer than a man. For example, the Human Development Report reveals that 'poverty has a decided gender bias.' In a similar vein, the Report of the South Commission explains that 'women suffer disproportionately from poverty, illiteracy and malnutrition.' The question is: proportionately with whom? The assumption is that the comparison is made with men (Patel, 1995, p. 62).

In the myriad statistics and reports, concerns regarding women with disabilities have often been ignored or they have received scant attention. Women with disabilities are more vulnerable to neglect, and physical, sexual and mental abuse. The media, women and organisations working for disabled persons are also indifferent to the discrimination faced by them. The issues concerning women with disabilities, thus, have to be seen in the larger and total context of society, 'where large sections of the population—male and female, adults and children—suffer under the oppression of an exploitative system' (Mitra, 1997). It becomes imperative to probe the concerns, problems and discrimination faced by women with disabilities from economic, social, cultural, political and psychological perspectives.

Women all over the world, in general, are victims of a discriminatory system. Why among them are *women with disabilities* conspicuously missing? What relegates them to the periphery? In the Indian context, what societal, cultural and historical factors are responsible for their invisibility, reticence and chronic neglect?

To begin with, disabled women do not have any history. They have not set any precedents, which some disabled men have, although like men they too have been projected in a very negative light. In Indian mythology as well as history, disabled people have been depicted as cruel and spiteful. One disabled woman in Indian mythology is Manthara, a one-eyed, orthopaedically impaired maidservant of Queen Kaikeyi in the Ramayana, who was responsible for the exile of Lord Rama. Another is Kubja, a hunchback *gopi* (cowherd) in Braj, whom Lord Krishna addressed as 'sundari', meaning a beautiful woman. Lord Krishna saw the inner beauty of Kubja, but the other gopis teased him for liking an impaired woman who appeared ugly owing to her disfigurement. There are other similar stories where women with disabilities are neglected by the gods. According to a *katha* (story) recited during the festival of *Kartik Poornima*, Goddess Lakshmi had an elder sister who could not marry because she was dark and disfigured. When Lord Vishnu proposed to Lakshmi, she expressed her inability to marry as her elder sister was still unmarried, and instead urged him to marry her sister. Lord Vishnu refused, saying there was no place for disabled people in heaven. However, he married off her sister to a *peepul* tree, which he said was another form of Vishnu.

Disabled men, on the other hand, have prominent positions in mythology. Examples are the visually impaired Dhritarashtra and the orthopaedically impaired Shakuni, both of whom sided with evil in the Mahabharata war. However, when we enter the realm of history, we find that disabled rulers are very few and far between. Taimur-e-Lang (1336–1405), also known as Tamerlane, a Mongol ruler who attacked northern India in 1398, is a rare instance. Taimur derived his name, Lang, from a malformed foot that made him walk with a limp. Though a powerful ruler, he is depicted as a brutal ruler. Such negative images have had a deep influence on the psyche of many Indians, who till today perceive disabled people either as objects of pity or as evil personified.

In a patriarchal society, there are different yardsticks for perceiving and judging disabled men and women, and the treatment meted out to them is definitely discriminatory. Women are often perceived as objects of beauty who bestow services to their husbands and families. Their contributions are seldom calculated in numerical terms. Their role as producers are overlooked and they are considered a burden on the family. It is this perception of non-disabled women as beautiful objects, delivering services free of cost, which interferes with the development of disabled women. The globalisation of the economy has also played a major role in strengthening patriarchy, as it has brought women to centre-stage of the sex market. A testimony to this fact is the increase in the number of beauty pageants held even in remote, small towns in India, a process that has aggravated the marginalisation of disabled women, as they are considered neither physically beautiful nor sexually marketable. In fact, they are considered asexual. Their disability makes them lose the quality of 'looked-at-ness', and also renders them inefficient, incapable, unwanted and undesirable.

Society's response towards disabled women is of utter neglect and the demanding of total submission. One can find this negative attitude in the media, which, however, acts not only as a mirror of society but also as a catalyst of change, bringing in new ideas, values and modes of perception. In a country like India, where 50 per cent of the population is illiterate, it is the visual media, especially cinema, which makes a powerful and lasting impact on the people. Indian film actors and actresses are not only matinee idols but also icons and role models who are imitated and emulated by the masses. In the movies, disabled people are often portrayed as dependent on society. Usually confined indoors, they pity themselves and cry for escape from their dysfunctional physical state. Popular Indian cinema (often called Bollywood) has always been inspired by Hollywood, and as Madeleine Cahill and Martin Norden have observed, like their American counterparts, Indian films reflect the discomfort of society in the company of the disabled.

In Indian films, one can see the difference in the construction of images of disabled men and women. Let us first observe the similarities.

In both genders, the disability is rarely congenital. It is always acquired later, making it easier for the masses to accept it. Usually, the disability is cured in the climax, which brings the disabled back into the mainstream of society. Both men and women lead dependent lives, without anyone to interact with except their immediate kin. They more or less belong to the upper strata of society, blessed with facilities—medical, financial, educational—which help them get integrated into society.

As in Hollywood, in Indian films, too, images of disabled men are more prevalent. In spite of their disability, which might interfere with their male ego, they are loved and cared for by non-disabled women. But the reverse image, of women with disabilities, is rare. Women are objects of beauty, gazed at and desired by mainstream males. This obsession with femininity makes the film-makers bestow them with impairments which do not interfere with their attractiveness. Those disabled women who have severe impairments are always placed in character roles such as mother or sister, and never in the lead role of the protagonist.

A brief analysis of some of the images of disabled women in Bollywood films, in contrast to those of men with disability, may be a proof of the way society responds to them. There are hardly any images worth analysing in the 1950s, as the disabled had only marginal roles then. They are portrayed as beggars or given other roles which were totally inconsequential to the main subject of the film. These films, however, abounded in images of blind mothers who were poor, miserable and were looked after by their only sons. Disability was simply unacceptable, and this made the disabled themselves negate their existence. For example, the 1958 film *Hum Dono* had Dev Anand starring in a double role. In one of the roles he is portrayed as a disabled war veteran, a situation so unacceptable to him that he asks his own look-alike to present himself as his wife's husband.

In the 1960s, there was *Aarzoo*, which had Rajendra Kumar in the lead opposite Sadhna. When he loses one of his legs in an accident, he tries to avoid the female protagonist, as he believes his disability would make her life miserable. She, however, continues to love him and, in order to convince him of her love, attempts to get one of her legs amputated. Such a sacrifice demanded from a non-disabled woman for a disabled man is never inverted. If a woman becomes disabled, she is left lamenting her plight all by herself.

The 1970s were a transitional period, and one finds quite a few physically impaired women in lead roles in Bollywood films. However, severe impairments were still the speciality of character actresses. Thus, we find Farida Jalal as the wheelchair-bound sister of Amitabh Bachchan in *Majboor*, and lower-limb paralysed Naaz as Rajesh Khanna's sister in *Sachcha Jhoota*. They are, no doubt, loved by their family members, but no effort is made to help them become self-sufficient. Their brothers try desperately, but in vain, to look for a suitable match who would accept them with their disabilities, and thus assume their burden too.

There were four more films depicting disabled women in the same decade: *Kinara*, which had Hema Malini in the role of a visually impaired dancer; *Man ki Aankhen*, which had Moushumi Chatterjee as a visually impaired orphan girl; *Koshish*, a sincere and honest effort by writer-director Gulzar, in which Jaya Bhaduri and Sanjeev Kumar played the role of a deaf-mute couple; and *Imtihaan*, in which Tanuja played the part of a locomotor-disabled woman. In *Kinara* and *Man ki Aankhen*, one finds the lead disabled women extremely charming, beautiful and bestowed with unusual artistic gifts. They are loved by Jitendra and Vinod Mehra, the male protagonists of these two films, for reasons other than their disability. Hema Malini is shown acquiring visual impairment as the result of an accident that was partially a responsibility of the male protagonist. For the first time, a mainstream commercial film like *Imtihaan* showed a disability in its female protagonist which interfered with her ability to be admired and therefore made her undesirable. In the film, Tanuja walks with a slight limp, although, once again, she is beauty personified. Vinod, the protagonist, pities her for her disability and loves her for her good and noble nature. A disabled woman, thus, cannot be average, moderate, independent or an underachiever. She must always be good to look at; else she will find no place in mainstream cinema.

Koshish was a pioneering, sensitive and true-to-life portrayal of a speech- and hearing-impaired couple leading normal lives, depicting their struggles, desires and interactions with non-disabled people. The film is a deviation from the run-of-the mill stuff of commercial cinema. However, here too a disabled father is shown imposing his will upon his non-disabled son, whom he forces to marry a girl with hearing and speech impairment, implying that disability is acceptable only by the disabled, and that the disabled do not have any place in the world of the non-disabled. In spite of having close encounters with the disabled in their immediate family, the non-disabled refuse to develop any empathy towards them.

In the 1980s, there were two remarkable films on disability, *Naache Mayuri* and *Sparsh*, one a commercial venture and the other considered a part of parallel cinema. *Naache Mayuri* was based on the real-life story of Bharatanatyam dancer Sudha Chandran who, despite losing one leg in an accident, achieved the heights of glory in her chosen field of classical dance with the help of an artificial limb, thanks to her grit and passion. Sudha Chandran played herself in the film. *Sparsh*, on the other hand, has Nasiruddin Shah playing a visually impaired principal of a school for the blind. He is fiercely independent, highly educated and despises any display of pity. Shabana Azmi plays a non-disabled teacher working in the same school who loves him. The two films suggest a contradiction in the projections of male and female disability in mainstream and parallel cinema, and cue the viewer as to what is expected of women in society. A woman without disability accepts disabled men without any qualms, but non-disabled men hardly have any compunction in rejecting women with impairments. The former aspect is exemplified in films from the 1990s, which have disabled men in abundance but disabled women rarely. Examples are: *Saajan*, in which Sanjay Dutt is a polio-affected man who is loved by Madhuri Dixit; *Chandni*, in which Rishi Kapoor suffers from spinal-cord injury but is finally cured; and *Dushman*, which portrays Sanjay Dutt as a visually impaired man. They are all desired in spite of their disability, whether congenital or acquired at some later stage in life.

The 1990s had two other films on disability. Both had a commercially viable cast of stars, yet both failed to draw in the crowds, and the experiment of bringing the disabled to centre-stage ended badly. *Khamoshi* is a sensitive portrayal of a deaf-mute couple played by Nana Patekar and Seema Biswas. They are shown languishing in their own silent world and as misfits in the world of hearing people. Their only contact with the outside world is through their non-disabled daughter, Anne, played by Manisha Koirala. As in *Koshish*, they are shown imposing their will upon their daughter and creating obstacles in the fulfilment of her dreams and ambitions.

Mann is a love story revolving around Dev and Priya, played by Aamir Khan and Manisha Koirala. Priya meets with an accident and loses both of her lower limbs. Like the 1960s film *Aarzoo*, she too feels unfit for love or marriage, and that she would be a liability on Dev owing to her disability. But Dev accepts her in spite of her disability. Again, a stereotypical male image has been projected here. Dev might not have fallen in love with Priya had she suffered from a congenital disability, as such a disability would have left her on the periphery of society. However, since she was already a part of mainstream life prior to acquiring the disability, it was possible to bring her back into the mainstream again.

It is these negative images which go a long way in the formation of attitudes towards disabled women. The abilities of disabled women are never or rarely projected. Disability, in a majority of the films, is either ridiculed in comedies or is pitied and patronised. Disabled women are shown as vulnerable and at the same time undesirable, which makes their integration with the mainstream world impossible. They have never been projected as economically self-sufficient or as making a positive contribution to the family income. Indeed, it is this aspect which helps in giving them a status at par with their non-disabled counterparts, who too lead dependent lives.

When women start contributing to the family income, it not only adds to their self-esteem, but also enhances their worth in the eyes of the other family members. But how can disabled women increase their self-worth when they are confined to the four walls of a house, their mobility curtailed because of their disability and limited financial resources? In a country like India, marriage is a major economic burden on the parents of girls. When this is combined with disability, the expenses increase manifold, resulting in neglect and deprivation of disabled women. For economic reasons primarily, they are denied access to education, vocational training, and other rehabilitative services and welfare programmes which can play a major role in their empowerment.

According to Sujata Goenka: 'Disabled or not, women are respected if they contribute their share to the earnings of the family. Even if women do not work outside their grooves, they support a large part of the world economy by "free services" in the home and the community. For reasons of bias and prejudice in statistical and conceptual analysis, much of the work women perform has been officially described as non-economic activity.... Women are producers of income and assets in every economy, but are frequently forgotten or dropped out of developmental and/or environmental strategies at all levels of national and international life' (Patel, 1995, p. 27). This observation is equally applicable to disabled women, whose contributions are not quantified in statistical terms, resulting in increased violence, abuse and discriminatory attitude towards them. They are supposed to work permanently for their families without any remuneration. Added to this is the assumption that a disabled woman is a permanent liability for the family. In this context, Komal Kamra observes:

> In our country, economic status plays a very major role in deciding social acceptance. Economic rehabilitation is perhaps the most difficult to achieve for the disabled, particularly for the disabled women. Economic freedom can provide her with self-confidence, which improves her independence, and therefore should be looked into with a great deal of involvement by society. (Kamra, 1996, p. 17)

But the question here is how can disabled women be assured of economic independence? The answer is: only by expanding educational and rehabilitative services and empowering disabled women by providing them with vocational training, especially in the rural areas of our country. Another requirement is to change the narrow mindset of the people. This is because education, even professional qualifications, may not guarantee the disabled person a suitable economic status, all other things being equal.

The economic aspect of empowerment of disabled women has to be necessarily seen from a cultural and social perspective, especially in a country like India. Our culture and society, unlike that in western countries, encourages dependence and subjugation instead of independence and self-sufficiency. This culture of dependence is a direct result of a society dominated by patriarchal attitudes. Disabled women are permanently caught in a vicious cycle of deprivations. They are 'subjected to deliberate neglect, verbal abuse, physical assaults and sexual harassment. There seems to be a conspiracy against women, almost an underground male agenda, resulting in the marginalisation and even victimisation of disabled women' (Baquer and Sharma, 1997). In rural areas, at least, there exists some kind of social watch, which is, however, absent in the urban environment. This makes disabled women more vulnerable to sexual harassment and victimisation in the cities. This vulnerability in turn compels disabled women to look for male protection and thus seek marriage. As Baquer and Sharma opine, society regards disabled women as non-sexual. They are not considered suitable for marriage. Even if marriage ever takes place, a number of compromises are made. They are married to either much older men or to widowers. In most cases, non-disabled men get married to disabled women, but the reverse is not true. The dowry demanded by men and offered by the families of the disabled women is exorbitant. Disabled women are considered incapable of bearing and rearing healthy children. Society undervalues a woman with disabilities. She is not considered an ideal child or adult; she is deemed unfit as an employee, unsuitable as a wife, and incapable as a mother (Baquer and Sharma, 1997, p. 193–94).

I can confirm this out of my personal experience. In spite of my disability being less severe than the prospective groom's, our economic statuses were at par (he was a doctor and I a lecturer), and I possessed above-average looks (something Indians are obsessed with), I was rejected in favour of a non-working, less-qualified, but non-disabled girl. Indian society and culture denies women with or without disabilities the right to decide for themselves. Ours is a culture which encourages dependence, especially of women. Ironically, women are considered as service deliverers, and their contribution is not economically quantified. Gender bias, discriminatory practices and low economic status combine to aggravate disabled women's subjugation, segregation and misery. It is an established fact that more than 80 per cent of disabled women remain single throughout their lives. Recently, I had the opportunity of talking to a visually impaired person who has been married for twenty-two years to a non-disabled woman. He disclosed three reasons for his insistence on marrying a non-disabled woman. First, he said, a disabled man should marry a non-disabled woman because that would give him services for a lifetime free of cost. Second, he feared the response of society. He felt that, had he married a disabled woman, the sarcastic remarks of his acquaintances would have isolated the couple. Last and most important, he confessed that although he himself had no hesitation in taking a helping hand from someone of the opposite sex, he would not have been able to tolerate his disabled wife being touched by another man. Thus, we see that even if a disabled woman does get married, the marriage would always remain precarious. Its success would depend on how much the bride can contribute and endure. The need to look at the ability of a disabled woman without forgetting her disability, and avoid comparison with non-disabled women, is never emphasised. This attitude, together with poverty, ignorance, illiteracy, malnutrition, male attitudes, and their own indifference towards their status and situations adds to the suffering and problems of disabled women.

The following two case studies of mobility-impaired women of different economic and educational backgrounds should help substantiate the point. Both are urban case studies: the first is of Kalpana from Gwalior, and the second is of Meera from Jaipur.

Kalpana is the second of four siblings. She belongs to a high-income group of society and has access to all the facilities. A postgraduate in English with a diploma in computer applications, she is today a broken-hearted divorcée. In spite of being highly qualified, she lacked the right guidance, and did not show any inclination to empower herself with a suitable job. Like a meek cow she agreed to be married off. Her parents gave huge sums as dowry, but the alliance was annulled after three months, as the degradation, alienation and abuses proved unbearable for Kalpana. She was constantly abused for her disability, but at the same time was considered a milch cow. Demands for more dowry payments continued unabated. She had no alternative but to escape from such a life. Today she is back at her parent's place, a victim of overprotection, looking for another partner on whom she can depend.

Meera, on the other hand, is a victim of utter neglect, whose dreams have been shattered to pieces. She is the only daughter of her parents, who belong to the lower-middle, semi-literate strata of society. Her mother has borne sole responsibility for her. Meera owes her education up to college to her mother. After the death of her father, her brothers stopped all financial aid, forcing her to discontinue her studies. She was pushed into doing household chores all day. The search is now on for a match who will accept Meera with her average looks and her impairments, so that she can be got rid of once and for all.

Thus, apart from the mindset, the denial of the right to become productive members of society results in greater handicapping of women with disabilities. The problems of women with disabilities are further aggravated due to the accordance of inferior status to them by others of their own gender. Disabled women also lack role models and powerful advocates of their rights and problems. They are inadequately represented in the disability sector, which is largely dominated by disabled men unaware of the specific concerns of disabled women. They do not have any representation in women's organisations and NGOs fighting against violence or for social empowerment, equality, rights and opportunities. Disabled women, thus, have to fight not only with their own disability but also against an insensitive society.

The complex problems highlighted above are common to both urban and rural disabled women. But rural disabled women face some particular problems which prevent them from enjoying the benefits of development. Data published by the World Health Organisation on women's health show that there are several blocks in the information flows of many countries. The inadequate or total lack of access to information, health care and rehabilitation services is compounded by much higher illiteracy rates, longer distances to services and facilities, and more severe conditions of poverty than in the urban areas. Disability creates and exacerbates poverty because of economic strain and isolation. However, because far fewer opportunities for productive work or gainful employment exist for a disabled woman than for a disabled man, she is perceived as a greater burden for the family (Mohit, 1996, p. 26).

The life of a disabled woman is beset with multiple challenges. But these challenges are not insurmountable. The solution lies in moving away from the traditional attitude of treating women as objects of worship, as this attitude makes them providers of services and deprives them of the right to procure anything on their own. More importantly, there is a need to empower women with educational and vocational skills so as to make them productive and thereby enhance their economic and social worth. More and more vocational training centres need to be opened, especially in rural areas, for this purpose. At the same time, it is the duty of educated and privileged disabled women to adequately voice the concerns of their less privileged and less fortunate disabled sisters. The onus of being vocal activists regarding gender-based disability lies on them. They must be role models and try to place themselves in strategically decisive positions. Further, a gender-based data of disabled people is necessary, as that would help in perceiving the true extent of the problems and discriminations faced by disabled women.

Finally, women as a group must be sensitised so that the issues pertaining to disabled women are seen in a wider perspective and get the attention they deserve.

References

Baquer, Ali and Sharma, Anjali. 1997. *Disability: Challenges vs. Responses*. New Delhi: Concerned Action and Now.

Ganai, N.A. 1994. 'Child abuse: The aetiology and prevention', in S. Sood and J.N. Choudhary (eds), *Marriage, Family and Socialisation in Developed and Developing Countries*. Jaipur: Ariant Publishing House.

Kamra, Komal. 1996, 'Social and economic rehabilitation of disabled women', in *The End of Long Silence*. New Delhi: National Association of the Blind-Community Based Rehabilitation Network, p. 17.

Mitra, Jyoti. 1997. *Women and Society: Equality Empowerment*. New Delhi: Kanishka Publishers.

Mohit, Anuradha. 1996. 'The problems of discrimination', in *The End of Long Silence*. New Delhi: National Association of the Blind-Community Based Rehabilitation Network, pp. 10–30.

Patel, K.A. 1995. *Women and Sustainable Development: An International Perspective*. New Delhi: Ashish Publishing House.

13

The Baby and the Bath Water: Disabled Women and Motherhood in a Social Context

Carol Thomas

INTRODUCTION

In highly industrialised societies today, childbearing is an option, not an inevitability, for most women. An increasing proportion of women in Britain do not give birth to children, and many are 'child-free' through choice. However, the majority of women do have at least one child, and for most the experience of bearing and/or rearing children is something they would not want to forego. Of course, some women who do want to conceive experience the problems and distress associated with their own or their male partner's infertility. Others choose to parent singly, or to parent in same-sex relationships.

A proportion of women in all of the above categories have physical or sensory impairment and first-hand experience of disability, but their experiences have been largely overlooked in sociological studies of pregnancy, childbirth and early motherhood. This paper reports on the analysis of data from 17 interviews with disabled women. These were conducted as part of a follow-up study associated with a much larger

Thomas, C. 1997. 'The baby and the bath water: Disabled women and motherhood in a social context', *Sociology of Health and Illness*, 19 (3): 622–43.

health authority-commissioned research project on the *maternity preferences* of women of childbearing age resident in one city. The disabled women who were interviewed were either contemplating childbearing, were pregnant, and/or had young children.

While the voices of disabled women are almost totally absent in sociological work on reproduction and parenting, there is a small but growing literature on disabled women's motherhood experiences springing from the disability movement itself (Finger, 1990; Morris, 1992; Morris, 1996). My interpretation of the interview data owes much to this literature, not least because I can relate to the issues at a personal level.[1] It is becoming clearer that disabled women's desires, decisions and experiences of childbearing and parenting are interlaced with additional concerns stemming from the disabilism they encounter, their personal experience of living with impairment per se, and their knowledge about the possible affects of reproduction on their bodies.

While the aim of this paper is to give an account of these women's experiences through a discussion of three of the themes which emerged in the analysis of the interview data, it can also be read as a contribution to the further development of a *sociology of disability*—in the Irving Zola tradition, perhaps? (Williams, 1996a)—as distinct from the well-established *sociology of chronic illness* (Bury, 1991). In other words, the analysis presented here is informed much more by a disability than by a chronic-illness paradigm. In relation to my usage of key terms, this means that in common with those writing from a disability-movement perspective, the meaning of the term *disability* is *not* the condition or functional consequence of being physically or mentally impaired. Rather, *disability* refers to the disadvantaging affects—referred to by many as the 'social barriers'—faced by people with impairments flowing from *disabilism*: the ideological antipathy to what is considered to be undesirable physical, sensory or mentally-related difference or 'abnormality' in western culture. Disability is a form of social exclusion and not a product of impairment per se. However, conceptualising disability as a social phenomenon is not unproblematic, and Gareth Williams has recently referred to the 'hotly contested terrain' of the meaning of disability (Williams, 1996b, p. 194).

[1] I was born without a left hand and now have a four-year-old child.

There are a number of dimensions to this contestation but, in conceptual terms, debate revolves around the place and nature of 'the social' in understanding disability. On the one hand, 'disability theorists'[2] and medical sociologists are engaged in debate about the 'divide' between the 'social model' approach (a touchstone of those writing from a disability-movement perspective) and mainstream sociological approaches (interactionist, phenomenological), which focus on the experience of living with chronic illness. For a review of this debate, see Barnes and Mercer (1996). On the other hand, disability theorists and writers are engaged in a debate among themselves (a notably gendered debate) about the place in the social model of both the 'personal experience of disability', and the 'experience of impairment' (see Oliver, 1996; Morris, 1996; Crow, 1996; French, 1993). At the heart of these debates are questions such as the following. Is disability entirely socially constructed/created as suggested by the social model of disability (Oliver, 1996), or is this an over-socialised view (Bury, 1996; Williams, 1996a)? Can/should the social model of disability be developed to take on board the *experience* of disability, and/or the *experience* of impairment (Morris, 1996; Crow, 1996; French, 1993), or would such a development be politically dangerous because it redirects attention back to the individual and away from the social barriers which really cause disablement (Oliver, 1996; Finkelstein, 1996; Campbell and Oliver, 1996)?

It is not my intention to explore these debates here, but against this backdrop it is necessary to outline my approach more closely. It is one which attempts to explore the *experiences* of these women in order to understand better the ways in which *disabilism* manifests itself in the reproductive arena. Much of the research in the sociology-of-chronic-illness tradition tends to concentrate on the issues of *identity and meaning* associated with 'living with' *particular* conditions (Bury, 1991). My approach differs from this in that I am interested in looking at the common *experiences of disability* of women who may have a *range* of impairments and chronic illnesses. Furthermore, there are disability

[2] 'Disability theorists' is a term which has come to be used to identify those academics, most of whom are themselves impaired, who are researching or writing about disability from a 'disability rights' or radical socio-political perspective. For example, see Swain et al. (1993), Oliver (1996), Barnes and Mercer (1996).

theorists who argue that personal experience (either of disability or impairment) has no place in social-model analyses (or disability politics), because it deflects attention away from the 'social barriers external to the individual'. My starting point is that the study of personal experience can powerfully illuminate aspects of these 'social barriers', and so point to areas for social change. This reaffirms the sociological position that the study of individual lives can very effectively illustrate the social (Evans, 1993; Plummer, 1995; Williams, 1996a).

So, what can these women's experiences tell us about the ways in which disabilism presents itself on the journey through conception, pregnancy, childbirth and early motherhood? The quotations and examples which are selected for use in this paper are those which best exemplify what I interpret to be manifestations of disability. To put it another way, they illustrate the problems and issues that the women faced, which were embedded in the social fabric of services and structures, and particularly in the social relationships in which they engaged. The manifestations of disability are considered in connection with the following themes which emerge from data analysis: first, engagement with the 'risk' discourse; second, the pressure felt by disabled women to demonstrate that they are, or could be, 'good-enough mothers'; and third, the experiences of receiving unhelpful 'help' from health- and social-care workers. While not the only themes yielded by the data, these are the ones reported here because of their particular sociological significance. They connect with much wider concerns within medical sociology: medical discourses and risk, the social construction of motherhood, and the social interaction between lay people and health professionals. Other themes, reported elsewhere, relate to issues of practical and environmental significance: for example, the design of maternity departments, the utility of equipment, and information needs. Evidence is presented which draws in particular on 11 of the 17 interviews, but exemplars relating to at least one of the themes could have been drawn from any of the interview transcripts. I make no pretence to be representing these women's experiences in their totality (and, of course, in many respects their maternity experiences are the same as those of non-disabled women documented extensively elsewhere). Following a discussion on methods, the three themes are considered in turn.

METHODS

The data from 17 interviews were the product of a study on maternity, motherhood and disability, which was a follow-up of a much larger research project on (all) women's 'maternity preferences'. In the wake of *Changing Childbirth: Report of the Expert Maternity Group* (DoH, 1993), the main *maternity preferences* study was commissioned in 1994 by a health authority in the north of England to gather information on the forms and features of maternity provision which women of childbearing age favoured. It involved a postal questionnaire survey in 1995 with an achieved sample size of over 1,400 women of variable parity, aged between 16 and 44 years, resident in one city. The questionnaire contained items about experiences and intentions in connection with: preferences about the place of birth, features of antenatal care, care during labour, and care and support in the immediate postnatal period. Through the medium of the questionnaire, women were invited to indicate if they would like to participate in a follow-up interview if they were disabled (that is, considered themselves to be disabled) and felt that this had affected or would affect their maternity-care needs. Attempts were made to contact all of the women who responded to this invitation by telephone and/or letter. (There were 17 responses in total; some women sent in only a name and phone number, others an address and phone number.) As a result, 10 in-depth semi-structured follow-up interviews were conducted. A further three interviews with disabled women were organised by 'networking' with a midwife and an occupational therapist. These two health professionals had worked with a number of disabled mothers, and they agreed to contact a few women on our behalf to ask if they would be willing to be interviewed by a member of the research team. Another two interviews were arranged with women who were known to the researchers. Also included in the analysis were the data from interviews with two more disabled women which had been conducted in the pilot phase of the maternity preferences study, again using networking/reputational methods to obtain names. Thus, there are interview data from a total of 17 interviews. This 'mixed method' of obtaining the sample of disabled women reflects, in part, the difficulties of obtaining a sample when no pre-existing sampling frame is available. It was fortunate that a broad range of experience was represented in the present sample, associated with differences in parity, age, the nature of the impairment(s), and the women's socio-economic status. However, it should be noted that all of the women were white.

The range of physical and/or sensory impairments represented in the sample is as follows, and included one woman with mental-health problems:[3] deafness (Janet, Susan); hearing and visual impairment (Sheila); arthritis in the spine (Helen); limb amputation above right knee (Fran); amputation below left elbow (Sarah); Crohn's disease (Sally); systemic lupus erythematosus (SLE) (Mary); diabetes (Ann); epilepsy (Penny); back injury resulting in chronic back pain (Rachel); asthma (Lorna); mobility problems associated with cerebral palsy (Pat); Addison's disease (Angela); back pain and mobility problems associated with dislocated hip at birth (Sarah); bilateral dysplasia and osteoarthritis (Clair); high levels of anxiety, panic attacks and agoraphobia (Terry). The names used here are not real names, and care has been taken to avoid the inclusion of identifying details.

The in-depth semi-structured interviews were sensitively conducted in a conversational style. The author conducted two 'pilot' stage interviews, and the rest were conducted by one interviewer recruited for the purpose and overseen by the author. With the women's permission, all interviews were tape recorded and transcribed. All covered issues to do with pre-conception plans and intentions, pregnancy, labour and delivery, the postnatal period, childcare, and 'being a mother', building on the areas covered in the postal questionnaire. However, because of the following variable childbearing histories, not all of these areas relate to the actual or past experiences of all the women:

- four were childless but were actively thinking about having a baby in the next few years;
- two were pregnant—one with her first child and the other with her second;
- four had one child each, ranging in age from nine weeks to seven years;

[3] While not an impairment as conventionally defined, mental-health problems are, nevertheless, associated with disability because they carry the medical label of 'mental illness' and, as such, give rise to the experience of social exclusion.

- six had two children each (children's ages ranging from 1 to 12 years); two of these mothers had been sterilised at the time of the interview;
- one woman had six children, the youngest of whom was 1 year old.

In relation to validity, I can claim, first, that the data-generation methods were well matched to my research question: what can disabled women's experiences tell us about the ways in which disabilism presents itself on the journey through conception, pregnancy, childbirth and early motherhood? Semi-structured interviews were an appropriate way to access experiences, allowing respondents to 'tell their stories' and recount their experiences in ways which were meaningful to them, with minimal researcher constraint. Second, I would defend the validity of my interpretation of the women's accounts in terms of disabilism. Essentially, these accounts did three things: (a) outline the nature of their impairment(s); (b) tell their reproductive story; and (c) reflect upon how (a) affected (b) and vice versa. The analysis of the interview transcripts involved cross-sectional indexing of all the data in the building up of 19 categories relating to aspects of experience and other social characteristics. It became apparent that these categories could be readily grouped into a number of substantive themes relating to the social, that is, to the problems and issues the women faced which were embedded in the social fabric of relationships, services and structures. Informed by a disability paradigm (as outlined above), it was possible to argue that these experiences/themes could be interpreted as manifestations of disability. While the number of interviews was small and the findings are not empirically generalisable, the arguments are theoretically generalisable (Mason, 1996), in the sense that the sample was not atypical of disabled women and that the analysis has a much wider resonance.

TAKING 'RISKS'?

The strongest theme to emerge from the data was that of 'risk', an issue of growing interest to medical sociologists more generally (Gabe, 1995). Most of the women interviewed had faced issues to do with reproductive 'risk', either to themselves or to their babies. Is the health and/or survival of the foetus 'at risk' because the condition is hereditary or because of drug treatments? Would their own health be placed 'at risk'? The women could not avoid a close encounter with a medical discourse which has at its core the belief that (1) if there is a risk of abnormality, or the risk of worsening an already abnormal bodily condition, then steps must be taken to avoid it; (2) genetic counselling outlining the 'risks' or suggesting/recommending termination should be given to those parents who are 'at risk' of producing a baby with a serious impairment; (3) women with impairments who are 'at risk' of worsening their condition through pregnancy should be advised not to bear children. Of course, all women who come into contact with maternity services during pregnancy experience this medical-risk discourse in some way (Lane, 1995), but for women whose bodies are already 'abnormal', the encounter is a particularly sharp one, and there may be heavy personal costs to be borne. In what sense can this experiential encounter with the risk discourse relate to manifestations of disability? Before exploring this question, let us look at the nature of the women's encounters.

In general, the women interviewed did not question medically defined reproductive risks, and tended to share in wider lay beliefs that 'passing on' or 'causing' impairment in a child was irresponsible and 'unfair' to the child (see also Parsons and Atkinson, 1992). Sheila, for example, had retinitis pigmentosa (a hereditary visual impairment, involving 'tunnel vision', caused by progressive degeneration of the retina) and deafness in one ear (not hereditary), and spoke in terms of risk about the decision to be sterilised some years after the birth of her two sons. Sheila herself had no signs of the visual impairment when her two sons were born. Now, she had marked impairment and her eldest son had signs of the condition, but it was too early to say whether her second son had this inheritance. She explained how the pattern of inheritance of retinitis pigmentosa cannot be predicted; it 'skips' some offspring, and others become merely carriers. Her GP had suggested that she should be sterilised because of the hereditary nature of the condition. Sheila reported that her mother, to whom she was very close, had strongly supported the GP's view on the grounds that, 'It's not fair, is it, on the children you bring through, cos you don't want them to suffer, do you?' This had clearly been an emotionally painful course of action for Sheila. She and her new partner wanted a daughter: 'Otherwise, I'd have kept going until I got a girl. ... I still pine a lot for a little girl, but it weren't to be so ... end of subject. You get over it.' What is particularly interesting about this woman's account is that the decision to be sterilised was made reluctantly in the context of pressure from trusted figures of authority (her GP, her mother), and in the context of considerable uncertainty about the likelihood that any additional child would in fact 'suffer' from the condition.

Another mother, Mary, with systemic lupus erythematosus (SLE, a chronic inflammatory disease of connective tissue, affecting the skin and various internal organs and requiring steroid and other drug treatments) had made the decision not to try for a second child because 'it wasn't worth the risk' either to her own health or that of the baby. When she became pregnant with her first child, the medical team responsible for the treatment of her SLE had refused to believe her claim that she was pregnant, because they were convinced that her prescribed medication would have prohibited conception. A scan had to be conducted to confirm her pregnancy to these specialists. The doctors advised her to continue with her medication at current levels throughout pregnancy. However, following a move abroad during her pregnancy, she was later told by doctors in the other country that 'because of the tablets I'm on he could be slightly deformed—fingers and toes or something.' She describes herself as having been 'fit and healthy' throughout the pregnancy, and that her son was born, prematurely, with no apparent 'deformities'. On her return to the U.K., she was referred to a consultant rheumatologist, who was the first doctor to give her detailed information about SLE, and in whom she developed much confidence.. Mary explained that she now knew that her steroid medication could and should have been reduced during pregnancy to reduce 'the risks' to the baby. She talked about how her health had deteriorated in the years following the birth of her son. At one stage, she had decided to try for another baby, and had been in contact with both her rheumatologist and the maternity hospital for advice about conception and pregnancy. She was given contradictory advice about 'the risks' associated with her medication. The rheumatologist told her that one of her drugs was contra-indicated and that an abortion would be absolutely necessary if she became pregnant while on this drug, but the doctors at the maternity hospital asserted that the drug was 'safe'. She had stopped taking this drug, but then had a 'flare-up' of her condition, 'so I decided, myself, that it's not worth the risk … there's no point in having another child if there's no mum there to look after them.' She knew of cases where mothers had died of SLE following childbirth. This decision not to have another child had not been an easy one to make, and the health services had certainly indicated a willingness to assist her with conception and pregnancy if she had wanted to persist in her attempts to have another child:

> I said to my husband, I've got to go through the grieving process, and he said, why? why? why? And I said, because I've made a decision. I said that I can't risk having another one. I said the maternal instincts are still there, so I sense, like, you've lost something; you've lost a part of you.… I've to go through the grieving process. I said you've got to give me time for that.… I mean, they told me [my son] was a miracle really, and at least I've got one. (Mary)

The issue of the risks to the woman of ceasing medication, or of reducing or increasing its levels, versus the risks to the foetus of continuing with pre-pregnancy levels of medication, was also a key one for some other women, particularly those with chronic back pain, epilepsy, diabetes, asthma or mental-health problems. Some of these women had experienced, or would expect, extra monitoring during pregnancy to ensure that the baby was developing 'normally' and that their own health was not being compromised. The balance was sometimes a very fine one. For example, Penny (with epilepsy), said that because her medication meant there was a slim chance of foetal deformity, it was kept to a minimum. However, she did have one fit during pregnancy because her medication dosage was too low. This had distressed her because she had read that the oxygen supply to the baby can be dangerously reduced during a fit: 'it can cause you to lose the baby.' Penny believed that the doctors were at fault for not increasing her medication in proportion to her weight increase.

Rachel, who had chronic back pain following an accident, talked about having a baby in the future as a kind of trade-off: living with increased pain during pregnancy in return for having a 'beautiful baby' at the end. She knew that her injections at the pain clinic would 'have to stop' during pregnancy:

> I know I'm going to be in pain. It's my decision to have a baby and I've got to weigh it up.… I can always think, 'Well, at the end of this I'm

> going to have a baby,' you know, and then I can go back to the pain clinic and have some more treatment and so ... I think that's the way I would have to look at it. (Rachel)

Terry, a respondent with mental-health problems (anxiety and panic attacks, agoraphobia, and depression) which had developed in the time since the births of her two children, agonised about the problem of medication and pregnancy. She experienced this as a real dilemma; she desperately wanted more children, especially with her new partner (she had two children by previous partners, both of whom had abused her emotionally and/or physically), but was terrified that she would not be able to 'cope' without her drugs (especially Prozac):

> I've been told I can't 'ave a baby on medication so ... I don't know if I've got the guts to actually start coming off them [the tablets]. I want to, but the fear of being how I were without them is stopping me. I really, really want to come off 'em. I'm so scared, I don't.... I think if I, if I were going to be like that, I wouldn't even attempt to come off 'em, no matter how much I wanted a baby. (Terry)

Terry had not felt able to seek help from health professionals about this, and clearly struggled alone with these tensions. In a life of considerable emotional hardship, she had gained tremendous satisfaction and self-belief through becoming a mother: 'Satisfaction of thinking they're a little human being and ... it depends on you for its care, and you giving it, and its thriving, and you think: Oh! You're doing something right.'

Two mothers, Sarah and Pat, did give birth to children who had impairments associated with hereditary conditions. Feelings of guilt after the birth of her first child were expressed by Sarah, a mother of six who was herself born with a dislocated hip, a hereditary condition which may or may not manifest itself in offspring:

> When my first daughter was born, they thought that she had a dislocated hips as well, and that was very sad. Well, it was a very sad time for me because I felt that I'd done it to her, you know.... They told me when she was a day old, when I think you are quite fragile anyway, and so that was a very bad time then for me because, you know, my beautiful new baby—and I'd made her not quite right. And then she had to have a harness when she was six months old, and that particular consultant thought she should

> wear it the whole time, so we never took it off for a bath or anything for six months.... There was a lot about our baby that didn't look normal and ... it was a big iron thing round her legs. (Sarah)

Sarah's fourth child, too, was born with the condition, but a different consultant suggested that a harness only needed to be worn at night. Sarah experienced this as much less problematic: it carried considerably reduced 'guilt'.

Pat's first child was diagnosed with a chronic condition as a baby. However, this child had cystic fibrosis (CF), which was completely unconnected to Pat's cerebral palsy. She and her husband were, unknowingly, carriers of the gene for cystic fibrosis. What is particularly interesting is her account of how some people made assumptions that her child's condition was a direct result of her own impairment (or, at least, of its visible manifestations: some difficulty in walking, in maintaining balance, and a weakness in one hand), with the unspoken implication that she was irresponsible to have this child: 'I've just had a couple of people say "Erm, is it related in any way to what you've got?", but that's, you know, their ignorance rather than anything else.' Pat admitted to feeling 'relieved' that her son's condition was not related to her cerebral palsy, and that his CF could not have been predicted. In fact, she had sensed some hostility from other people when she was pregnant:

> I do think that sometimes they thought that I shouldn't be pregnant. You know, nobody actually said anything, but, and it wasn't anybody I knew or anything like that, but if I went on public transport and things like that. Not all the time, just once or twice, well, they'd probably think that whatever I'd got, the child has got a chance of being the same, and they wouldn't know that what I'd got wasn't passed. (Pat)

Pat talked about her decision, made with her husband, to have a second child. She described this as 'murderously difficult.' They wanted another child, and thought their son should have a sibling, but they had to weigh this up against what they saw as other factors to take into consideration: the chances of a second child having CF or a different impairment, the effects that an early death of the first child would have on the second, her assessment of the impact of her own impairment on her ability to manage another child, especially one with CF, 'cos you get less capable of doing things as you get older.' She did have a second child, and it did not have CF. Six months after this birth, she decided to be sterilised: 'You can't have any more taking those risks, can you, I thought, with all the odds against us.'

From the above we can see that considerations of 'risk' were an important feature of the women's reproductive journeys, and we can also see that disabled women often share, albeit sometimes ambivalently, in the wider social and medical discourses about what constitute reproductive 'risks'. Having a child with an impairment is seen as something to be avoided, and if it occurs, is experienced with feelings of 'guilt', which spring from the knowledge that their actions in having a child are widely seen as both irresponsible and 'unfair' to the child. Such women often face very difficult decisions about whether to take the 'risk' of childbearing if they have a hereditary condition which might be 'passed on', or if they are on medication which may 'damage' the foetus, or if their own condition may be worsened through reproduction. The women's accounts bear witness to the considerable 'emotion work' involved in personal encounters with the risk discourse: worry, anxiety, guilt, lost hopes, unfulfilled dreams and spoilt identities.

But is this emotional burden simply an inevitable feature of the 'personal tragedy' of living with 'impairment'? Of course not. These individual experiences are shaped by encounters with wider discourses about personal responsibility, which accompany all women on the journey into motherhood, coupled with encounters with disabilism. The key point is that the risk discourse is not a neutral one. What is and is not judged to be an acceptable risk hinges not just on life or death questions, or on purely biological criteria, but on social assumptions about the quality of life and intrinsic value of children and adults with impairments. As Freidson pointed out so well, medical knowledge about illness (or impairment) is social, and as such is 'inevitably evaluational' (Freidson, 1988, p. 208). Despite its seeming 'scientific objectivity', medical knowledge inevitably draws on deep-rooted cultural antipathy for, and prejudices about, people with 'abnormalities'. Jenny Morris (1991) has argued that, in our society, judgements are made about the quality of life of people with impairments which equate physical impairment (particularly severe impairment) with 'lives not worth living', and that impairment is considered in abstraction from the social, economic, cultural and spatial circumstances which really do determine the quality of life. It is noteworthy that medical sociologists who have considered the reproductive-risk discourse (for example, Parsons and Atkinson, 1992; Lane, 1995) have described lay encounters with it in connection with impairment and disability, but have not commented upon or questioned its disabilist character.

Drawing on Morris' work, and a wider literature springing from the disability movement, it is clear that a minority of disabled women have rejected the socio-medical discourse about risk, and see it as part of an all-pervasive disabilist ideology. They know that there are medically defined 'risks', that is, probabilities of impairment effects for self or the baby, but they do not necessarily evaluate these risks negatively. Impairment *per se* is not equated with 'the problem'. Their perspective is clear: the problem is disability—the social barriers which socially exclude. Micheline Mason (1992), for example, has written about her great joy and sense of achievement in becoming a mother (a single parent), and about her decision to continue with an unplanned pregnancy, though she knew that her child would inherit her own condition—'brittle bones' (osteogenesis imperfecta), giving her a tiny stature, deformed limbs, and the need for assisted mobility:

> Once I had made the decision to choose life, and whatever that may bring, the confirmation that the baby did indeed have brittle bones only seemed to make the initial decision more meaningful and special. (Mason, 1992, p. 115)

Micheline Mason, who describes herself as a disabled activist, has been able to throw off disabilist attitudes about the 'tragedy' of having a child with an impairment, and, rather, to celebrate it and to demand that the disabling social barriers, which are the real source of the disability experienced by disabled children and mothers, are removed.

To see the 'risk discourse' as disabilist (something of significance for all women) requires a change in consciousness, which Morris (1991, 1996), Mason (1992), Anne Finger (1990) and others have made. The women in my study, like most disabled women, had not travelled that journey, or, perhaps, had not had the opportunity to do so. This does not lessen, however, the power of their personal accounts to 'tell of disabilism'. I would argue that, in some very fundamental ways, their engagement with the medical risk discourse was an engagement with disabilism, and that the considerable personal costs to be borne were one important aspect of the 'manifestations of disability' they faced. To put this another way, that is, in 'disability rights' terms, the powerful medical (and wider) discourse on reproductive risk acts as a social barrier, in the sense that it plays an important part in 'restricting activity'; in its light, decisions are made not to have a child/another child, or to be sterilised, or to terminate a pregnancy.

'GOOD ENOUGH' MOTHERING?

A second theme which emerged strongly in the data analysis revolves around the fear of being judged inadequate as a mother, and of the consequences that this might bring. Again, all women who become mothers (and particularly those in pilloried groups such as 'single mothers') experience this to a greater or lesser degree, especially in these times, when public and professional discourses highlight concern for 'children at risk'; but this study suggests that disabled women are particularly vulnerable. A number of the women lived with this fear, believing that they might be seen by others—representing either the powers of the state (health visitors, community midwives, doctors, social workers and so on) or the power of the wider family—as having failed to live up to being a 'good mother'. Two women had actually experienced threatened or actual loss of their children, not, perhaps surprisingly, as a consequence of action by 'officials', but as a consequence of family members taking unofficial action against their wishes. For example, Jane, who had lost her left arm below the elbow as the result of an accident, described the way in which her own mother wanted to 'keep' her two-year-old daughter (born before the accident) because she believed that Jane would not be able to cope. Jane's mother had become involved in sharing the care of the child while Jane was in hospital having a series of operations, over a number of months, following the accident:

> I actually then had to ask solicitors to get involved, because mum decided she wanted to keep [my daughter]. So mum went to the solicitors to try and ... there was an argument over access, because I was quite happy for mum to see her whenever. It was over coming home at night custody, really.... I think, looking at it from her point of view, now, she just decided that because I'd only got one arm I couldn't cope ... [that I] should be sat there in my rocking chair, almost, you know, in a wheelchair, and

> give up on everything.... I just said to mum, 'You can see her whenever, but I can cope,' and I think that's what actually made us decide we'd like another child. Just to sort of prove that we could cope. (Jane)

The other respondent who had experienced a struggle over custody was Terry, who had mental-health problems. While she was going through a divorce with her first husband, he took their child without Terry's consent to live with his own parents. Terry reports that these grandparents 'tried to make me out to be mentally unstable,' and only allowed her to visit her son for one hour per day over an eight-month period until the custody case finally came to court. On one such visit, she had been physically assaulted (requiring hospital treatment) by the grandmother when she tried to take her son out of the grandparents' house. She got legal assistance through the intervention of health-care workers, and was finally granted custody of her son by the court. Her fears about her children being removed from her care were ever present, and certainly not helped by her own mother's refrain: 'If you don't get better, they'll take your children off you.'

The fear of losing her children had begun to creep into Sarah's mind after the birth of her sixth child. She had begun to experience a lot of difficulties in walking and bending, and had discomfort and pain associated with residual impairment, having been born with a dislocated hip:

> It's very hard to think that I can't look after my own children. It's a very hard thing to come to terms with, really. And I'm not quite at the point of saying, 'Look, I can't really do this,' but if I was, I don't really know what would happen. I suppose the children get taken into care, don't they, when the parents say they can't cope? But, you know, that's a very frightening prospect, really, so it's easy just to think of treading along. (Sarah)

These fears had been heightened by a health visitor with whom Sarah had been discussing a future hospital admission for a hip-replacement operation. Sarah was worried about child-care arrangements, because she would need some kind of help during the hospital stay and for some months afterwards while she was relatively immobile. The health visitor's reply was quite astonishing to Sarah:

> She said, 'Well, the children won't all be able to go into care together, you know,' which wasn't what I was asking for, because I wouldn't want

> my children to go into care, you know. I mean, who would? What a response! (Sarah)

Living with the fear of losing the right to care for their children forces some mothers to go to great lengths to 'present' themselves and their children as managing 'normally', often at significant personal cost in terms of comfort, and emotional and physical well-being. One consequence is that assistance may not be requested when it is needed because the mother feels that her request may be interpreted to mean that she is not capable. Clair, a woman in the study with quite severe impairment (a wheelchair user from a very young age), spoke about her joys at giving birth to her son, but also about her anxieties that other people's prejudicial judgements might lead to her child being removed from her care, particularly as she was a single parent:

> I felt that it was going to happen very soon, that maybe the prejudice of someone who lived around me [a neighbour] would make them think that they'd got to ring up social services and that an investigation would start.... It terrified me, it really did. I don't think I relaxed into motherhood until he was bout 18 months or two years old, I really don't think I did.... I would love to have those months again, cos I was so scared, tidying the house, cos I knew somebody was coming who was from authority, you know, that when he was asleep.... I was too busy doing jobs rather than enjoying him and relaxing. (Clair)

Jane, too, worried about professionals' judgements that she might not be able to manage. Despite having some practical difficulties in getting her new baby dressed and undressed several times a day for nappy changing while she was adapting to life without her left arm below the elbow, Jane struggled on with the dressing routine in the early weeks in order to 'present' herself to others and to herself as a 'fit' mother:

> I felt that she had to be dressed every day, and I had to ... otherwise people would think that I couldn't do it, cos,... certainly for the first six or eight weeks I felt that I ... was letting her down, because I couldn't get her back dressed properly, but after that I just got to the point where I thought, well, she's warm, she's healthy, as long as she's clean it doesn't matter. (Jane)

Jane noted that, after the birth of her first child, before her accident, she had not worried at all about always having the baby dressed, because she had 'felt in control of things much more'.

These accounts testify to the particular vulnerability that many women with impairments feel when they become mothers, or if they become impaired while fulfilling the socially defined obligations of motherhood. This feeling of vulnerability and insecurity is caused, in part, by their own concerns about managing some of the practical child-care tasks because of the impairment, but in the main it is caused by disabilism: the prejudicial attitudes of others and the failure to provide appropriate assistance to disabled women on their own terms. While the majority of non-disabled parents can take it for granted that the quality and character of their 'parenting' is their own business, although this may be increasingly illusory (Abbott and Sapsford, 1990), disabled women really do feel under surveillance, and this feeling is usually well founded because disabled women are often assumed by professionals and lay people (often including close relatives) to be incapable unless they can prove otherwise: guilty until proven innocent.

Given the strength and widespread nature of disabilist ideas which doubt the ability of women with impairments to be 'good mothers', to be able 'to cope', it is not surprising that many disabled women, especially those with a recently acquired impairment, have to overcome doubt about their own capacity to become mothers, or may privately share in some of the social anxieties about the welfare of the children of disabled parents. Once again, the personal costs involved, including the actual loss of the right to parent, are in fact the consequences of the way that disability manifests itself, rather than as something inherent in being impaired.

WHEN 'HELP' IS NOT HELPFUL

The third but closely related theme concerns the women's experiences of receiving inappropriate or inadequate 'help' from health professionals and social-care workers. At issue here is the nature of the social interaction between professionals and disabled patients/clients in contexts where the professional maxim, 'we know what is in the patient's best interests,' finds full expression. Once again, a large literature on the medicalisation of childbirth suggests that many women experience a sense of loss of control over their bodies during pregnancy and childbirth as doctors and other health professionals 'take over' (Roberts, 1981; Oakley, 1981; Garcia et al., 1990). However, this experience of loss of control can be intensified when 'disability' is an additional factor in the lay-professional encounter. Now, from a professional perspective, it is not just the 'management' of the pregnant woman and new mother that is of concern, but the management of women with the additional problems that come with 'being disabled'. A number of women in the study gave accounts of individual health workers who, although well intentioned, had 'taken over', had been unhelpful, or had lacked the information or skills they required. However, it is important to point out that all of the women said that some midwives, doctors (particularly some GPs), health visitors, 'home helps' and others were 'brilliant', 'great' or 'wonderful'. Similarly, some friends and relatives were 'great', 'always there for me' (often this was their own 'mum') or a 'real safety net'; but others were 'hopeless', 'fussing', 'over-protective' or 'taking over'.

Jane's experiences illustrate this theme particularly well (she had lost her left arm below the elbow). She reported her well-meaning GP as saying: 'Right, we'll get someone in, they can bath the baby and dress the baby, give the baby to you and you can sit there and nurse it, and if you want, we'll get someone in to help you bath.' The first time the baby had needed a bath in hospital, the midwives had said 'we'll do this.' Jane went on to explain that what she had really wanted was for someone to assist her with tasks like bathing the baby, but not to do it for her. Her experience of professional assistance was a largely disempowering one. It had been a source of distress, and had undermined her self-identity as a mother: 'When people wanted to take over, I found I was getting really cross, and I didn't want to get cross with the nurses. I'd take it out on [my husband] later: "they said they're going to bath that baby!".' 'Taking over' also occurred in relation to breast feeding:

> I just really felt that I was being left out of the important decisions, you know, and as if ... I did start feeding her myself, and then felt it just wasn't ... there was always someone fussing around me and, you know, 'you can cope?' and 'you'll have to put the head further into the crook of your arm,' and it was always ... wanting to prod and poke and 'are

> they all right?' I mean, I only stuck with it about four or five days and then started feeding her with a bottle, because I could do that myself. You know, they used to bring the bottle with the teat on, and I could do that. (Jane)

One midwife had said:

> We'll come everyday and put the baby on the breast ... They've got this vision of it all being so awful.... I must admit it didn't feel, being a mum didn't feel as natural with [my second]. Everything seemed much more difficult, and I did get depressed.... (Jane)

Jane thought there should be 'more emphasis on helping, not doing it helping mum not doing it for the baby'. By the time the health visitor had started to call at home: 'I'd already started saying, "Right, I can manage that," and she went the other way and said "Oh, you can cope, you're managing really well and you can do this."' In short, Jane's experience was largely one of inappropriate help or no help.

For other women, who had taken the risk that they might be signalling their inadequacy as a mother by asking for 'help', there were further personal costs to be borne. For example, Sarah, who had problems with walking and bending after the birth of her sixth child, had to endure being 're-assessed' by the home-help organiser in connection with a service she received, which involved a home help transporting her older children to and from school:

> She [the organiser] turned up just before my daughter's first birthday party, which was a bit difficult, really, and she only saw me sitting down, and her line was, 'Why are we only doing this for you two days a week?', you know, and I said I could manage the other days, and she said, 'Well, perhaps we should stop then?' I found that very difficult, really. I thought afterwards, perhaps I should have got up and showed her how difficult it was for me to walk, but there's something really horrible about that. Well, that's something I've had to do for doctors all my life, really, and I found that quite demeaning, I didn't actually want to do that. (Sarah)

Sometimes, technological aids were required, and what women wanted was information about, and access to, appropriate aids. For example, the three hearing-impaired women in the study mentioned the use of aids such as 'alarms' to indicate that the baby was crying, antenatal information videos for hearing-impaired people, and adapted telephones, doorbells and other equipment. In some instances, these women found out about aids by chance, or more often through meeting with other deaf mothers. This form of practical assistance was rarely offered by professionals in the health or social services; it was a case of repeatedly asking for and pursuing information. Another disabling barrier experienced by these hearing-impaired women was associated with face-to-face communication with health professionals. Most professionals encountered did not know how to communicate effectively. For example, midwives rarely knew any basic sign language (and signing was not always wanted, anyway). Susan reported having repeatedly to ask the midwives to 'slow down' so that she could follow what they were saying by lip-reading. Janet was very angry when unwanted 'help' was thrust upon her when she was in labour. The hospital midwives had arranged for an 'interpreter' to be present at the birth to assist with communication. Janet felt that she did not want a stranger present at such a private time. In fact, she did not feel that an interpreter was needed at all, and that if anyone needed to interpret, then it could be a close family member she had chosen.

Pat, who had mobility and balance difficulties, would have appreciated help with some housework tasks, both during her pregnancies and while her two children were small. She had also found bathing her babies difficult, although her husband helped with this. Additional assistance with housework and other tasks was not asked for, in part because she did not believe that such services would be available, but mainly because she felt that asking for help makes 'you feel a burden.' This feeling was a common one among the women interviewed; you just had to 'get on with it' and 'do the best you can.' As Sarah said, 'I think it's very, very difficult to ask for help.' As noted previously, this is partly associated with the need to be seen 'to cope' without additional help, to be a 'good mother', but it is also because women feel they 'should' be able to cope, that women always do have to cope. As in Pat's case, disabled women may also assume that there is no entitlement to assistance, or they may lack information about the services available.

What unites the accounts of inappropriate or inadequate assistance is that nobody appears to have asked the women themselves in the first place what assistance, if any, they really wanted, and how assistance could best be given. Professionals (and non-disabled lay people) assumed that 'they knew best.' It can be argued that this is a classic feature of disabilism: the impaired person is constructed as 'dependent', as reliant on the wisdom and help of expert others. Jenny Morris has written powerfully about disabilism constructing disabled women as the 'cared for', ignoring and excluding them as 'care givers' (Jenny Morris, 1991, 1995). There is no recognition that dependency, which is a feature of everybody's life to some degree, is socially created. So pervasive is this view that non-disabled feminist writers have reproduced (and reinforced) it in their critique of community-care policy in the U.K. (Morris, 1991, 1995, 1996; Keith, 1992). In this critique, the characterisation of disabled women as cared for rather than as care givers is taken as given.

In fact, what is striking about the situation of the disabled women interviewed in this study is that their care-giving role was fundamental to the physical and emotional maintenance of others in the household, and that, even where a male partner was present, disabled women were, or continued to be, the *main* carers of children and other family members. The traditional sexual division of labour was very much intact, whether or not the women needed any assistance over and above the help that women 'normally' get within families. Furthermore, these women's self-identities and aspirations were very firmly tied in with being a successful mother and running a home. Like many other disabled women, their personal fight in the face of disabilism was fundamentally about the *right* to be mothers and home makers.

Nevertheless, it seems that the normative assumption that disabled people are dependent profoundly colours the way in which 'help' is offered to women with impairments, both by well-meaning professionals, and often by friends and relatives as well. Non-disabled people generally *assume* that disabled women will need particular forms of help, and that they know best how to give it. In reproductive contexts, where maternity services already construct women as patients to be cared for by expert others, many disabled women receive a double dose of dependency creation. However, it is certainly not always the case that assistance is needed or wanted. Where it is, for example in the form of practical help with child-care tasks, the 'help' which is offered is quite likely to be inappropriate and/or conditional, or it may not be offered in any guise. Where 'help' is unwanted but forced upon disabled mothers, or is inappropriate in its form, it can be experienced as a threat to the right to parent (as we saw in the previous section), and/or as intrusive and disempowering. These are some of the 'manifestations of disability' that are faced. No help, or the wrong help, is the common lot of disabled women.

CONCLUSION

This paper has reported on the experiences of 17 disabled women who were at different stages in their reproductive journeys at the time of interview. It has explored the ways in which disabled women's decisions about, and experiences of, childbearing and motherhood are interlaced with additional concerns which originate in the social fabric of services and structures, and, particularly, in the social relationships between themselves and others. It has focused on three themes which emerged from an analysis of the interview transcripts: engagement with the medical 'risk' discourse; the pressure felt by disabled women to demonstrate that they are, or could be, 'good enough mothers'; and the experiences of receiving unhelpful 'help' from health- and social-care workers. The interpretation of these personal-experience narratives has taken place against the backdrop of current debates about the nature and meaning of disability, and the emphasis has been on what these women's accounts tell us about the manifestations of disability, or disabilism, which women with impairments face when they think about having a child, become pregnant, come into contact with maternity and related services, and when they become mothers.

Disabilism was evident in a number of ways, including in the women's close encounters with the medical 'risk' discourse, with its unspoken evaluative assumptions that, for example, to give birth to an impaired baby is to give birth to a life of less worth. This could entail living with the fear that one might be judged to be an inadequate mother, and that actions might follow involving the denial of the right to be a mother. Furthermore, there might be disempowering encounters with (usually well-meaning) health- and social-care workers, who frequently offered inappropriate help informed by a professional ethic of 'we know best.'

The paper has highlighted those features of the women's accounts which tell us something about the 'differences' disability brings. It suggests that disabled women's reproductive journeys are strewn with social barriers of an attitudinal, ideological and material kind. I hope to have demonstrated that the exploration of these women's *experiences* can provide a deeper insight into the nature of these 'social barriers'. In doing so, I also hope to have made a contribution to a sociology of disability which, while starting out from the experience of individuals, allows the examination of the social manifestations of disabilism, rather than pursuing an ever deeper exploration of the 'subjectivity of experience' (Williams, 1996b, p. 202). The point of it all it is not, however, to generate knowledge for its own sake, but to inform those engaged in disability praxis.

References

Abbott, P. and Sapsford, R. 1990. 'Health visiting: policing the family?', in P. Abbott and C. Wallace (eds), *The Sociology of The Caring Professions.* London: The Falmer Press.

Barnes, C. and Mercer, G. 1996. (eds) *Exploring the Divide: Illness and Disability.* Leeds: The Disability Press.

Bury, M. 1991. 'The sociology of chronic illness: a review of research and prospects', *Sociology of Health and Illness*, 13 (4): 161–82.

———. 1996. 'Defining and researching disability: challenges and responses', in C. Barnes and G. Mercer (eds), *Exploring the Divide: Illness and Disability.* Leeds: The Disability Press.

Campbell, J. and Oliver, M. 1996. *Disability Politics: Understanding our Past, Changing our Future.* London: Routledge.

Crow, L. 1996. 'Including all of our lives: renewing the social model of disability', in C. Barnes and G. Mercer (eds), *Exploring the Divide: Illness and Disability.* Leeds: The Disability Press.

Department of Health. 1993. *Changing Childbirth: Report of the Expert Maternity Group.* London: Her Majesty's Stationary Office.

Evans, M. 1993. 'Reading lives: how the personal might be social', *Sociology*, 27 (1): 5–13.

Finger, A. 1990. *Past Due: A Story of Disability, Pregnancy and Birth.* London: The Women's Press.

Finkelstein, V. 1996. 'Outside, inside out', *Coalition*, April: 30–36.

Freidson, E. 1988. *Profession of Medicine.* Chicago: University of Chicago Press.

French, S. 1993. 'Disability, impairment, or something in between?', in J. Swain et al. (eds), *Disabling Barriers, Enabling Environments.* London: Sage.

Gabe, J. (1995). (ed.) *Medicine, Health and Risk: Sociological Approaches.* Oxford: Blackwell.

Garcia, J., Kilpatrick, R. and Richards, M. 1990. (eds) *The Politics of Maternity Care Services for Childbearing Women in Twentieth-Century Britain.* Oxford: Clarendon Press.

Keith, L. 1992. 'Who cares wins? Women, caring and disability', *Disability, Handicap and Society*, 7 (2): 167–75.
Lane, K. 1995. 'The medical model of the body as a site of risk: a case study of childbirth, in J. Gabe (ed.), *Medicine, Health and Risk: Sociological Approaches*. Oxford: Blackwell.
Mason, J. 1996. *Qualitative Researching*. London: Sage.
Mason, M. 1992. 'A nineteen-parent family', in J. Morris (ed.), *Alone Together: Voices of Single Mothers*. London: The Women's Press.
Morris, J. 1991. *Pride against Prejudice: Transforming Attitudes to Disability*. London: The Women's Press.
———. 1992. (ed.) *Alone Together: Voices of Single Mothers*. London: The Women's Press.
———. 1995. 'Creating a space for absent voices: disabled women's experience of receiving assistance with daily living activities', *Feminist Review*, 51 (Autumn): 68–93.
———. 1996. (ed.) *Encounters with Strangers: Feminism and Disability*. London: The Women's Press.
Morris, V. 1996. *Lives Worth Living: Women's Experience of Chronic Illness*. London: Pandora, Harper Collins.
Oakley, A. 1981. *From Here to Maternity: Becoming a Mother*. Harmondsworth: Penguin.
Oliver, M. 1996. *Understanding Disability*. London: Macmillan.
Parsons, E. and Atkinson, P. 1992. 'Lay constructions of genetic risk', *Sociology of Health and Illness*, 14 (4): 437–55.
Plummer, K. 1995. *Telling Sexual Stories: Power, Change and Social Worlds*. London: Routledge.
Roberts, H. 1981. (ed.) *Women, Health and Reproduction*. London: Routledge and Kegan Paul.
Swain, J. et al. (eds), *Disabling Barriers, Enabling Environments*. London: Sage.
Williams, G. 1996a. 'Irving Zola (1935–1994): An appreciation', *Sociology of Health and Illness*, 18 (1): 107–25.
———. 1996b. 'Representing disability: some questions of phenomenology and politics', in C. Barnes and G. Mercer (eds), *Exploring the Divide: Illness and Disability*. Leeds: The Disability Press.

PART 4

Technology and Rehabilitation

Introduction

Stuart Blume & Myriam Winance

Artificial limbs, wheelchairs and other 'compensatory technologies' have a very long history. By the nineteenth century, specialist manufacturers of artificial limbs were to be found in many industrialised countries. At the end of the First World War (1914–18), hundreds of thousands of servicemen who had lost a limb in battle returned home. They were amputees, but also heroes whose reintegration into social and economic life was a matter of national concern. In Britain, for example, the government guaranteed each returning amputee an artificial limb of good quality. It was the status of the amputees as ex-servicemen who had lost a limb serving their country that was seen as justifying a collective effort at helping them reintegrate into the community. War has been a major stimulus to subsequent developments in prosthetics. It has influenced the organisation of the industry, the technologies available for prosthetics production, and, above all, it stimulated the emergence of rehabilitation medicine as a specialised approach to treating people with disabilities. With the emergence of rehabilitation medicine in the 1950s and 1960s, care and treatment moved into specialised medical centres. The objective was to provide patients with both restored function and a place in society. A more critical interpretation is that rehabilitation practices and technologies are there to ensure conformity with social and aesthetic norms and values.

Many professions collaborate in these specialised rehabilitation centres, and they make use of a wide range of technologies. Though a medical doctor is typically its senior member, the rehabilitation team may also include an occupational or physical therapist, a social worker, and a prosthetist or specialist technician. It is the physician, usually but not always a specialist in rehabilitation medicine, who advises the patient about the kind of assistive device he or she requires. In recent years, increasingly sophisticated medical and engineering sciences have contributed to the design of new prosthetics and other assistive technologies. Advances in materials science, in computing and information technology, and in physiology and neurology, all have played a part. Some researchers have found that rehabilitation engineers have different ideas about this than people with disabilities. Engineers tend to like 'high tech' solutions that are not always user-friendly. They may resent users' attempts to modify the device, or use it in unanticipated and creative ways. On the other hand, there are examples of organisations of people with disabilities having major influence on the design and production of devices tailored to their own desires and aspirations. Wheelchairs designed specifically for the use of sportsmen and sportswomen with disabilities are an example.

The question of how the western model of prosthetics services and rehabilitation medicine became established outside Europe and North America is a complex one. Relatively little has been written about it. In some cases, colonial relations played a part. For example, the first orthopaedic appliance workshop in Malaysia was established in 1937 by a British doctor. It became part of the National Leprosy Control Centre. Quite differently, an orthopaedics and prosthetics service was established in Vietnam in 1947 during the war against the French colonists. In more recent years, international NGOs have often played a key role, sometimes at their own initiative, and sometimes after being approached by the government of a developing country.

In the 1970s, people began to question the organisation of rehabilitation. Perhaps institutional care, separating the disabled person from his or her family and community, was not the best approach. It was at this time that the World Health Organisation introduced a new approach to disability prevention and rehabilitation known as Community-Based Rehabilitation (CBR). Its aim was to make rehabilitation services available to all people with disabilities, using the resources of the local community, with more specialised services available at the district level and in national referral centres. Gradually, influenced by debates about disability taking place in the west, the meaning of the concept changed. In 1994, three UN agencies agreed on a new definition of the term:

Community-based rehabilitation (CBR) is a strategy, within community development, for the rehabilitation, equalisation of opportunities, and social integration of all children and adults with disabilities. CBR is implemented through the combined efforts of disabled people themselves, their families and communities, and the appropriate health, education, vocational and social services.

The emphasis now was on the achievement of full participation, and a much wider range of barriers to participation had to be tackled. Persons with disabilities themselves, and organisations active on their behalf, were to be involved in planning the services needed. The term 'rehabilitation' was seen by some as too medical and too narrow for the new approach. In many developing countries, it proved difficult, if not impossible, to involve people with disabilities in the rehabilitation process, partly, it is said, because of continuing medical dominance. Some critics have argued that essentially western models and technologies did not achieve their expected effects because local values and traditions were not respected. Thus, Ingstad (see Further Reading) explains that CBR failed in Botswana because the ideological preconceptions on which it is based—an ideology of equal rights and of state responsibility for the weak—were not those of Tswana society. The western rehabilitation discourse, she explains, is based on the idea of individuals having equal rights. By contrast, and hindering the adoption of rehabilitation programmes, was the hierarchical nature of Tswana society, 'with some people being ranked higher than others by virtue of descent and wealth.' Ingstad suggests that when technically-inclined experts argue that modern information and computer technologies can bring about the integration of people with disabilities in developing countries, they totally fail to understand the role that culture plays. Technology and rehabilitation medicine have an important role to play, but it is a role that cannot be understood independently of the social and cultural characteristics of the society.

Just as questions were raised about the appropriate organisation of rehabilitation services, so they were raised also about the technologies of rehabilitation. How well could, and did, assistive devices developed and produced in 'northern' countries meet the needs of people with disabilities in 'southern' countries? It is partly a question of resources: the cost, the materials available, and the maintenance that a sophisticated device requires. But it is also a question of the compatibility of a device with local work routines, geography and ways of life. Considerable discussion has ensued regarding local production of 'appropriate' assistive technologies suited to local conditions, resources and ways of life. Perhaps the most famous example of an 'appropriate technology' is the Jaipur foot, initially developed by Professor P.K. Sethi in the 1960s and 1970s. Today, variants of the original rubber foot and the original aluminium prosthesis for below-the-knee amputees are produced in many developing countries. Imported wheelchairs, too, failed to meet the needs of many users in developing countries. It was local innovators, often working with local associations of disabled people, or with NGOs, that began to develop and produce mobility devices fitted to rural surroundings, or durable enough for village life, or at the right height for women accustomed to cooking at ground level. This is not to say that an easy consensus emerged. In areas where many national and international NGOs are active, each may have its own favoured technology.

Although prosthetic technologies play an important role in rehabilitation medicine, the ways in which people incorporate the technologies into their lives involve more than the formally defined purposes of rehabilitation. People with disabilities ask themselves, 'What are now my possibilities?' Both imaginatively and practically, they try to work out how the new device can best be incorporated into their lives. These issues are discussed in detail in Part 4 in the articles by Kurzman and Kohrman, both anthropologists. Steven Kurzman, speaking from personal experience, explores how amputees and prosthetists, using the language of biomechanics, manage to communicate with each other in the fitting of a prosthesis. Matthew Kohrman's paper discusses how a technology not only helps individual people with disabilities change their own lives, but can also serve to project a different—more empowered or competent—image to society at large. Finally, Susie Miles, who has practical experience with an international NGO, discusses a number of crucial issues regarding CBR. While focusing, in particular, on problematic relations with organisations of people with disabilities, Miles' article at the same time points to the issues that will be presented in Part 5 of this Reader.

14

'There's no language for this': Communication and Alignment in Contemporary Prosthetocs

Steven Kurzman

This essay is about how contemporary lower-extremity amputees and prosthetists communicate with each other during the process of fitting and aligning a prosthesis in a clinic. Amputees approach the use of prostheses from a subjective perspective, while prosthetists speak about fitting and aligning prostheses in the language of biomechanics. Since fit and alignment are essential to using a prosthesis, prosthetists and amputees must find ways to communicate with one another about prostheses and the subjective experience of using them. This essay describes how they collaboratively invent a language to do this. I explore the clinical language, silence, and experience of prostheses in an effort to imbue this text with a flavour of these two perspectives, and to show how they are in embodied dialogue with each other. I am both a cultural anthropologist and a below-knee amputee, and this dialogue also expresses my own peculiar position during my dissertation fieldwork in the prosthetics field in Chicago. Ultimately, I believe that juxtaposing the subjective experience of using a prosthesis and the clinical work of constructing bodies has potential to disrupt our habitus (in Marcel Mauss's terms), or learned techniques,

---

Kurzman, S. 2002. 'There is no language for this', in K. Ott, D. Serlin and S. Mihm (eds), *Artificial Parts, Practical Lives*. New York: New York University Press, pp. 227–48.

of how we think about, talk about, and use our bodies for walking and able-bodiedness (Mauss, 1992).

'THERE'S NO LANGUAGE FOR THIS'

The process of fitting and dynamically aligning a prosthesis is integral to making and using one, and Kevin and I were ready to start. Kevin is a certified prosthetist who, during my fieldwork, worked at a prosthetics shop that served as one of my field sites. We were working on an informal experiment, a prototype for an inexpensive, easy-to-use below-knee prosthesis intended for geriatric amputees. It was a collaborative project in which Kevin designed the limb and did most of the fabrication, while I tested it and offered feedback. And now it was time to align the check socket.

As we entered the fitting room and closed the sliding door behind us, we shifted our roles from prosthetist and amputee/researcher to clinician and patient. Half kidding and half serious, Kevin began to speak in a more clinical tone, addressing me as 'Mr Kurzman' and giving me gentle but authoritative descriptions and instructions about how to use the new prosthesis. After removing my everyday leg, I pulled on silicone and cloth stump socks and donned the prosthesis. I stood up, shifted my weight around, and began to walk in the parallel bars. I didn't get very far, though, before the fibreglass tape binding the check socket to the pylon ripped with a loud cracking sound. After a quick repair, I walked in the bars for a few minutes and, quickly getting a feel for the limb, moved out of the fitting room and started trotting up and down the hallway. I tried to walk evenly and smoothly, looking straight ahead, and paying attention to where my body was and how it was moving. How were my feet rolling over during the gait cycle? Was my trunk leaning after heel-off? Meanwhile, Kevin gazed intently at my feet and body, asking himself similar questions, while Noah and Milton, the two shop technicians, cracked jokes about the prosthesis hurting.

After a few minutes of this, I informed Kevin that the prosthesis didn't feel right. He posed questions in an effort to pinpoint the problem: Where does it hurt? Does it feel like you're walking up a hill? Does it feel like you're walking into a hole? We moved to the workshop in the back of the facility, where I doffed the prosthesis and he made some adjustments. I was soon pacing the hallway again and we repeated the cycle of walking, feeling, observing, questioning and readjusting. My attention focused on my legs and the effort of thinking about what it feels like to walk and how to articulate this feeling, while Kevin alternately observed my legs, face and body language. We repeated the process over and over again, grinding out tight areas of the socket, plantarflexing or dorsiflexing the foot, adducting and a-b-ducting the socket, and toeing the foot in and out.[1] 'Is that better or worse now? Or the same?' he asked after each adjustment.

Finally, we reached that moment when the prosthesis just felt right and I stopped thinking about walking because it no longer felt remarkable. I began walking at a faster pace and stopped looking at my feet. My face exuded the expression of one who has just figured something out. Kevin noticed this, as did Noah and Milton, especially when I cheered and raised my arms like a goal post. We got it right: the socket was comfortable and the prosthesis was aligned. Back in the fitting room, we were chatting about the process and its difficulties when Kevin remarked thoughtfully, 'You know, there's no language for this....'

COLLABORATION

What Kevin meant was: there is no shared language available with which amputees and prosthetists can communicate about aligning or using a prosthesis. Kevin's comment indicates the importance of communication in the prosthetics clinic, and, implicitly, the importance of amputees' subjective experience in the process of alignment. The process is so fascinatingly nuanced, so intimately customised, and the communication often so difficult, it was amazing that we could fit and align a prosthesis at all. A full day at a prosthetics shop participating in clinical situations usually left me completely stunned, and a lasting impression I carry from fieldwork is that it is a minor miracle that anything actually works in prosthetics.

[1] Plantarflexing is bending your ankle to point your toes downwards, and dorsiflexing is pointing your toes upwards. Abduction and adduction are movements away from or toward a midline or reference point, respectively. Prosthetists frequently spell out the 'ab' sound of abduction as 'a-b-duction' to avoid confusion with the similar sounding 'adduction'.

Thus, the purpose of this essay is to explore how anything does work in a prosthetics clinic. I argue that lower-extremity amputees and prosthetists collaboratively communicate, and that amputees' subjective experience, whether communicated verbally or through performance, is crucial to this collaboration. Alignment itself is an important ritualistic performance of integrating or embodying a prosthesis, and the ability to communicate during and about the alignment process is a key to understanding how anything works in prosthetics, both inside the clinic and out.

Medical anthropologists often approach clinical communication in terms of the dichotomy between subjective experience and objective biomedical authority, and the difficulty of describing the experience of illness, pain and suffering from within this dualism. In their essay, 'The Mindful Body: A Prolegomenon to Future Work in Medical Anthropology', Schepper-Hughes and Lock (1987) argue that the Cartesian dualism of mind and body is so strongly embedded in biomedicine that it colours our attempts to describe the experience of illness. They note that there is no language to describe this: 'As both medical anthropologists and clinicians struggle to view humans and experience of illness and suffering from an integrated perspective, they often find themselves trapped by the Cartesian legacy. We lack a precise vocabulary with which to deal with mind-body-society interactions, and so are left suspended in hyphens, testifying to the disconnectedness of our thoughts.'

It is indeed difficult to escape the material dualism of body and technology that permeates the prosthetics clinic, and, as Kevin pointed out, amputees and prosthetists do lack a shared vocabulary that fully describes body-prosthesis interactions. But amputees learn how to articulate their experience of prostheses, and good prosthetists tacitly recognise the importance of the subjective component of prostheses and often rely on their patients to help them understand problems in which the technical and the experiential blur together.

This may be due in part to a notable difference between the epistemologies of the biomedical clinic and the more biomechanical prosthetics clinic. Although the experience of aligning a prosthesis may involve pain and suffering for new amputees being fitted for their first prosthesis, the subjective experience of the prosthetics clinic is generally not about illness, but rather about integrating and embodying technology. As Martin (1994) describes it, biomedicine has long conceptualised the body as a fortress, or a closed system under attack from external contaminants. But prosthetists tend to consider bodies as biomechanical systems in conjunction with prostheses, and are generally more interested in the interface between bodies and prostheses as a system, rather than in the body itself. They work within a tension between the claimed objectivity of biomechanics and the acknowledged relativity of prostheses to amputees' bodies. The technical and scientific influence of biomechanics is a key part of the increasingly medical and clinical quality of prosthetists' work, and is also important to speaking authoritatively to patients about treatment. But prosthetists believe that prostheses are relative to amputees' bodies and must be integrated into the subjective experiences of bodies and mobility. Since most prosthetists have not had this subjective experience, clear communication greatly facilitates this process.[2]

Prosthetists talk about bodies in terms of anatomy and physiology, and walking in terms of gait cycle and biomechanics. Many older prosthetists have learned gait analysis and alignment through apprenticeship and practice rather than formal education, but younger prosthetists learn these ideas as a didactic element of their increasingly medical prosthetics certification course as well as clinical practice. These terms are extremely precise and descriptive for discussing gait, but they obviously don't describe the subjective experience of walking. For instance, you can say that a foot is too plantarflexed, resulting in the patient vaulting over the foot and the trunk leaning medially, and you can say that dorsiflexing the foot will probably help normalise gait. But this does not capture the feeling of walking over a plantarflexed foot, of trying to roll over toes that feel strangely resistant, or of vaulting over the foot and momentarily feeling your body catapulted just a bit higher, with just a slightly better view of things, and then falling back down onto your other foot. And while prosthetists would spot this particular example in their own terms, they rely on amputees at other times for subjective feedback in fitting and alignment.

[2] There are actually a number of jokes in the field about whether amputee prosthetists are the best or worst prosthetists as a consequence of having had this experience. One opinion is that they are likely to be good, out of empathy and the embodied knowledge that comes with wearing a prosthesis. The other side jokes that amputee prosthetists are horrible clinicians, because they are jaded and don't communicate with, or listen to, their patients.

Amputees frequently have great difficulty articulating this verbally. The subjective experience of using a prosthesis disrupts language. This is especially true of new amputees, for whom an amputation is still a great shock to the body. Stumps are perplexing and delicate new body parts, and phantom limbs are somewhat disconcerting, distracting, and often painful at first. Compounding this problem, wearing a prosthesis is initially very uncomfortable. Part of your body, which was not evolutionarily designed to bear weight, is suddenly bearing your weight in motion, while your stump is encased in cloth socks and plastic. It is all so supremely alien that it is extremely difficult to describe the sensation at all, much less respond to the question as to whether it 'feels right'. Longer-term amputees learn from experience what feels right and what they like, and maybe even how to communicate that to their prosthetist. But for newer amputees, it's often frustratingly difficult to know, not to mention to articulate to the prosthetist, how it should feel. And yet, despite the fact that 'there's no language for this' or, perhaps, that there are two languages for this, every time a prosthetist and amputee meet clinically, they must invent a way of communicating about the prosthesis and how it feels. Alignment and clinical interactions, in general, are interactive performances through which amputees and prosthetists communicate. The communication is important not only because fitting and alignment are crucial to a prosthesis being comfortable and easy to use, but also because such communication helps to negotiate clinical roles, bodily boundaries, and working rapport.

The vitality of clinical communication is most apparent when it goes wrong. In addition to Kevin's shop, I also did fieldwork at another prosthetics shop, which was more working-class in flavour.[3] Don was working with a new patient named George, and felt that his previous prosthesis, which had been made at another shop, was too short and caused gait problems. So he made his new prosthesis taller, at what he

[3] Prosthetists make a subtle differentiation between themselves and practitioners. Practitioners are 'old school', often having learned in apprenticeships, or grown up working in their fathers' shops, while prosthetists are more academically trained. This also translates into a difference of emphasis on technical skill and craftsmanship versus theoretical knowledge and clinical skills, and a class division between working-class limb shops and more middle-class prosthetics clinics.

believed to be the correct height. George felt adamantly that his new leg was too tall, but couldn't elaborate a more specific reason for not liking it. It didn't hurt; it was just too tall and didn't feel right. They were both getting a bit crabby when Don turned to face me and two physical therapy students visiting the shop for the day and hissed, 'Half the difficulty of prosthetics is understanding *what the [expletive]* the patient is talking about.'

This sentiment is sometimes mutual for amputees, and I will turn to a discussion of alignment in order to explain how they do manage to understand each other. Alignment refers to how a prosthesis is positioned and moves in relation to an amputee's body. It is the process of locating a prosthesis relative to an amputee's body and mechanically manipulating that relationship in order to facilitate the amputee's ability to comfortably integrate and embody the prosthesis. The mechanics and physical construction involved in integrating this technology into bodies are as important as the physical foundation of embodying prostheses. In other words, alignment involves physical as well as discursive construction of bodies.

ALIGNMENT

The alignment of joints and limbs to each other is, to a certain degree, embodied in common sense: it's difficult to walk with your foot pointing backward, and it's hard to feed yourself if your forearm is too long. Although dynamically aligning prostheses is basically a process of getting the foot pointed in the right direction, it is much more nuanced than this sounds. In theory, as prosthetists learn during their training, alignment is based on biomechanical principles and the concept of normal gait. But in the clinic, normal gait is more a guideline for how to observe patients and arrive at a gait that is 'good enough': an amalgam of normal gait, symmetry, and subjective comfort and satisfaction.

If we had gone through a formal patient exam, Kevin would have inquired as to my age, height, weight, cause and date of amputation, general health, illness complications, and physical activity level. Then he would have palpated my stump, checking for a number of physical landmarks and characteristics. On a below-knee amputee, for example, a prosthetist checks for stump shape, bony prominences, skin type, and other characteristics that figure into prostheses in terms of what areas of an amputee's stump will bear weight, what areas won't accept pressure without pain, and which kind of socket and suspension (method of keeping the prosthesis on the body) will best fit the person. For example, bony prominences such as the tibial tubercle and the fibular head are areas that suffer pain under pressure. Areas such as the patellar tendon, tibial flare, and interosseous region will comfortably support weight. Neuromas or 'trigger spots' (balled-up nerve endings near the end of the stump) are very intolerant of pressure.

The patient exam for prosthetists is a tactile process of mapping stumps and marking reference points to get to know the body. This tactile knowledge becomes a basis for deciding what the most appropriate type of prosthesis is for the patient, especially with regard to the socket and suspension. Bob, another prosthetist, one day pointed out to me how patients' bodies either 'indicated' or 'contra-indicated' certain styles of sockets and suspension. I didn't fully understand what he meant until later, when we were on a house call to one of his patients. Mr Gambino was having difficulty donning his prosthesis. He was an above-knee amputee with a suction socket, which requires a good deal of pulling effort to don. You don a thin stump sock and then essentially pull your stump into the socket by pulling the sock through the socket and out a hole in the bottom. Bob pointed out that Mr Gambino's effort to pull his stump into the socket was inappropriate because he had a heart condition and shouldn't be exerting himself that heavily. His health 'contra-indicated' this type of prosthesis, but the doctor, who lacked any expertise regarding prostheses, had written a very specific—and inappropriate—prescription.[4]

Since Kevin and I were already acquainted, and even had a design in mind, we omitted the patient exam, normally the initial step, and proceeded directly to casting. Casting is a continuation of the exam, and is basically an opportunity for the prosthetist to make a visual and tactile

[4] Prescriptions, which can be worded specifically or generally (e.g. left below-knee prosthesis), are *de facto* necessary for prostheses because third-party payers require a prescription for reimbursement. Prescriptions also create a line of communication between prosthetists and doctors, and, increasingly, a rehabilitation-clinic team.

inspection of his or her patient. Mapping landmarks prior to casting is essentially a way of knowing the body, reading its terrain in a very tactile sense, and then mapping it. Kevin had me don a thin cloth sock, called a casting sock, and made measurements of length and circumference at intervals along the length of the stump. Then, using a grease pencil dipped in water, he marked and defined landmarks on my stump. The pencil marks on the casting sock transfer to the inside of the cast and serve as guides for later modifications. He grabbed a couple of rolls of plaster of Paris bandage and, unwinding one and dipping it in warm water, began wrapping my stump and knee in warm plaster. When the cast had dried, we pulled it off and checked to ensure that the grease-pencil marks matched up with their corresponding landmarks inside the cast. Casting is important because it's surprisingly easy to mistakenly make bad markings or take wrong measurements, which can add to the difficulty of making an accurately fitting socket. It's an uncomfortable moment of crossing bodily boundaries: prosthetists and technicians have to learn to touch people in a way that would otherwise be inappropriate, and amputees have to get used to having their stump palpated, squeezed and caressed. But it's also crucial to the process of knowing and mapping stumps and bodies and how they experience these tactile sensations.

Kevin filled the finished cast with plaster and, after it hardened, gave me the tedious chore of stripping the embedded plaster of Paris, leaving a solid, positive impression of my stump. He then modified the cast into a desirable negative image of the socket, using rasps and other tools to do the sculpting. The shop technicians made a check socket, or test socket, by wrapping the cast in an oven-heated piece of polyethylene plastic and applying a vacuum. They 'broke out' the socket by using an airhammer to remove the plaster, and Kevin attached a pylon (a hollow pole) and foot, and put the limb in bench alignment, a generic position for prostheses. We were ready for dynamic fitting and alignment.

I donned the prosthesis and stood up, shifting my weight back and forth to gauge the height and try to gain a sense of balance. I thought about how the socket felt and where it bore my weight as I shifted onto and off it. Kevin, sitting on one of the stools on caster-rollers that seem to occupy every prosthetics shop fitting room, checked my height, first visually and then by digging his fingers uncomfortably into the flesh above my hips. As I stood still, he scooted around me to check the pylon, making sure it was vertical in both sagittal and coronal planes. I began walking between the parallel bars. I focused on trying to walk consistently, and paid attention to how the socket felt. Kevin hunkered down on his stool at the end of the bars and watched me walk toward him, looking at where the pylon was at mid-stance, when the foot was flat on the floor bearing my weight. Then he scooted to the side and watched the pylon from the sagittal plane to ensure that it was vertical at mid-stance from this view.

After a few minutes, he had me sit down and doff the prosthesis. I peeled off the layers of socks and silicone, and Kevin inspected my stump for redness, a sign of excessive pressure and friction. He also used the back of his hand to check skin temperature on the weight-bearing areas. The fit was fine but the alignment was off, so Kevin made the adjustments using his Allen wrench. In common endoskeletal prostheses, the socket and foot are connected using a hollow aluminium pylon and a pair of titanium pyramids, or mounts, one at either end.[5] By adjusting hex screws in the mounts, the prosthetist can move the foot and socket in relation to the body. The processes of casting, fitting and alignment are physically customised techniques, intimately connecting bodies with prostheses.

COMMUNICATION

Whenever I have been fit for a prosthesis, whether in the United States, India or Cambodia, the first question is always something to the effect: 'Does it hurt?' Prostheses may be uncomfortable on occasion, especially at first, but they aren't supposed to hurt. Pain may be the fragmentation of language, but it is the opening of communication about how a prosthesis feels (Scarry, 1985). If pain is 'the unmaking of the world', alignment is one way of remaking the world for new amputees. They know when their prostheses hurt, and will call it to the attention of their prosthetist even when they are unable to articulate the cause. If they don't say anything, they still communicate through their performance on a painful socket.

[5] An endoskeletal prosthesis is an assemblage of the socket and connecting hardware, which may be covered with cosmetically shaped and coloured foam and skin to resemble an organic limb. An exoskeletal prosthesis is a plastic shell incorporating the socket within the shell.

For example, an unwillingness of amputees to put their weight fully on the limb is often a sign of pain or of not yet trusting the prosthesis.

Although most lower-extremity amputees are interested in walking well and passing as non-amputees, they don't speak in terms of normal gait. From an amputee's perspective, dynamic alignment is about making sure the prosthesis feels right, learning how to walk again, and, on some level, beginning the process of embodying and habituating to a new limb. Amputees often speak metaphorically about their prostheses to describe what they feel like. The ultimate metaphor for many new amputees is their previous organic limb, particularly as it functioned and enabled them when they were younger. Lance, one of Kevin's patients, often compared his prosthesis to his organic leg, but differentiated between cosmesis and feeling. He and his wife were happy that his prosthesis resembled his leg, but he had difficulty adjusting to it, partly because it didn't feel like his old leg. In a variant on this, longer-term amputees often compare their new prosthesis to their last one. Amputees become strongly habituated to their prostheses, particularly to the fit of the socket and the style of suspension. This is an important issue for older men who lost limbs during the Second World War and the Korean War, many of whom still prefer the style of limb they started wearing in the 1940s or 1950s. It is also a problem, as older practitioners retire and are replaced by younger prosthetists who lack the woodworking and leatherworking skills to continue in this tradition. And both of these metaphors put prosthetists in somewhat of a bind, since no one can adequately replace an organic limb, nor can they exactly recreate the idiosyncratic fit of a previous prosthesis.

Longer-term amputees also share a few stock metaphors with prosthetists, who reproduce them in prosthetics school and in the clinic. For example, the feeling of 'walking into a hole' corresponds, for prosthetists, to excessive dorsiflexion in the foot. Imagine that you are walking down a steep hill, and think about the feeling of walking heavily on your heels and having your foot quickly slap down flat when your foot rolls down the hill: that is the feeling that 'walking into a hole' describes for amputees. Likewise, the feeling of 'walking up a hill' corresponds to excessive plantarflexion. Think about the feeling of walking up a steep slope and how you're pretty light on your heel, but spend a lot of time on your toes, maybe even actively pushing yourself off as you roll over your toes. This is the feeling described as 'walking up a hill' by amputees, and it means the prosthetist needs to dorsiflex the foot. These metaphors are interesting, not only because of the easy correspondence between feeling and foot position, but because they make use of our common, nearly intuitive experience of walking on these terrains. Obviously, there's not actually a slope in the clinic, but the position of the foot comes to embody the landscape, and the prosthesis becomes a hill or a hole.

Other metaphors describe prostheses in terms of parts of the foot that may not even physically exist in the structure of the prosthesis, such as heel and toes. Both amputees and prosthetists often speak of prosthetic feet as having or not having toes, or as having soft or stiff heels or toes. During alignment, toes can also be turned too far in or out, giving one the odd sensation of rolling over a foot that isn't pointing in the right direction. At the prosthetics school where I conducted fieldwork, students gave professional patients a wide variety of feet in order to solicit diverse opinions from their patients during critique. One of the patients was trying a new brand of foot called Flex-Foot for the first time. Flex-Foot feet are renowned for their springy quality, because they are basically a long keel of carbon fibre. The patient commented that he liked the foot because 'it has toes.' But this is always relative to the person using the component. Brian, an engineering graduate student at the lab and a bilateral above-knee amputee himself, didn't like the same brand of foot because he felt it had 'too much toe' and made it difficult for him to roll over the foot.

Amputees are remarkably inventive in creating their own metaphors to describe prostheses, fit and alignment. One of the professional patients at the prosthetics school, a young man who worked in construction, gave a funny running commentary one day on the practice prosthesis his student had just made for him. As he paced back and forth between the parallel bars during critique, he described why he didn't like a certain new, lightweight prosthesis (which was interesting, because lightness in a prosthesis is often equated with better quality). 'It's like forks, you know? My normal leg, it's like a silver fork. It's solid, sturdy; you can really feel it when you pick it up. But this thing,' he waved the new leg dismissively, 'just feels like a plastic fork. Like it might snap in half if I walked too hard on it.' Upon completing his critique, the senior instructor took the opportunity to point out the importance of occupation (and, implicitly, class as a factor influencing choice of occupation and physical activity level) as a consideration for prosthesis design.

This raises the issue of how to talk about feet. Longer-term amputees often compare different prosthetic feet using these metaphors, but this is largely a personal preference depending on many factors. While writing this essay, I realised that I've never actually had an extensive conversation with another long-term amputee about feet, because we always speak in shorthand, metaphors and nods. For example, I've heard people refer to a model called a SACH foot as 'dead' or feeling 'like a doorstop', and understood exactly what they meant: that the foot had no spring, and rolled over with a particularly inactive feeling. I first became aware of the difficulty of describing what a foot should feel like while participating as a subject in an engineering experiment. Andy, one of the graduate students, was collecting data on the alignment of four different prosthetic feet for his M.S. thesis. Many trials were involved, requiring me to walk on four very different feet, which Mark, the senior instructor at the prosthetics school, worked to align. Following the first trial, I wrote in my field notes:

> The Flex-Walk was intriguing, but not very appealing to me. It feels like a giant spring; I could feel it load and compress when I stepped onto the heel, and then could feel it unload and propel me when I rolled over onto the toe. It didn't feel at all like a foot. This makes me think that the function, and the sensation or experience of walking on a particular foot, are two different things. The Flex-Foot is functionally attractive, but doesn't feel like a foot should feel, which I found disconcerting. Mark asked me if I felt like 'the foot is walking me,' and I said yes. It felt as though it was propelling me, and I felt compelled to walk faster. Part of this wasn't just the spring loading and unloading, but the very quick roll-over.

I borrowed the Flex-Walk and learned how to use it for walking and cycling. I grew to like it and, following the second trial, wrote in my notes:

> I also had a surprising reaction to the Flex-Walk this time: I liked it. I remember that I didn't like it last time because of the bounce, which was so severe that I felt a bit out of control of the foot. For whatever reason, the bounce wasn't that bad this time. In neutral, it did have a real strong kick to it, where my knee felt as though it were being pushed up and the foot

> kicked straight out when I was rolling off the toes. Apparently too much toe, but after Mark moved the knee and toed it out a bit, it felt pretty good. The bounce was nice and controllable, and worked together with a smooth roll-over to feel somewhat like a foot. Got some crazy compulsion to run on the thing, and had a great time running in the halls and on the E. Superior sidewalk. I can totally understand why athletes use Flex-Feet; it was amazingly easy to run on. I sort of glided along on this very smooth foot, with subtle heel and toe. After occasionally clomping along on my Carbon Copy 2, it was really fun.... My favourite overall would have to be the Flex-Foot, but how would I explain this turnaround in opinion? It definitely feels different from other prosthetic feet—I remember thinking this during the previous trials—and I think I was able to use that difference to my advantage this time, rather than be annoyed by it. I didn't feel a distinct heel or keel or toe on it, whereas the other feet all have these identifiable foot characteristics. In some ways, it may be hard to judge as a prosthetic foot (e.g. there is no discernible keel).

At first, I had to resort to the concepts of spring from biomechanical engineers, and roll-over from gait analysis, to describe how the foot felt. I was at a loss for embodied language, except that it didn't feel like a foot and it felt external to me. After some practice and thought, I was able to describe how my body moved with the foot and why it didn't initially 'feel like a foot should feel.'

PERFORMING ALIGNMENT

Despite all these ways of talking about prostheses and how they feel, amputees are frequently rendered inarticulate about their prostheses. I have been in that position myself, and it is frustrating to walk back and forth, knowing that something just doesn't feel right, but not feeling able to describe what doesn't feel right. During one of my first days in the field, I observed a clinical interaction between Mr Mitchell, a retired steel-mill worker, and his prosthetist, Mark. Mr Mitchell was actually Kevin's patient, but Mark was aligning him on his new prosthesis because Kevin was out of the shop. While Kevin is remarkably skilled in communicating with patients in lay terms, Mark deals with his patients much more clinically.

The contrast was striking as he addressed Mr Mitchell in clinical language, while the latter responded in lay language about how his body felt. He felt the pressure in the back of the prosthesis was too tight, right where the shelf of the prosthesis presses against the gastrocnemius muscles, a key weight-bearing area. He couldn't pinpoint a problem but simply felt it was too tight, just a bit uncomfortable, and continued to pace back and forth between the parallel bars, muttering to himself. Mark was uninterested in grinding out and irrevocably loosening the socket so soon in the process, feeling that a new prosthesis was bound to feel a little snug. There was a stalemate, in which Mr Mitchell paced and muttered, while Mark stood with his arms crossed. Though there was no mutually satisfactory resolution, Mr Mitchell eventually agreed to give the prosthesis a spin in the outside world and return the following week.

Alignment and gait analysis are always performative, but even more so for inarticulate patients such as Mr Mitchell. When the communicative performance of walking and analysing gait breaks down, amputees and prosthetists utilise other means to perform alignment. One of these means is donning, using, and doffing the prosthesis. One day, Bob and I went out on a house call to the home of Mr Gambino (the same man mentioned earlier, whose heart condition contra-indicated his prosthesis), who was having difficulties donning his prosthesis. The first thing Bob did was have Mr Gambino doff his prosthesis and then go through the process of donning it, standing and walking on it, and then doffing it again. Bob noticed that, because Mr Gambino failed to pull his stump deeply enough into the socket, the prosthesis wasn't totally secure. So he reviewed instructions on how to don it, and guided Mr Gambino tactilely through the performance of donning his prosthesis correctly.

Another form of performance is much less conscious—on the amputee's part at least—and involves the prosthetist reading the amputee's body. Prosthetists read body language, facial expressions and walking speed to gauge their patients' comfort with their alignment, and the colour, texture and temperature of skin on a stump to gauge socket fit. In an important sense, amputees' bodies perform and communicate through touch and without active intention.

TECHNOLOGISATION

Prostheses are an important idiom for expressing emotions of loss, fright and joy, and negotiating issues such as body image, physical function and the ability to live independently. Kleinman uses the concept of somatisation to describe the use of bodies as an idiom for expressing personal, interpersonal and social distress (Kleinman, 1995). The analogous concept in the more biomechanical world of prosthetics is technologisation, which describes how amputees and prosthetists use prosthetics technology as an idiom for expressing and dealing with personal and social distress. In fact, much of alignment and clinical interaction is about technologisation, in which the prosthesis becomes a common ground for amputees and prosthetists to work through non-technical issues.

An important factor in all of this is emotion. The majority of amputees I met in clinical situations were there for their first prosthesis, which meant they were also learning to walk again. This is an emotionally charged moment, especially for older amputees, many of whom, irrespective of amputation, have concerns about balance and stability and are afraid of falling. These concerns are exacerbated by the fact that they are essentially walking on stilts now. For example, Lance told me that walking was actually not the hard part for him, but getting his balance while standing: 'getting his motor going,' in his words. Once he started to walk, it became easier, but he still remained fearful.

Yet fright is often mixed with nervous excitement and joy. Mr Konner, a patient of Don, was still fairly young but had a particularly brittle case of diabetes, which had led to bilateral below-knee amputations in his forties. He had spent an extensive postoperative recovery period in bed, and had recently started physical therapy. He was openly scared that he wouldn't be able to walk, because it had been so long since he had been on his feet. Nervous, excited questions for me bubbled out of him as Don worked on his prostheses in the workshop. Do they leave the legs unfinished like they are now, or will they look more like real legs? When does it start to feel less weird and more comfortable? How long will it take to learn to drive a car again? Will I be able to walk up stairs again? Don sensed his nervousness and was firm with him, and commanded him to stand up and walk. As Mr Konner stood and took his first steps, his face was beatific and beaming, and the electricity of his excitement at being able to walk was palpable in the room. Don was also pleased by the success, and I began to suspect that the thrill of enabling people to walk for the first time—again—is a powerful emotional draw for prosthetists.

Alignment and clinical interactions were highly emotional experiences for me, too. Prior to my fieldwork, I had forgotten how horribly uncomfortable prostheses are initially, how little sense it made to learn to adjust them, how alien they feel, and how disembodying it can be, during the first disoriented months following an amputation, to pull a sock, first try, onto a foot that is no longer there. Over the course of nearly a year and a half of fieldwork for my dissertation, I participated in dozens of these interactions, and spent extensive periods of time with elders who had undergone recent amputations. I accompanied their prosthetist and dressed professionally, and fell into the role of 'expert amputee'. Nearly everyday, I had to counter people's expectations for their prostheses by explaining to them that I walked relatively well because I was young enough to be their grandson and had had a decade of practice. I found this emotionally exhausting and frustrating. While many ethnographers face the classic challenge of how to get inside their field sites, I often faced the opposite challenge when working with other amputees: how to gain some distance from the outpouring of emotion. Technologisation is a syncretic mixture of somatisation and medicalisation. Somatisation, borrowed from Kleinman, describes the use of bodies and, in this case, prostheses, as an important idiom for expressing individual and social distress. But prosthetics-clinic interactions are also about the medicalisation of amputation, and how distress becomes the object of treatment. It is not so much a dialogue as it is a mode of communication about this experience that is expressed through verbal and physical performance. In a sense, technologisation is about the embodied dialogue between the experience of prostheses and the observation of their biomechanical interaction with bodies, and how prosthetists and amputees communicate across this gap.

References

Kleinman, A. 1995. *Writing at the Margin: Discourse between Anthropology and Medicine*. Berkeley: University of California Press.

Martin, E. 1994. *Flexible Bodies: Tracking Immunity in American Culture from the Days of Polio to the Age of AIDS*. Boston: Beacon Press.

Mauss, M. 1992. 'Techniques of the Body', in J. Crary and S. Kwinter (eds), *Incorporations*. New York: Zone.

Scarry, E. 1985. *The Body in Pain: The Making and Unmaking of the World*. Oxford: Oxford University Press.

Schepper-Hughes, N. and Lock, M.M. 1987. 'The Mindful Body: A Prolegomenon to Future Work in Medical Anthropology', *Medical Anthropology Quarterly* 1 (1): 16–41.

15

Motorcycles for the Disabled: Mobility, Modernity and the Transformation of Experience in Urban China

Matthew Kohrman

INTRODUCTION

In September 1994, I flew from Boston to Beijing, a city where I studied for two years in the mid-1980s but subsequently barely visited. My goal that September was to interview people and officials at the Far East and South Pacific Games for the Disabled (FESPIC), and to begin my second year of dissertation research in Beijing on the social construction of disability in contemporary China.[1]

In spite of its size and pageantry, the first few days of FESPIC were ethnographic disappointments. So, by the fourth day, I was thinking of leaving the games behind and starting in earnest my second year of community research. But that afternoon, just as I was exiting a ping-pong stadium and beginning to trek across a pavilion towards another of the

Kohrman, M. 1999. 'Motorcycles for the disabled', *Culture, Medicine and Psychiatry*, 23: 133–55.

[1] Because official and local Chinese discourse rarely uses the conceptual distinctions made by the World Health Organisation (1980) between 'impairment', 'disability' and 'handicap', I do not deploy them here.

Asian Games Village's towering athletic facilities, something happened that fundamentally altered my fieldwork.

It started with a rumbling din. Then, before I knew it, I was enveloped by the deafening sound of small engines as a convoy of thirty motorcycles zoomed around the ping-pong stadium and shot across the pavilion, the riders whooping and waving as they raced by. In the twenty seconds or so it took them to pass, I realised these people were like no 'bikers' I had ever seen before. Rather than black leather, these motorcyclists wore polyester pants, bright white T-shirts and yellow-brimmed baseball caps. And instead of Harley-Davidsons, each rode a very unusual vehicle that possessed three wheels (one in front and two in the back), a seat shaped like a straight-back chair, and a chassis and fenders painted vermilion. Adding to the confusion and oddity of the sight was the fact that, next to most of the drivers was a set of crutches, precariously lashed. 'Who are all these people?' I wondered to myself. 'And why are they all driving these motorbikes?'

When I reached the other side of the pavilion, most of the riders had already dismounted and were starting to make their way into the stadium with cane or crutch. I introduced myself to a few of them and learned that these sports fans, mostly men, were all from Beijing and had been organised months earlier into a cheering squad (*la la dui*) by the China Disabled Persons' Federation, the powerful state organ run by Deng Pufang, Deng Xiaoping's paraplegic son. When I told these cheering squad members I was fascinated by their motorcycles and noted they must possess the only vehicles of this kind in Beijing, my interlocutors' faces shifted from smiles, to blank looks, to unbridled laughter. 'The only ones in Beijing? You haven't been here very long, have you?' one man said between the group's collective guffaws. 'Look around. These bikes are everywhere. There are thousands of them in this city.'

The next day, rather than attend more FESPIC events, I decided to follow this man's advice. I borrowed a friend's bicycle and spent the day pedalling through central Beijing, visiting many of the neighbourhoods that I had developed fond feelings for in the mid-1980s. On my ride, I counted more than fifty of the three-wheeled vermilion motorbikes, some parked in front of stores amidst a jumble of bicycles, some cruising Beijing's wide boulevards. Nearly all the drivers I saw were men, and more than a few of them travelled with a pair of crutches. Many of their bikes bore symbolic markings of disablement: license plates or decals with the international icon of disability (a stick drawing of a person on a wheelchair).

Thus, there in Beijing was something I had never expected, and it contrasted vividly with the picture of disability I had painted in my mind based on my first year of fieldwork, conducted in rural Hainan province (located east of Vietnam). During that earlier research (1993–94), I never saw anybody using a wheelchair, motorised or otherwise. Nearly all my disabled Hainanese acquaintances, who might have benefited from such conveyances, got along by using homemade crutches, by hobbling or, in some cases, by crawling. Just as significant was the fact that very few of my Hainanese informants ever articulated any sense of connection with a domestic—let alone an international—disability movement. Moreover, most people in the village where I conducted research were unaware of either Deng Pufang or his Federation.

The purpose of this article is to discuss the role these motorcycles have played in shaping people's understandings and social experiences of disability in Beijing and, by extension, other metropolitan areas of the People's Republic of China (P.R.C.). In doing so, this paper seeks to provide concrete illustrations of important transformations underway in contemporary China. The discussion to come is framed around the following three questions. What historical forces have fuelled the development of motorcycle technologies for the disabled? How have these technologies contributed to the production of new understandings and responses to disability among Chinese people? How have users' lives been affected by the technology?

FORDISM AND THE RISE OF THREE-WHEELER TECHNOLOGY

To understand how three-wheeled motorcycles have been implicated in framing 'disability' in contemporary urban China, one must begin by highlighting larger processes that have led to these vehicles' introduction and proliferation. The emphasis in this first section, consequently, will often centre more on the 'social life of things' (Appadurai, 1986) than on the people who use the 'things'.

In modern China, as in many societies, the development of wheeled devices has been linked to issues of power and modernity. Several North

American and European scholars have demonstrated that, in their countries, the proliferation of mass-produced wheeled mechanisms has been tied to a regime of accumulation which they have called Fordism (see, for example, Gramsci, 1971; Harvey, 1990; Martin, 1992). Named for the American industrialist, Henry Ford, Fordism has several features. One of the most important is *time-space compression*: the idea that power—both institutional and monetary—can be expanded by harnessing technology to *speed up* human actions so that the temporal and geographic distances of productive tasks are reduced. Time-space compression, scholars of Fordism state, involves a dramatic transition, not only in the way people approach labour, but also how they experience the self and the body, changes that are held to be emblematic of our increasingly globalised post-modern times.[2]

Fully detailing Fordism's rise outside of China is obviously not possible in this paper. Nor is it possible for me here to scrutinise all the transnational and domestic processes that have shaped Fordism and post-Fordism in the People's Republic (see Ong and Nonini, 1997). However, I would argue, to understand the growth of mobility aids for 'disabled people' in China, it is necessary that we give careful attention to how Chinese society has incorporated time-space compression into national, institutional and individual agendas, as well as examine how this incorporation has affected both the definition and experience of disability.

Chinese people have, for centuries, considered speed of great value.[3] But it was not until the twentieth century and the rise of Chinese nationalism that using speed to compress time and space became a paramount agenda of the state. Mao's Cultural Revolution (1966–76) notwithstanding, a perennial goal of the Chinese Communist Party (CCP) has been to speed up human activity so as to catapult China and the Chinese people to the forefront of world modernity. After 1949, one of the first ways the CCP symbolically and pragmatically pursued the modern was by building urban roadways. By crisscrossing cities with clean, wide, surfaced roads,

[2] Antonio Gramsci stated that Fordism has entailed 'the biggest collective effort to date to create, with unprecedented speed ... a new type of worker and a new type of man,' with a new mode of work 'inseparable from ... living and thinking and feeling life' (quoted both in Martin, 1992, p. 122 and Harvey, 1990, p. 126).

[3] In 500 B.C., after all, Sun Tzu declared, 'Speed is the essence of battle.'

the Chinese leadership was at once facilitating faster urban movement and symbolically pronouncing to the nation and the world that 'New China' was quickly advancing. Until recently, though, it was only the *dictatorship of the proletariat*—the CCP's largely male leaders—who were permitted to use motorised sedans on either the newly built urban boulevards or on China's thousands of kilometres of unpaved roads. For most urbanites during the first few decades of the People's Republic, the only motorised devices available were overcrowded busses.

One type of non-motorised transportation that was increasingly visible on city roads after 1949, carefully rationed to 'urban workers' through a coupon system, was the bicycle. Bicycle rationing gradually enabled more and more city workers to move across urban landscapes at speeds that were, collectively, far faster than anything ever achieved before in China. Not surprisingly, owing to its speed, its scarcity and the banning of rickshaws after 1949, the standard black bicycle was a coveted status symbol during the early years of the People's Republic, a status symbol that was enjoyed mainly by an elite, and again predominantly male, sector of society. The cachet associated with possessing and riding a bicycle, particularly one with a good brand name, remained strong until the early 1980s, when production finally caught up with demand and bicycles became a ubiquitous part of urban residency for both men and women (Gaubatz, 1995, p. 43).

The bicycle's initial status and eventual ubiquity among city dwellers contributed significantly to the notion of the urban resident (*shi min*) during the Maoist and early post-Maoist epochs. To be a rightful and respectable urbanite, one was expected to operate a bicycle. Indeed, pedalling a bicycle became an enunciation (De Certeau, 1984) of the modern person: an individuated being who possessed the ability (*neng li*) to use technology to speed up society. Likewise, bicycle usage became an embodied statement about personal privilege and the right to belong in the highly desired and tightly restricted metropolitan setting.

THE HAND-CRANK TRICYCLE

Deng Xiaoping's reforms, in particular, greatly expanded bicycle usage. Profit-seeking manufacturers, in the early 1980s, increased the production and varieties of bicycles, including bicycles for women, children's bicycles and, eventually, mountain bikes. In addition to these, there was at least one more type of bicycle that began to appear in large cities during the early 1980s, one which served a highly specialised domestic market. This was the 'hand-crank tricycle' (*shou yao san fun che*), the first widely used 'disability' conveyance in China.[4] Initially, most hand-crank tricycles were built at home by men out of old bicycle parts, and were only later produced in small numbers by factories.

Who used hand-crank bikes and what attracted them to the technology? Anecdotal observations, formal interviews and discussions with local residents indicate that the vast majority of people in Beijing who have used hand-crank tricycles over the years have been men whose lower bodies cannot provide the balance and propulsion needed to operate a bicycle. Many of these men, although not all, have been polio survivors. Polio was a major scourge in the P.R.C. during the 1950s and 1960s, striking people of all class backgrounds. Today, the lion's share of people who live with the paralytic effects of polio are adults between the ages of 30 and 45. These men and women can be found in nearly every community in the nation.

In China, polio survivors and others with weak or damaged legs are frequently called *que zi*. A close English-language equivalent to que zi is 'the lame'. But such an English gloss is incomplete, because it underemphasises two crucial characteristics of the term. First, while in earlier historical epochs que zi was used to signify those with either a 'sick hand or foot' (*shou jiao bing*), since the Qing dynasty (1644–1911) it almost exclusively has designated those who have trouble 'moving' (*dong*) (Lu and Dao, 1996, pp. 10–12). Second, que zi is an intensely pejorative idiom.

The disapprobation encoded in the term que zi is a reflection that, today and in the past, Chinese people with certain bodily differences have persistently undergone what Kleinman and others call 'intersubjective delegitimation' (1995, p. 1328). Through complex processes, Chinese citizens have relentlessly objectified polio survivors and others with

[4] Before the twentieth century, wheelchairs in China were extremely rare and usually home-built. Four-wheeled wheelchairs of western design were uncommon in China until recently, and were generally found only in hospitals. Most of these were imports and thus costly, and they also had the problem of being too large for many Chinese homes.

supposed corporal defects, transmuting their so-called spoiled bodies (*shen ti*) into flawed social and moral status (*shen fen*).[5] As a consequence, polio survivors and others viewed as que have for centuries been denied educational opportunities, discriminated against in jokes, shunned as potential marriage partners, and treated with paternalism or bureaucratic indifference. Such delegitimation and discrimination has occurred in part because of the importance Chinese culture has long placed on bodily perfection as an indicator of moral and spiritual standing (Hansson, 1988).[6] But, to be sure, Chinese people have also considered the lives of que zi spoiled because the que are understood to be lacking in the ability (neng li) to traverse space.[7]

In recent years, it would seem that the evolving regime of Fordism has played a significant role not only in this second type of delegitimation but also in the transformation of the que zi category from denoting someone with a 'sick hand or foot' to denoting 'the immobile'. In particular, the proliferation of bicycle usage has greatly amplified the perception that the

[5] See Brownell (1995, p. 16) for a discussion of the terms shen ti and shen fen.

[6] The most frequently noted source for how Chinese society has historically emphasised bodily perfection is Confucianism. Key here is an oft-cited passage of the *Book of Filial Piety*, where Confucius is described as stating that all children have the filial duty to preserve the body given them by their parents, and that they must avoid even their hair or skin being injured.

[7] Given the pejorative meanings attached to the term que zi and the pain its usage regularly inflicts on many Chinese, I am reluctant to invoke it. On the other hand, one of anthropology's central goals is to examine culture's culpability in the production of suffering, and this can only be done by direct observation. I am further inclined to use the term que zi rather than depend on euphemistic terms like 'disabled' or 'handicapped' because, as the American polio survivor and author Leonard Kriegel notes, the latter terms do 'little more than further society's illusions about illness and accident.... For, to be 'disabled' or 'handicapped' is to deny ... the rage, anger and pride of having managed to survive as a crippled (1991, p. 61).' Lastly, I am inclined to use the category que zi here because many of my informants, who community members recognise by the term, regularly invoke que zi when speaking. Therefore, my solution, however imperfect, is to follow literary convention and place que zi in quotation marks. By doing so, I hope readers will be alerted continually to the power and pain attendant on the term.

que have difficulty moving. As noted above, bicycle usage in China after 1949 became an enunciation of social rank, personhood and belonging. But because bicycles were engineered to be powered by legs of a specific sort, they were of little use to most polio survivors and others like them who were unable to produce the necessary syncopated leg movement. Rather, these sorts of people often found bicycles to accentuate their moral, political and economic decline. As a Beijing polio survivor named Meng once told me, 'The sudden growth of bicycles in China didn't help us a bit. They just made people like me slower, more incompetent *(geng bu neng gan) and* more que.'

Curiously, the delegitimation that bicycle proliferation visited on people such as Meng contributed significantly to their ultimate adoption of cycle technology. 'To *keep up* with everyone else, to participate in the quickening pace of social development,' remarked an older so-called que zi named Zheng, 'we had to devise something to help us move around, and to help us move around independently.' Transforming bicycles into hand-crank tricycles, and later buying disability motorcycles, became a way for many people like Zheng to keep up. Hand-crank tricycles allowed them to move around alone at speeds far faster than ever possible before.

But why, over the years, have so many male and so few female que zi adopted tricycle technology, be it hand-crank or motorised? Why is it that, in 1995, at one of Beijing's largest retailers of three-wheeled conveyances for the disabled, the staff were unable to remember ever selling a vehicle either to or for a woman? Granted, reported cases of polio paralysis in China have been predominantly male, to the degree that, in 1987, male survivors outnumbered females 3 to 2 (Ministry of Civil Affairs, 1993). Yet, such figures alone cannot explain the near absence of females among the ranks of tricycle owners in the mid-1990s. Thus, forces typically beyond the purview of most epidemiologists must be at play.

One of these forces, which has become closely tied to Fordism in modem China and elsewhere, is the evolving politics of gender. Gender is about many things. But something it is consistently about, in almost every culture, is the power to traverse and control space (Bourdieu, 1990, pp. 77–78). Today in China, nearly all men and women of working age are willing, if not eager, to venture away from home to earn a better living. The existence of more than 100 million 'floating' migrants evinces strongly that Chinese society has come to increasingly define personal status, for males and females alike, in terms of the ability (neng li) to project oneself out of the home and local community and into public arenas.

But the way men and women move across the Chinese topography differs in at least one important way. While both men and women increasingly use gasoline-powered instruments of time-space compression, the people who control and operate these machines—much like most bicycle operators of the 1950s and 1960s—are nearly all male. Whether it is tractors or trucks, motorcycles or cars, ships or trains, buses or airplanes, those piloting gasoline-powered conveyances today are predominantly men.

A number of authors, writing on cultures other than China's, have discussed how sexual identity and gender inequality are refracted by the way people use technologies of time-space compression (Bolton, 1979; Bourque and Warren, 1987; Mosse, 1985; Connell, 1995; Scharff, 1991). While cultural differences obviously exist, it would seem that, in contemporary China, such technologies have come to play an important role in distinguishing the so-called 'idealised man' (*nan zi han*) from its 'female' counterpart; and that, unlike womanhood in China, manhood is increasingly equated with controlling conveyances of speed in order to demonstrate and generate status.

This has been echoed frequently in discussions I have had with Chinese people from all walks of life over the last decade. So too has its female converse. Some of the most poignant comments on the latter have come paradoxically from a small number of female taxi drivers. When asked why it is so rare to see women at the wheel of motorised vehicles (*ji dong che*), female taxi operators have consistently said that driving is 'unsuitable' to women because it challenges their socially prescribed role as 'keeper of the home', and because venturing alone from the hearth is 'more dangerous' for women than men.

That female que zi have adopted tricycle technology so infrequently is no doubt connected to this stereotypical gendering of public and private space.[8] Less obvious, though, is how the male-female discrepancy in tricycle

[8] See Strathern (1988) and Bray (1997) for discussions of the relationship between power, gender and inside-outside distinctions within the China context and elsewhere.

usage is closely related to intersubjective delegitimation. Living with a lower-body impairment is excruciating for Chinese—whoever they are. But the locus of pain seems to undergo significant gender differentiation. For men, the most difficult aspect seems to be immobility. For females, however, the pain appears to centre on bodily imperfection.[9] This juxtaposition is strongly supported by informants' comments regarding tricycles. Many women have told me they would never drive a hand-crank or motorised tricycle because it would only draw attention to their appearance (*wai mao*). As Ms Cai says, 'Women like me, who have trouble walking, are less able to endure people's looks, and comments about our appearance, when we go out in public. We're much happier staying at home.' Many men who drive three-wheelers, by contrast, articulate sentiments similar to that of a Mr Lin: 'Sure, the stares hurt. But, what hurt even more was, in the past, when I was young, being closed up in the house. I'm never going back to that kind of life.... I'm not going to be a hermit because people look at me.'

CHANGING DEFINITIONS OF DISABILITY

The fusion of all of these forces—gender, Fordism and delegitimation—is also closely reflected in changing definitions of the term *can ji* (the term which is regularly translated today as 'disability').[10] Documents indicate that, during China's long existence, people tended to use the ideogram

[9] See Mark (1995) for a discussion of contemporary urban Chinese women's emphasis on beauty and bodily perfection.

[10] Until the creation of the Disabled Persons' Welfare Fund in the early 1980s, can ji was not used much in institutional or popular discourse. Still, like its two main Chinese language cognates—*can fei* and *fei ji*—can ji dates back deep into antiquity. Contemporary dictionaries define the ideograms that make up these three couplets as follows: *can*, as a verb, means to injure, to spoil, to destroy, to oppress; as a noun it denotes remnant or residue; *fei*, as a verb, means to do away with, to abrogate, to waste, to destroy; as an adjective it denotes useless, wasted, or abandoned; and *ji* is a noun meaning sickness, disease or pain. Because of the particularly pejorative meanings associated with the ideogram fei, China's party-state stopped using the terms can fei and fei ji in the mid-1980s and pressed for can ji to be used in their place.

can to represent a male's[11] bodily injury and disease.[12] Today, while many Chinese citizens continue to use can ji in this gendered and physiological way, they additionally associate it closely with the idiom que zi, which, as noted above, has increasingly come to denote 'the immobile'. The contemporary linkage between can ji and immobility came across strongly during my fieldwork. When requested to describe everybody can ji in their natal communities, the vast majority of respondents talked about 'men', who they characterised as having a 'lame foot' (*que jiao*), 'unable to walk' (*bu neng zao lu de*), or 'immobile' (*dong bu hao de*). In other words, it would seem that the paradigmatic popular image of 'the disabled person' has become the very sort of person that, in the 1970s, most often adopted three-wheeled hand-crank tricycles.

ENTER THE MOTORISED TRICYCLE AND FEDERATION

By the late 1980s, these paradigmatic disabled people found a new transportation device available to them. This was the machine I first observed outside the ping-pong stadium. Chinese citizens usually refer to such gasoline-powered tricycles as three-wheelers, disability bikes, or motorised tricycles. For the informed P.R.C. observer, the machines

[11] One example of how, in the past, the ideogram *can* was linked to men comes from China's imperial censuses. Starting as early as the Han Dynasty (206 B.C.–A.D. 220), Chinese sovereigns required local magistrates to count men under their control (Rockhill, 1904, p. 659). Men counted by censuses were recorded under the title *ding*. Starting in 1391, imperial documents directed local magistrates to stop counting as ding the following males: can ji, 'the aged', 'children under ten', 'widowers', and 'migrants' (Zhao, n.d., p. 4.2a–2b; also cited in Ho, 1959, p. 11). A more recent example of linkages between can and males comes from the military arena. In 1950, the Chinese government established graded criteria for identifying and compensating 'revolutionary crippled veterans' (*ge ming can fei jun ren*).

[12] According to Wieger (1965), the earliest meanings associated with the radicals that comprise the ideogram *can* were 'destruction', 'broken bones', and 'male skeletal remains'. *Matthew's Chinese-English Dictionary* (1931) states that the English equivalents for *can ji* and *can fei* are: maimed, crippled, or deformed. *The Large Chinese Dictionary (han yu da ci dian)* (1989) offers similar definitions, but adds that *can ji* may also denote ailment or disease.

appear to be a cross between at least three pre-existing and predominantly male devices of time-space compression: the hand-held tractor, the police motorcycle with side-car, and the hand-crank tricycle.

From where have three-wheelers emanated, and how has their proliferation related to the forces described above? These machines are the product of the Disabled Persons' Federation. And, in order to outline their genesis, something more must be said about the term can ji and the Federation.

In the 1980s, the Chinese state began attempting to do two things to the term can ji: (1) broaden its meaning in relation to the transnational term 'disability';[13] and (2) give it society-wide significance as a welfare entity. As many readers will know, the person in China who has done the most to bring about these changes has been Deng Xiaoping's eldest son, Deng Pufang. Less known, however, is the degree to which time-space compression has influenced not only Deng Pufang's life-course but also how his institution, the Federation, has framed disability in the post-Mao period. As a youth, Deng Pufang took avid interest both in operating conveyances of speed and in utilising high technology for national development. He regularly pedalled a bicycle to and from school—something which his biographer says made him 'extremely cheerful' (*kuai huo*, literally meaning 'fast with life')—and he coaxed his father's drivers to teach him how to operate a car (Qin, 1992, pp. 132, 123).

Pufang lost the ability to control either a bicycle or an auto at the beginning of the Cultural Revolution, a period when Mao dictated that class purity, not developmental speed, was to be the nation's key concern. In the spring of 1968, while under incarceration by Red Guards, who demanded he denounce his father as a 'capitalist roader', Deng threw himself from an upper-storey window of a building at Beijing University, where he was a graduate student in nuclear physics. After Deng Pufang experienced several years living isolated and immobilised in a dilapidated welfare facility on the outskirts of Beijing, Mao agreed to let him rejoin his family. Three years after Mao's death, Pufang re-injured his unstable

[13] The Chinese government today recognises five categories of disabled people: physically disabled, mentally ill, mentally disabled, blind, and deaf. These five categories and their corresponding criteria were created and codified by the Chinese government, initially, for the 1987 National Sample Survey of Disabled Persons.

spine, probably as a consequence of propelling himself by wheelchair. His family (once again at the apex of the Chinese political system) used their special access to devices of time-space compression to fly Pufang to Canada for types of surgery unavailable anywhere in Asia. After his surgery, as Pufang lay recuperating in Ottawa, he decided to cut short his treatment and rush back to his homeland in order to become an advocate for China's disabled (Qin, 1992, p. 244).

On his return to Beijing, Deng's initial project was to build a facility like the Ottawa Civic Hospital and have it serve as a flagship for the speedy development of rehabilitation medicine (*kang fu yi liao*). To raise funds and enlist high-ranking advocates for the centre, Deng Pufang and a handful of other 'crippled'[14] men of elite rank established the Federation's precursor, the China Disabled Persons' Welfare Fund. The hospital was built during the mid-1980s. It is called the China Rehabilitation Research Centre (CRRC) and is located in south-western Beijing. Much to the Disabled Persons' Federation's chagrin, the CRRC has been as much a locus of controversy as a source of care since its opening.[15] The Federation, however, has strongly supported the CRRC throughout the hospital's rocky history and, today, promotes other large, technology-laden rehabilitation centres elsewhere in China. Two reasons the Federation has so ardently followed this path have been: (a) the way Deng Pufang initially embraced the western medical model for disability (i.e. that to aid disabled people one must heal them through clinic-based rehabilitation medicine); and

[14] I employ the word 'crippled' here because it is the term used by Deng Pufang's official biographer, Qin Van (1992), to describe Pufang and his colleagues during this period.

[15] One conflict has been over the CRRC and Deng's umbrella organisation controlling and dictating the development of rehabilitation medicine in China. Primarily a battle over resources, the conflict has involved the Ministry of Public Health doing such things as denying insurance coverage (*gong fei yi liao*) for many kinds of rehabilitation treatment, sponsoring competing rehabilitation centres and projects, and challenging the Federation's right to co-author documents with institutions of ministerial rank (*bu ji*) or higher. Another systemic issue centres on whether the Federation could better spend its resources developing more community-based rehabilitation programmes, rather than capital-intensive, technology-laden facilities like the CRRC (see Henderson, 1989; World Bank, 1992).

(b) the way Pufang oriented his rehabilitation goals around his father's national developmental agenda of using technology to speed up the Chinese economy. Regarding the latter, Pufang has regularly represented Federation work, and rehabilitation efforts in particular, as follows: that their mission is to employ scientific means to help the sort of people, who would otherwise fall behind, to keep up and contribute actively to the rapid changes his father had set in motion across China (see, for example, Deng, 1988).

There is another reason why the Federation has been so anchored to quick-fix technology and institution-based rehabilitation. After its founding in 1988, the Federation began a massive expansion programme. In addition to its central Beijing offices, the Federation established chapters in every major city and provincial capital, and began working to create independent offices in all county seats and major metropolitan city districts. The Federation also applied to the State Council for full ministerial status. What was driving all this rapid expansion? Death. Deng Pufang and his staff were in possession of a moribund treasure: filial ties to China's paramount leader. They consequently were racing to convert this treasure—this symbolic capital (Bourdieu, 1984)—into a powerful and durable institution. The more symbolic capital they could convert to bureaucratic structures before Deng Xiaoping's death, they calculated, the better chance the Federation would have at continuing its existence long into the future.[16] Indeed, it could be argued that, for Deng and his staff, the regime of time-space compression was simply a tool for accruing the more traditional, more inertia-bound, more typically Chinese form of power: bureaucracy.

Yet, to stimulate wide-scale support for bureaucracy building, Federation leaders needed more than ties to Deng Xiaoping. They needed to create tangible proof that they were improving the livelihood of people, and they needed to publicise this proof. Rehabilitation medicine was at the heart of this public relations campaign. In its first few years of existence, the Federation used rehabilitation techniques to treat hundreds of thousands of people across the country, and they orchestrated a steady flow of local

[16] In explaining their sense of urgency to me, Central Federation officials repeatedly invoked a Chinese aphorism, *shi zai ren wei*, which can be translated as 'tasks can only be accomplished when you have the right person on your side.'

and national media reports about individuals being transformed by the humanitarian efforts of the Federation.[17]

THE BUREAUCRATISATION OF THREE-WHEELERS

How do motorised tricycles fit in here? The vehicles were the first 'rehabilitation products' designed by the CRRC's Rehabilitation Engineering Institute. That the Federation produced these devices and, through the mid-1990s, continued to guarantee their right to exist, not only related to the Federation's institution-building agenda, but reaffirmed the cultural link between can ji and the idea of immobility.

Currently, motorised tricycles can be found in greatest concentration in China's highly structured metropolitan transportation landscape. To anyone visiting China for the first time, urban traffic there might seem anything but structured. But despite the growing malady of vehicular gridlock, state control of urban roadway usage is often tight, which means getting around urban China by any method besides foot, human-powered bicycle or mass transportation remains very much a privilege and a mark of status.

The fact that three-wheelers have enjoyed such a privilege stems from their institutional and symbolic link to Deng Pufang. In the beginning, the Federation, vehicle manufacturers and users barely had to emphasise that connection in order to keep traffic authorities in major cities from restricting three-wheelers. But this changed in the early 1990s, when the numbers of three-wheelers started to surge, such that, by 1995, Shanghai officially had over 12,000 of them and Beijing had more than 30,000

[17] High ranking Federation officials have told me that the kinds of treatments they usually provided—cataract surgery, polio-correction surgery, and oral language training for deaf children—were chosen: (a) because the Federation leadership saw these treatments as the quickest and the most effective procedures for aiding three out of the five Federation-recognised categories of disability; and (b) because the procedures were viewed to be public relations-friendly ways for the Federation to assist the disabled and garner more resources. Federation leaders chose the two surgical procedures, in particular, because China's military had a ready supply of surgeons familiar with the procedures, and because the military was willing to deploy those surgeons at almost no cost, owing to Deng Xiaoping's longstanding ties with China's military leadership.

(*Liberation Daily*, 19 March 1995; *Beijing Evening News*, 21 February 1995).

One force behind the exponential growth in three-wheelers was their unregulated status and speed, both of which made them extremely useful tools for entrepreneurs, be they disabled or otherwise.[18] Another force was the increase in supply. At the retail level, Federation chapters were the primary purveyors of motorised tricycles. Initially, when supplies were limited, chapter staff created waiting lists and limited sales to only those people who they viewed as demonstrably disabled. But, as supply grew, Federation chapters began selling three-wheelers to anyone who wanted them, in order to generate greater earnings. By the mid-1990s, selling motorised tricycles had become a big business for Federation chapters, and a primary way many were augmenting their incomes.[19]

In 1994, a number of city governments—alarmed by the growth of three-wheelers and their unbridled use of public space—banned them. The result was protest by men who called themselves can ji. These men first acted locally, demanding that their city governments lift the bans. When that failed, many brought their grievances to the eastern edge of the Forbidden City, to 44 Beichizi Road, the home of the Central Disabled Persons' Federation. A senior Federation official, who recounted these events to me under condition of anonymity, said the most ardent of the regional protesters was a group of men from the north-eastern industrial city of Shenyang. These people travelled to Beijing twice in 1994, requesting that Deng Pufang intervene. Deng responded by inviting Shenyang's mayor and Liaoning province's governor to 44 Beichizi for extensive meetings with himself and top Federation officials. But before the meetings had a chance to get very far, the Federation's main office in Shanghai began reporting that similar protests were breaking out there.

[18] It is now common for motorised tricycle drivers to earn sizeable incomes moving consumer goods and transporting people. This has become particularly common in cities where standard motorcycles are banned.

[19] Like nearly all state agencies throughout China, Federation chapters receive most of their funding from local city, county and district governments; and the chapters are expected to bolster their budgets by pursuing entrepreneurial activities. Prices in Beijing for the most popular type of three-wheelers, produced by the motorcycle manufacturer Jia Ling, hovered around 3,500 yuan in 1995.

Realising he had a national problem on his hand, Deng took action. He contacted one of the men with greatest administrative authority over public space in China, the Minister of Public Security. Deng and the minister met several times during the spring and summer of 1995. Their meetings were paralleled by lengthy discussions between high officials from both the Ministry and the Federation. Ministry staff took the position that three-wheelers needed to be banned because they were dangerous and disruptive to public order. Deng and his Federation cadres countered with a detailed set of arguments.

After only modest resistance, the Ministry of Public Security agreed in early 1995 to nearly all the Federation's points and signed a detailed set of regulations. The staff at 44 Beichizi were jubilant. It is easy to understand why. Besides being an important revenue source to local chapters, the vermilion tricycles were quickly becoming the most visible icons of the Federation and its constituency—disabled people—to be found on a daily basis in urban China. Local government attempts at banishing three-wheelers were direct challenges to both the Federation and its constituencies' attempts to speed up, to amass more power.

Assessing how the Federation-Public Security agreement will affect popular definitions of disability across the country is difficult. But, based on my time in Beijing, where similar regulations have been in place already for a few years, I believe the agreement will intensify the linkage between the term can ji and the concept of immobility. For one, it requires a major and very public bureaucratisation of three-wheelers. Now, to avoid fines, people must register as a legal owner-operator, and to do this they must cross a series of administrative barriers and subject themselves to intensive institutional scrutiny.[20] Also, if Beijing is representative of the future, motorised tricycle drivers nationwide can expect police to more closely monitor their movements vis-à-vis disability status; that is to say,

[20] In Beijing, where city-level regulations began to appear as early as 1989, the barriers include: (1) getting registered as a disabled person, (2) buying a vehicle, (3) getting the vehicle and oneself licensed, and (4) registering for commercial status. Each of these steps has numerous sub-steps, many of which require that owner-operators must visit hospitals and government offices to have their bodies measured along a host of axes (e.g. national identity, residential status, age, psychological competency, physical functionality and impairment level).

police are increasingly likely to stop tricycles and evaluate the credentials and bodily status of their operators.[21]

For these reasons, I expect that an increasing number of people across the country will come to understand what kind of people constitute the disabled, in the way that ever larger numbers of people came to do during my stay in Beijing. As one of many people told me shortly before I left: 'Oh can ji? They're the ones the police permit to drive three- wheelers. You know, que zi. People who can't walk.'

THE EXPERIENCE OF AUTOMATIC TRICYCLE USE

Now that I have described some of the history surrounding three-wheelers, I will switch gears (so to speak) and discuss ways these vehicles are shaping the experiences of people who regularly use them. Because the goal of this section is to understand how motorised tricycles have been influencing China's emergent disability construct, the discussion here will not cover all tricycle drivers, but only 'legal' owner-operators, most of whom have been male polio survivors.

Given the moral, gender, political, economic and institutional forces at play, what is it like for such men to buy and use three-wheeled devices of time-space compression? Let me first elucidate this with excerpts from interviews conducted with two Beijing polio survivors. The first excerpt comes from a man named Mr Peng, who today runs a CD store.

Peng: The old hand-crank tricycles were remarkable. They let disabled people like me have concrete contact with society, often for the first time.

[21] In March 1995, for example, I witnessed Beijing's Fourteenth Automatic Tricycle Rectification Campaign. One hundred police teams spread out across the city stopping three-wheelers either lacking a license plate or operated by anyone the police suspected was an illegal driver. A similar campaign in 1994 resulted in police fining 16,330 riders and impounding nearly 6,000 vehicles (*Beijing Evening News*, 21 February 1995). Oddly though, campaigns like this have done little to stem the number of illegally operated three-wheelers. The main reason is the cost-benefit issue. The fines given during the campaigns are paltry when compared to the potential earnings for using bikes illegally. According to several Beijing government acquaintances, the reason fines are kept low in the capital is because of the tremendous influence the Federation wields there.

I got my first hand-crank tricycle in 1985, when I was 22. I started working at a factory a little less than a year afterwards. It was an utterly transformative event getting a tricycle. With it I was able to leave home and go out and see the multicoloured world. Before then, I rarely had contact with anyone. I was closed out.

I purchased my first disability motorcycle three years later. I was still at the factory then, so I was able to pay for most of the three-wheeler by myself. The initial feeling of driving a hand-crank bike and driving a disability motorcycle was very different. My initial impression of my first motorbike was how much quicker it was than a bicycle. The second impression was that, without any force, I could go incredibly far. At first, I was spooked by it being so much faster than a bicycle. I was scared to take it out on the big boulevards and drive quickly with all the cars. Coping with this fear took a long time. I didn't dare drive more than 20 km an hour back then. Not like now. Now I'll go 50.

Getting a three-wheeler, at first, gave me a deep sense of satisfaction. I can't drive a car, but I have the ability (neng li) to drive this sort of motorcycle. That gave me a real sense of power and vanity (*xu rong xing*). I think all men have this sort of vanity. That I could drive this kind of vehicle really boosted mine. My heightened feeling of vanity has pretty much disappeared, however. Now, after six years on the road, I just look at my three-wheeler as a transportation tool. It's something I can't survive without. If I walk out the door, I must use it. I couldn't live, or run my business, without it.

As I see it, there are clear pros and cons to motorised tricycles. My scope of activity is much greater. That's one pro. I've driven as far as 150 km to a tourist spot in Hebei with a bunch of disabled friends. Another is that it has given me the ability to open my own business and start supporting my parents. A con is, physically, I'm nowhere as strong as when I used a hand-crank bike. Before, I was strong enough to crank myself 10 km in less than 25 minutes, about as fast as a bicycle. Now, I probably couldn't crank 10 km an hour. Another con is the danger of accident. That's why I wear a helmet. If I crash and become more disabled, I'm done for. As an independent businessman, I have no national health insurance, no nothing. If I have a serious accident, I'm dead.

The next man, Mr Liu, is 39 years old. At age four, Liu contracted polio, which left his legs so weakened that, today, he cannot walk without leg braces and crutches. Mr Liu rarely left his house before 1988, when, with the help of his parents and siblings with whom he lives, he purchased his first disability motorcycle. Five years ago, Mr Liu opened a tobacco store. Mr Liu makes a good living from this shop, and contributes more to the family's finances than his retired parents combined.

MK: Can you tell me about getting your first three-wheeled motorcycle?

Liu: I purchased it from the factory, very near the Rehabilitation Research Centre. The quality was dreadful. It's funny. The first thing I did after buying that motorcycle wasn't learn how to drive it, but go out and purchase a manual and study automotive repair. [Laugh] Everyday I had to fix something, the carburettor, the wheel bearings, the brakes. It was fun learning how to fix a motorcycle, but it was also a real pain in the ass. The big advantage was that, when I'd go out on the road and the bike broke down, I didn't need others' help. After so many years depending on people—my parents, my siblings—I just want to take care of myself. That motorcycle, as horrible as it was, allowed me to become much more self-sufficient.

The second motorcycle, the one I'm still using, I got at the Disabled Persons' Service Centre [run by the city Federation]. It's a Jia Ling. Jia Ling has become the most popular brand of motorcycle among disabled people because it has a Japanese-designed engine. I got my Jia Ling by pulling a nice little trick. It's quite an interesting story. At first, the only place to get a Jia Ling was the Service Centre, and the boss there was a real bastard. He'd take your money for a new motorcycle, but he wouldn't hand over the bike for months. So, when I'd saved up enough money, I spoke to one of the boss' men. I told him, 'Sir, I don't have a motorcycle and I need one right away because the government has just moved the factory where I work to the suburbs.' The guy was sceptical. He thought I was going to resell the vehicle for a big mark-up. So he had me write and sign a guarantee I wouldn't do that. Afterwards, he said, 'OK, you're a disabled guy. You deserve to have a motorcycle.' Later that day I drove my Jia Ling home. [Laugh]

But the truth is, I really didn't like lying to that guy. In general, I never lie. Well, almost never. Sometimes, if I'm giving a person a ride and the police stop me, I'll fool the cop by saying I'm on my way to do some business and my passenger is coming along to carry me up the stairs to the office I must reach. I think lying to a cop in that way is OK.

MK: Have you always been this bold?

Liu: [Laugh] No. I was pretty childish before. I was just like an infant, always at home, always needing others to do things for me. Once I started to get out of the house, once I set up my own store, I became much more pushy. My parents frequently urge me to be more cautious, particularly when I drive. Going out on the Beijing streets on a three-wheeler is very, very dangerous. But what choice do I have? To make a living, to help the family, I need to drive one of these bikes. Still, it's hard not to think about the fact that an accident might leave me even more crippled (can fei).

Several points stand out from these excerpts. Mr Peng's and Mr Liu's access to devices of time-space compression has altered their lives enormously, and their transformations have been framed by a paradoxical mix of sensations. Buying tricycles and travelling alone at increasingly higher speeds has been, to a large degree, a joy for Peng and Liu. It has bolstered their sense of self-worth and given them the power—or ability (neng li)—to expand their experiential and economic reach. This joy, however, has been dampened by deep feelings of fear and dependence. Peng and Liu clearly state their lives and businesses are at once contingent on, and threatened by, their access to three-wheelers. To sustain their current situation, they need the speed of motorised tricycles. Yet they and their families worry—and for good reason—that such speed might either kill them or cause an injury that will worsen their disablement.[22]

LIVING A PARADOX

There are several ways men like Peng and Liu have been responding to the paradoxical mixture of feelings (pleasure, fear, dependence) entering their lives as a consequence of motorised-tricycle usage. Before concluding, let me outline three.

[22] Whether in Beijing or elsewhere, most three-wheeler accidents likely go unreported to traffic authorities because so many of the devices are illegally operated. Nonetheless, according to the police, there were 40 motorised tricycle accidents in Beijing during 1994, resulting in 31 injuries and seven deaths (*Beijing Evening News*, 21 February 1995).

One response has been to enter into active relationships with the Federation. These relationships have been closely akin to patron-client connections. As Walder (1986) has described, patron-client relations are a key feature of rulership in Communist China, and are built around government agencies, like the Federation, exchanging privileges for client loyalty. The primary way tricycle drivers articulate such loyalty is by being public relations figures. As stated earlier, the Federation, even before its formal founding, has required easily recognised and highly functional 'disabled people' to participate in the public events it has regularly mounted over the last decade as it races for ministerial rank. More often than not, these 'disabled people' have tended to be men, similar to the ones enlisted by Beijing's city Federation to work as FESPIC Games cheerleaders.[23] For people such as Liu and Peng, working intimately with Federation offices has been a way to guarantee that the joys entering their lives as a result of three-wheelers will not be eroded but instead enhanced. Many drivers like Liu and Peng give time and deference to the Federation and its staff in exchange for informal assistance with a host of things like dismissal of traffic fines, career advancements, housing assignments, residence permit transfers, enrolment of children in choice schools, and tax reductions.

A second way men, particularly those in Beijing, have responded to the paradoxical feelings associated with three-wheeler usage has been by developing identities more strongly connected to the category of disability (can ji). To a certain degree, this connection is the result of contact with the Federation. But, more importantly, it stems from interactions with other so-called *que zi* (interactions which have been made increasingly possible by motorised tricycles). Through these interactions, drivers have developed tightly knit circles (*quan zi*) of what, in Beijing, they call 'disability brothers' (*can ji ge mer*). At the heart of such circles is the idea of mutual assistance. Disability brothers treat one another to meals at restaurants and homes. They exchange professional services. They act as matchmakers. Disability brothers go on trips together. They pool

[23] Another example of this comes from my eastern Hainan field site. Between 1989 and 1995, more than ninety percent of 'disabled advisory members' attached to the Wenchang county Federation office were male, and nearly all of them were polio survivors.

finances when one falls on hard times. They share instrumental contacts. And disability brothers provide emotional support when trouble strikes. The intensity and importance of these circles is strongly reflected in a statement uttered by a man while he and I shared a home-cooked meal with a bunch of his brothers and some of their wives: 'The only people I really trust, the only people with whom I'm willing to express my honest feelings, are my disability brothers. When I'm away from them, when I'm with others, say my parents, people at work, I'm a fake.'

A third way survivors have responded to three-wheeler usage has been collective action. Obvious examples are the protests that popped up across the country when city governments tried to ban motorised tricycles. Collective action, however, has extended beyond petitioning Federation officials for protection from top-down modes of state-sponsored delegitimation. Disability brothers have also joined together to criticise the Federation itself, and to challenge non-governmental sectors of society. For instance, in late 1994, a group of disability brothers in Beijing sent a letter to the mayor in which they accused the city Federation's main tricycle dealership, the Service Centre, of financial improprieties. On another occasion, in early 1995, a group of disability brothers I know blockaded a company office for several hours until they received accident compensation. The day before the blockade, a driver in one of the company's cars had sideswiped a brother as he was heading home with his wife. Both husband and wife were injured in the collision and their tricycle was badly damaged.

CONCLUSION

While studying epilepsy in interior China, Kleinman et al. (1995, p. 1327) found few signs that Deng Pufang's disability-advocacy work had significantly affected people's lives. As noted at the beginning of this article, the research I conducted in rural Hainan (prior to the Beijing portion of my fieldwork) largely confirmed Kleinman's and his co-authors' findings.

What is transpiring in places such as Beijing and other large metropolitan areas like Shanghai, Changsha and Shenyang seems to be more complex, however. In these environments, certain individuals' lives are being radically transformed, in large part because of Deng Pufang's quickly growing Federation, and because of macro processes of modernity that have predated and framed Federation development. How are these transformations to be assessed?

What is occurring currently to people like Mr Peng and Mr Liu and their disability brothers, on first blush, might be called legitimation or re-legitimation. By gaining access to modes of time-space compression, Peng and Liu are projecting themselves out of their homes and creating financial and community structures. In doing so, they are making social enunciations to themselves and those around them about their value and social status: that they are not only members of a group but competent (*neng gan*) individuals.

But, on closer examination, it is probably more appropriate to think of these processes as a sort of quasi-legitimation. For, in as much as disability motorcycles are allowing some people to radically transform aspects of their lives, people like Peng and Liu continue to undergo unrelenting discrimination. Whether it is in the area of business, government work, education, housing or marriage (Kohrman, 1999), people regularly consider men like Peng and Liu as 'damaged' or 'useless', and thus undesirable as potential colleagues, students, spouses or neighbours. To a degree, this discrimination is being dampened by the Federation's propaganda, the vaguely worded *Disability Protection Law* (which the Federation pushed through the National People's Congress in 1990), and by the aggressive attitudes of people like Peng and Liu. But, until more systemic efforts are made—either to (1) change people's attitudes that mobility and ability are coterminous, or (2) make the built-world within China more accessible for all people who have difficulty walking—the discrimination will no doubt continue.

We must recognise also that men like Peng and Liu constitute only a small fraction of the millions of people in urban, let alone rural, China who fall within the Federation's overall criteria of 'disability'. In recent years, the lives of the less-visible majority—including the blind, the deaf, the mentally ill and the mentally disabled—have *not* been experiencing re-legitimation or even quasi-legitimation anywhere to the same degree as the disability brothers. Evolving cultural prescriptions, like those blocking females from using motorcycles, compounded by the Federation's institution-driven emphasis on quick-fix rehabilitation, are causing significant disparities in how people under the Federation's aegis are served.

To that extent, it could be argued that contemporary China is fostering a class system within its emergent disability sphere. For those people living in urban China today whose bodies fall within certain government-drawn parameters (i.e. having only a specific kind of lower-body impairment), there exists the possibility for some social advancement via motorcycle-assisted entrepreneurship. For those whose bodies do not fall within the parameters, however, such advancement is far more illusory.

Unless radical changes occur within the Federation and Chinese society, it seems that this sort of class disparity will continue to grow. Some observers, no doubt, might think that the mounting force of the disability brothers will invariably lead men like Mr Peng and Mr Liu to become disability 'activists' similar to the wheelchair-bound men who directed the disability-rights movement in the United States between 1970 and 1990 (Shapiro, 1993). Unfortunately, this seems unlikely. The disability brothers' interests are largely provincial, primarily focused on dealing among themselves with the paradoxes attendant to driving three-wheelers. And other than the disability brothers, there are few networks of people in China today who identify strongly enough with the concept of disability that they might try to significantly change the current course.

References

Appadurai, A. 1986. *The Social Life of Things: Commodities in Cultural Perspective.* New York: Cambridge University Press.

Bolton, R. 1979. 'Machismo in Motion: The Ethos of Peruvian Truckers', *Ethos,* 7: 312–42.

Bourdieu, P. 1984. *Distinction: A Social Critique of the Judgment of Taste.* Cambridge: Harvard University Press.

———. 1990. *The Logic of Practice.* Stanford: Stanford University Press.

Bourque, S. and Warren, K.B. 1987. 'Technology, gender and development: Incorporating gender in the study of development', *Daedalus,* Fall: 173–97.

Bray, F. 1997. *Technology and Gender: Fabrics of Power in Late Imperial China.* Berkeley: University of California Press.

Brownell, S. 1995. *Training the Body for China: Sports in the Moral Order of the People's Republic.* Chicago: University of Chicago Press.

Connell, R.W. 1995. *Masculinities.* Berkeley: University of California Press.

De Certeau, M. 1984. *The Practice of Everyday Life.* Berkeley: University of California Press.

Deng, P. 1988. 'Speech Given to the China Disabled Persons' Federation Leadership Group and Implementation Committee on the Launching of the Three Rehabilitations Project', *Voice of the Deaf and Mute*, 67: 6–8.

Gaubatz, P.R. 1995. 'Urban transformation in post-Mao China: Impacts of the reform era on China's urban form', in D. Davis et al. (eds), *Urban Spaces in Contemporary China: The Potential for Autonomy and Community in Post-Mao China*. Washington, D.C.: Woodrow Wilson Centre Press, pp. 28–60.

Gramsci, A. 1971. *Selections from the Prison Notebooks of Antonio Gramsci*. New York: International Publishers.

Hansson, H. 1988. *Regional Outcast Groups in Late Imperial China*. PhD Thesis. Harvard University.

Harvey, D. 1990. *The Condition of Post-modernity*. Cambridge: Blackwell.

Henderson, G. 1989. 'Issues in the modernisation of medicine in China', in D. Simon and M. Goldman (eds), *Science and Technology in Post-Mao China*. Cambridge: Harvard University Press.

Ho, P.T. 1959. *Studies on the Population of China*. Cambridge: Harvard University Press.

Kleinman, A. et al. 1995. 'The Social Course of Epilepsy: Chronic Illness as Social Experience in Interior China', *Social Science and Medicine*, 40: 1319–30.

Kohrman, M. 1999. 'Grooming Que Zi: Marriage exclusion and identity formation among disabled men in contemporary China', *American Ethnologist*, 26: 890–909.

Kriegel, L. 1991. *Falling into Life*. San Francisco: North Point Press.

Lu, D. and Dao, S. 1996. *The History of Persons with Disabilities in China* (*zhong gho can ji ren shi*) (in Chinese). Shanghai: Xuelin Press.

Mark, R. 1995. 'On the Beauty of Beijing', in The Feminist Press Travel Series. *China for Women: Travel and Culture*. New York: The Feminist Press.

Martin, E. 1992. 'The end of the body?', *American Ethnologist*, 19: 121–40.

Ministry of Civil Affairs. 1993. *Information on the Physically Disabled* (*zhi ti can ji ren cai liao*) (in Chinese). Beijing: Ministry of Civil Affairs Press.

Mosse, G. 1985. *Nationalism and Sexuality: Middle-Class Morality and Sexual Norms in Modem Europe*. Madison: University of Wisconsin Press.

Ong, A. and Nonini, D. 1997. 'Chinese transnationalism as an alternative modernity', in A. Ong and D. Nonini (eds), *Underground Empires: The Cultural Politics of Modern Chinese Transnationalism*. New York: Routledge, pp. 3–33.

Qin, Y. 1992. *The Deng Pufang Road* (*deng pu fang de lu*) (in Chinese). Hong Kong: Kai Yi Press.

Rockhill, W.W. 1904. 'An Inquiry into the Population of China', *Smithsonian Miscellaneous Collection*, 47: 659–76.

Scharff, V. 1991. *Taking the Wheel: Women and the Coming of the Motor Age*. New York: Free Press.

Shapiro, J. 1993. *No Pity: People with Disabilities Forging a New Civil-Rights Movement*. New York: Times Books.

Strathern, M. 1988. *The Gender of the Gift*. Berkeley: University of California Press.

Walder, A. 1986. *Communist Neo-Traditionalism: Work and Authority in Chinese Industry*. Berkeley: University of California Press.
Wieger, L. 1965. *Chinese Characters: Their Origin, Etymology, History, Classification and Signification*. New York: Paragon.
World Bank. 1992. *China: Long-Term Issues and Options in the Health Transition*. Washington: World Bank.
World Health Organisation. 1980. *International Classification of Impairments, Disabilities and Handicaps: A Manual of Classification Relating to the Consequences of Disease*. Geneva: World Health Organisation.
Zhao, G. (n.d.) (ed.) *Hou-Hu Chi* (microfilm). Taibei: National Central Library.

16

Engaging with the Disability-Rights Movement: The Experience of Community-Based Rehabilitation in Southern Africa

Susie Miles

INTRODUCTION

The prevailing tendency among rehabilitation workers is to dismiss the strength, and thus the value, of engaging with the disability-rights movement. In so doing, they risk both missing out on an essential part of their education and alienating disabled people's organisations (DPOs) because of their reluctance to relinquish control of the rehabilitation process. The transition from omniscient professional to facilitator in the community requires an enormous shift in thinking, and, too often, institutional attitudes are carried over. I will argue here that community-based rehabilitation (CBR) is in danger of repeating the mistakes of institution-based rehabilitation (IBR) if it does not enter into genuine consultation with DPOs.

The World Health Organisation (WHO) formalised CBR into a strategy for developing countries in 1976. Since then the concept of CBR has spread rapidly, though implementation strategies are diverse. Twenty

---

Miles, S. 1996. 'Engaging with the Disability-Rights Movement: The experience of community-based rehabilitation in Southern Africa', *Disability and Society*, 11: 501–17.

years on, CBR is no longer considered to be a blueprint or ready-made solution; instead, it is a philosophy which can be tailored to suit the cultural context in which it is applied. Greater attention is now paid to the informal CBR support networks which predate WHO's initiative, and the need to validate indigenous practices is increasingly recognised.

In southern Africa, the disabled people's movement is relatively strong, and the enfolding philosophy of CBR in the region has been well seasoned with disability rights. CBR implementers are struggling to achieve a balanced perspective between delivering quality services and empowering disabled people and parents. This struggle has been observed and documented by the Save the Children Fund (SCF), and it forms the basis for this article. In 1994, SCF brought together staff and partners working in disability programmes in 17 different countries to exchange experiences (SCF, 1994). SCF's global disability work can be divided into three categories: CBR, Integrated Education, and the support of consumer organisations. A follow-up meeting was held in southern Africa to establish areas of common interest between CBR and disabled people's and parents' organisations, develop a mutually supportive relationship, and agree on a more coordinated way of working. The ideas and views expressed here are both a reflection of observations made by myself, as SCF's Regional Disability Advisor, and of the discussions held at the meetings.

The first section of this paper outlines some of the problems with IBR, describes in general terms the content of CBR, and stresses the need to reconceptualise CBR in the context of African communities and the collective way in which they operate. This is followed by a brief look at the way in which key writers on CBR view the role of disabled people and their organisations.

CBR is both a philosophy and a strategy for providing rehabilitation services in the community in a more equitable, sustainable and appropriate way than can be provided in a health or educational institution. Institution-based rehabilitation (IBR) in developing countries is expensive, often inappropriate, and only available to a 'lucky' few. Rehabilitation services are not considered a high priority by most African governments; even if they were, the cost of providing high quality rehabilitation institutions for those who require such services would be prohibitive. More importantly, the type of rehabilitation available in a highly professionalised institution is unlikely to be of benefit to the majority of people, whose home environment is in stark contrast to that of the institution. Furthermore, limited places means that IBR is beyond the reach of the majority, and the cost of travelling long distances to and from centrally located institutions makes IBR unaffordable for impoverished families.

CBR was pioneered at a time when many rehabilitation professionals were beginning to question the validity of their institution-based work, often as a result of visiting disabled people in their communities on an outreach basis. In many cases, such visits provided professionals with the information and experience required to launch CBR programmes, though many so-called community-based programmes have continued to function as outreach programmes.

There are arguably as many different types of CBR as there are programmes in existence. Most CBR programmes, however, include the following activities: the selection and training of village-based CBR workers; the identification, assessment and referral, where appropriate, of disabled children and adults; the design of aids and appliances by local craftsmen; and the teaching of simple rehabilitative techniques to family members for use with their disabled child. Awareness raising, public education, counselling, multi-sectoral collaboration, community development, and the promotion of integrated education are also key ingredients of CBR programmes. CBR services may be integrated into existing health, education or social welfare structures, or they may be vertical programmes run by NGOs. Increasingly, CBR services are being developed at village level as part of community-development programmes, with relatively little input from rehabilitation professionals. Although a CBR programme may contain some or all of the ingredients discussed above, its flavour will depend upon the cultural context in which it is implemented. Each programme is therefore unique. Differences exist not only between CBR programmes in different cultures, but also between villages in one geographical area.

CBR AND THE TENSION BETWEEN THE INDIVIDUAL AND THE COMMUNITY

It is very important to place the development of CBR in Africa in the context of a collective consciousness. In Africa, the needs of the collective, or community, are paramount, whereas in the west it is the individual whose needs come first. Although the true essence of CBR does not conflict with this cultural principle, CBR has been packaged and marketed from a western, individualistic perspective, and there tends to be a strong focus upon correcting or minimising the impairments of individual disabled people. Focusing exclusively upon the rehabilitation needs of individuals is likely to be counterproductive unless the informal support networks and the basic needs of the whole community are recognised and addressed. Serpell et al. (1993) contrast the emphasis in the west on the promotion of autonomy or independence with the tendency of African parents to cultivate social responsibility in their children, and discuss the implications of this when working with the families of children who have learning difficulties. This tension between the community and the individual, between Africa and the west, would perhaps render the already contentious concept of independent living inappropriate in the African context. Interestingly, however, centres for independent living in the U.K. are aiming to achieve a degree of *interdependence* which is closer to the African concept than to the western principle of independence (Barnes, 1993).

Vanneste (1995) cites a disturbing example of a CBR programme which effectively destroyed the pre-existing informal mutual-support network upon which a family had depended. A neighbour had been helping the family of a severely disabled child, but when a CBR worker began to visit the child, the neighbour withdrew her support. Later, when the CBR worker stopped visiting, the neighbour refused to resume her visits, leaving the child and her family in a worse situation. This could have been avoided if the traditional coping or CBR mechanisms had been respected.

Ideally, the CBR implementer or animator should unlock and place value on indigenous knowledge about disability, and balance the local expertise with sensitive application and adaptation of knowledge gained outside the community. CBR can be seen as a vehicle for the exchange of information between communities and governments, and between disabled community members and national DPOs. If CBR workers are to fulfil this role for disabled people's groups, and if they are to develop a coordinated way of working, a level of commitment to the disability-rights philosophy is desirable.

A range of attitudes and ways of working with disabled people and their organisations is reflected in the CBR literature. Implementers of CBR programmes increasingly recognise the importance of involving disabled people in the CBR process, rather than seeing them as recipients of services. However, the extent to which disabled people and their organisations are actively involved in the process is difficult to determine. The Zanzibar and Mauritania CBR programmes were set up by national DPOs whose leaders are well known in the international disability movement, but, unfortunately, these are isolated and little known examples. Definitions of CBR have developed and changed in response to field experience, and there is an arguably healthy lack of consensus. Unfortunately, though, disabled people's voices, especially those from the 'south', are rarely heard in the CBR debates or reflected in the literature.

The recent joint statement on CBR by UNESCO, ILO and WHO (1994) emphasises the importance of partnership with disabled people as individuals, by stressing that CBR should be implemented through the *combined efforts* of disabled people, their families and communities, and the appropriate government services. Helander (1993) recognises the value of working with local parents' and disabled people's groups, but bemoans the fact that DPOs too often develop top-down rather than from the grass-roots level.

Some writers place more emphasis on the family, rather than on disabled people. This is especially true of programmes that prioritise children, and particularly children with severe disabilities, whose experience and needs tend to be neglected by the disability-rights movement. O'Toole (1994) asserts that the greatest resource in developing countries for helping disabled persons lead lives which are fulfilled and productive is a well-advised and supported family.

The International Labour Organisation (ILO) is concerned about broader issues such as integration. Although the main focus is on service provision, the ILO acknowledges the increasing importance of the disabled people's movement.

A new development, which also makes its way gradually into rural areas, is the emergence of associations of disabled people. This development will, sooner or later, replace a patronising form of planning for disabled people by a planning process which involves the target beneficiaries (Momm and Konig, 1989, p. 6). David Werner goes a step further and argues that disabled people should be in control, that involvement is not enough. He recognises that families of disabled people have an equally important role to play. His views are substantiated by his experience, both as a disabled person and as a staff member of Project Projimo in rural Mexico. This is run and almost entirely staffed by disabled villagers, and maintains high standards of appropriate and affordable rehabilitation. Only when programmes for disabled people are led and controlled by disabled people (and/or their families) are they likely to help disabled persons gain self-determination and a respected, equal position in society (Werner, 1993, p. viii). It is worth noting that Werner is one of very few disabled spokespersons on CBR. Sadly, there appears to be very little cross-fertilisation of ideas between CBR writers and implementers and the disabled people's movement, and so attitudes tend to remain unchallenged. In southern Africa, however, interaction between CBR programmes and DPOs has led to the development of a more consumer-focused approach to CBR.

THE SOUTHERN AFRICAN CONTEXT AND SCF'S INVOLVEMENT

This section will focus on the role of Save the Children Fund (SCF) as facilitator and provider of technical and financial support for the work of both governmental and non-governmental initiatives in disability and development work. The nature of the support varied according to the national and political context in which it was provided, and these will be briefly described. This section will also highlight the role of the Southern Africa Federation of Organisations of the Disabled (SAFOD) as *agent provocateur* and ally in SCF's journey from service provision to politics. This journey, or process, has involved a redefining of rehabilitation needs through community consultation, and a greater focus on the empowerment of parents and disabled people.

The disability-rights movement in southern Africa has its roots in Zimbabwe. In the mid-1970s, a group of physically disabled people began to organise themselves in the institution in which they lived and worked. Charlton (1993) has charted this development through a series of interviews with key individuals, one of whom, Joshua Malinga, became the main link with Disabled People International (DPI) from its inception in 1981, and was later elected its chairperson. The disability movement in southern Africa was therefore strongly influenced from its early stages by international disability politics. Malinga was instrumental in establishing SAFOD in 1986. SAFOD is the umbrella body to which all national DPOs have become affiliated, and, in turn, it is affiliated to DPI. SAFOD's original aims were to support the formation of DPOs, both local and national, to strengthen existing ones and to promote leadership training.

The southern Africa region has been fraught with political conflict, drought and an unequal distribution of resources, and it has not been easy to foster the development of altruistic and committed leaders in this context (Leaman and Fricke, 1991). Although the struggle against apartheid in South Africa has had a profoundly negative effect on the whole region, it has provided a revolutionary context from within which the disability-rights movement has emerged and with which it has identified its own struggle. The relative cohesion of the region, which, ironically, is partly due to South Africa's political and economic influence, is one of the factors contributing to SAFOD's success as one of DPI's regional bodies.

It would have been conceivable, though arguably unethical, for SCF to have supported the development of CBR initiatives without reference to the disability-rights movement. SAFOD was, however, a rich resource upon which to draw in the late 1980s, when CBR was a little-understood concept in southern Africa. SCF's involvement began in 1988 with the appointment of a Regional Disability Advisor, whose responsibility was to act as an information broker, to develop south-south networks, and to support the development of innovative community-based initiatives which would provide models for evaluation and training (Saunders, 1987).

To date, SCF has supported 10 programmes in Mozambique, Zimbabwe, South Africa, Swaziland and Lesotho. These include a national Integrated Education programme run by the Ministry of Education in Lesotho; five CBR programmes, four of which are health-based and a fifth which is located in the Ministry of Social Action in Mozambique; two institution-based outreach projects run by a local NGO in Zimbabwe, which preceded the regional disability programme; and development programmes run by two DPOs. Interestingly, only three of the 10 programmes have a national brief and are run by government ministries; only one of these is a Ministry of Health programme. This programme has stimulated thinking on disability issues in Swaziland, as has the Integrated Education programme in Lesotho, but policies have not yet been developed. The Zimbabwean government has taken the issue of disability seriously ever since it came to power at Independence, and a disability act has been passed recently. In both Mozambique and South Africa, disability policy is currently being developed. SCF has only employed two expatriates in southern Africa, both of whom were requested by government ministries: the Ministry of Social Action in Mozambique and the Ministry of Education in Lesotho.

Historically, the dividing line between SCF-supported CBR programmes and DPOs was their target groups, with SCF focusing on children and DPOs on adults. However, this proved to be a naive and unrealistic distinction, as implementers of CBR programmes were faced with the changing needs of the children as they grew into adulthood. It was crucial, however, to define the CBR workers' relationship with disabled adults so that they were not simply seen as an extension of the client group, but instead as valuable participants in the CBR process.

The ILO has stressed the importance of establishing the different needs, and therefore the different types of assistance, required by disabled adults (Momm and Konig, 1989). Whether assistance means access to services or help with the establishment of self-help groups and/or empowerment, it is important to recognise the very different nature of the relationship between CBR workers and adults from the one that is likely to exist between CBR workers and children. Children do not have a voice and tend to be passive recipients of services, whereas disabled adults are either recipients of services, potential leaders of programmes, or they may choose not to be involved at all. The difference in the relationship is arguably more crucial than the different type of assistance required.

Assuming that a more equal relationship develops, opportunities for greater involvement of DPOs in CBR will increase. The need for positive adult role models for disabled children in CBR has prompted CBR implementers to challenge DPOs to become more involved with children's and parents' issues. However, many of the region's DPOs lack the capacity to involve themselves in anything other than the development of their own organisations. Others are reluctant to get involved because of their uneasiness about the underlying philosophy of rehabilitation, which places the power firmly in the hands of the professionals.

The continued use of the word 'rehabilitation' is, in itself, a source of conflict and debate. The following section will examine the difficulties arising from the word 'rehabilitation', and will describe the development of programmes in Lesotho and South Africa which prioritise disabled people's access to education and employment, rather than to medical rehabilitation.

CBR WITHOUT THE 'R'

The ideas represented by the term CBR have sparked off disability initiatives in communities in most countries in Africa and Asia, and the term has been interpreted in many different ways (Miles, 1993). For those projects that work in partnership with disabled people, it would be preferable to find a term that encapsulates the idea of a community-based strategy which promotes equality of opportunities. It should reflect the fact that disability is not only a health or social-welfare issue, but also one of politics, economics, development and human rights. Community-based support (CBS) for disabled people is an example of an alternative term. It was adopted by the Ministry of Social Action in Mozambique as a deliberate move away from the medical model, which emphasises the treatment and rehabilitation of impairments (Miles and Medi, 1994). In the meantime, the term CBR will continue to be used here as a catch-all, but it is accepted that it may outlive its usefulness.

The adoption of a more consumer-focused approach to CBR, by the Scott Hospital CBR team in Lesotho and the Amawoti Disabled People's Association in South Africa, has enabled disabled people and CBR workers to work together on a more equal basis. By approaching disability as a community-development issue, disabled adults and parents of disabled children have become active participants in the CBR process. This has resulted in a type of CBR which places less emphasis on the 'R' and instead prioritises education and employment issues.

I will now briefly describe the context in which the Scott and Amawoti programmes are working, the main aspects of the work, and the similarities between the two. This will be followed by a discussion of the role of home visiting and multi-disciplinary teams in CBR. It is argued that when disabled people and parents are actively involved in CBR, the programme is moulded by the skills and interests of the people involved, rather than by prescriptive manuals and the received international wisdom on the issue.

Scott is a mission hospital serving a sparsely populated rural community of approximately 170,000 people in the foothills of Lesotho. In the mid-1980s, Scott pioneered a Home Nursing programme which targeted elderly people and those who had suffered a stroke. The need to address disability as an issue in the community arose both from the Primary Health Care (PHC) team's consultation with the Village Health Committees and from the nurses' growing awareness of disability through the Home Nursing programme. Lessons learnt from mistakes made in the implementation of PHC ensured that the PHC team entered into genuine consultation with the community in order to establish community ownership and involvement in the disability work.

The long-term goal of SCF's support for this CBR programme was to provide Lesotho, and the Ministry of Health in particular, with a model for evaluation and training. This has proved to be a very slow process within Lesotho, but the impact of Scott's work has been felt both regionally and internationally through SCF's dissemination of lessons learnt. However, the Ministry of Education's Integrated Education programme, which is also supported by SCF, is also taking the lead in promoting disability issues at a national level. Amawoti is an informal peri-urban community situated 30 km north of Durban in South Africa. With a population of 100,000, it is a community marked by poverty and an associated lack of services (Philpott, 1995). The Amawoti Disabled People's Association grew out of the concern of one of the local civic committees about the needs of disabled people in their area. Support was provided by the staff of a community-based PHC project in Amawoti, which viewed health not as a medical problem but as a broader question of access to power.

Prior to South Africa's first elections in 1994, all pioneering work in the field of disability and development was carried out by NGOs, although between 1990 and 1994 dialogue was initiated by the government. Since 1994, however, considerable progress has been made by the government, with the support of the national DPO, to develop a comprehensive policy on disability.

Scott and Amawoti are small projects which have pioneered a different approach to CBR and have had an impact on the development of thinking in the region about community disability work. Despite their very marked differences, they have the following aspects in common:

- Disabled people and parents have been involved from the beginning, many as volunteer CBR workers.
- Disabled adults are seen as partners in the CBR process rather than potential clients.
- The disability work has emerged from PHC and has a strong community-development focus.
- Medical rehabilitation has not been the main priority, with education and employment issues taking precedence.
- Poverty alleviation is considered to be an essential part of CBR.
- Attitude change in the community is seen as crucial.
- The pace is necessarily slow.
- Home visiting is carried out when necessary, but is not a routine activity.

Home visiting, together with attitude change and the empowerment of disabled people, has always been thought of as one of the cornerstones of CBR. Home visits provide a crucial, though time-consuming, therapeutic and support service to those disabled people and their families who would otherwise be unlikely to have regular access to rehabilitation services. While not wishing to devalue the efforts of CBR workers to provide therapy and support to individuals, I would argue that, in some cases, home visiting is in danger of becoming an institutionalised activity which has lost sight of its original purpose. Interestingly, home visiting is given much less importance in the Scott and Amawoti projects. Some of the possible reasons are as follows:

- Home visits take place naturally as part of everyday life rather than as scheduled activities.
- Disabled adults and parents are so involved with the running of the programme that they no longer feel so isolated, and are therefore in less need of home visits.
- Disabled adults and parents are learning the skills they need in other situations, for example, at community meetings, in support groups, crèches, or while knitting in the income-generating groups.

Although the projects have prioritised attitude change, income-generating projects and empowerment, home visiting has not been ruled out. In fact, home visits were made in the initial stages in order to identify disabled children and to train key workers. Parents in both projects are beginning to express their interest in learning simple rehabilitation techniques in order to reach disabled people and their families who are not already involved in the programme. If home visiting is adopted as one of their strategies, it will be an activity defined and controlled by the community, rather than one performed or monitored by outsiders.

Similarly, roles and responsibilities in Scott and Amawoti have been defined according to the abilities and priorities of those involved, and this has led to the development of a multi-disciplinary team approach. These are not the multi-disciplinary teams associated with highly trained professionals and case conferences, but a collection of committed individuals with a variety of skills to offer. Tasks are assigned according to the abilities and interests of the individuals, in contrast to the WHO approach of training a cadre of workers who each carry out an agreed set of tasks.

In Amawoti, a conscious decision was made not to train individual CBR workers, but to assign tasks according to need. The Scott project has abandoned the CBR worker strategy in favour of supporting the development of parents' and child-to-child support groups, from which key individuals have emerged as resource persons and leaders. A variety of specialist services are on offer in both programmes, including literacy teaching, crèche facilities, examination of newborn babies, knitting-machine instruction, income-generating activities, the manufacture of aids and appliances, and the child-to-child approach in schools. Further training in these specialist areas will be sought, where possible, for the key individuals who have shown the greatest commitment.

DEVELOPING A MUTUALLY SUPPORTIVE RELATIONSHIP

The move towards a consumer-controlled approach to CBR has necessitated the formalisation of the working relationship between CBR programme implementers and their DPO counterparts. This process is far from complete in southern Africa, but initial discussions have been held to establish common areas of interest, while clarifying potential sources of conflict and differing priorities, for example, between adults' and children's issues. CBR workers tend to have more contact with the families of disabled people than with the disability-rights movement, especially in programmes which prioritise the needs of children. Therefore they do not necessarily feel that they should be accountable to DPOs. They may have contact with disabled adults as individuals, or they may be involved in facilitating the development of self-help groups of disabled adults, but this does not necessarily bring them into contact with the disability-rights philosophy, and they may never be forced to confront their own negative attitudes. Similarly, there is a tendency for DPOs to assume that rehabilitation workers are not interested in disability-rights issues, and for the two to be perceived as being mutually exclusive or incompatible, as illustrated by the following quote:

> Service providers would not be interested in the philosophy and objectives of the Movement. They suspect the Movement is there to sabotage them. (Mbewe and Lee, 1991, p. 30)

However, the movement sees itself as a watchdog whose responsibility it is to monitor the quality and availability of services. Furthermore, disabled people feel they have a duty to educate rehabilitation workers and transform them into supporters of the movement (Charlton, 1993).

In response to proposals for funding from SAFOD, SCF produced a discussion document (Miles, 1992) to clarify SCF's disability policy and funding capacity, and to open up discussion on common areas of interest with a view to developing and formalising a mutually supportive working relationship. In 1992, SCF secured funding for two DPOs which aimed to develop stronger links between themselves and CBR programmes. These were the Amawoti Disabled People's Association and the Lesotho National Federation of Organisations of Disabled people (LNFOD)'s development activists' training programme, whose impact will be examined later.

How best to work with DPOs had become a major issue for CBR workers throughout the region, and attitudes to this varied enormously. The need to consult and confront DPOs about the role of CBR in the disability-rights movement came about through discussions between project staff and SCF's advisor, which culminated in a series of meetings held both regionally and globally (SCF, 1994) to review SCF's disability work. An interesting comparison was made at the final regional meeting between the very similar aims of the CBR programmes and the DPOs represented. A sharing of resources and the development of a more coordinated way of working seemed the obvious way forward, but first, differences in philosophy and approach needed to be discussed as honestly and openly as possible. From the CBR perspective, it was felt by some that DPOs tended to be undemocratic, disorganised and led by elite groups of physically disabled people. It is difficult to encourage the development of decentralised and egalitarian DPOs when their membership and agendas are urban-based and largely middle-class (Werner, 1995). The tendency was to bypass them, or to inform them of CBR activities, but not to enter into genuine consultation about the needs of their common target groups. An example of a more coordinated approach to the needs of rural disabled people follows.

WHERE THERE IS NO CBR: THE ROLE OF DEVELOPMENT ACTIVISTS

This section highlights the role that DPOs can play in promoting the concept of CBR in the absence of CBR programmes. The mobilisation of disabled adults living in rural areas through LNFOD's development activists' training workshops has resulted in their increased confidence and motivation. A good working relationship between LNFOD and the CBR and National Integrated Education programmes in Lesotho has ensured that disabled children's issues are high on the agenda.

LNFOD is a cross-disability national umbrella organisation, and since 1993 it has consisted of four member organisations, representing people with physical, visual and hearing impairments, and those with learning difficulties (and their parents). Over a three-year period, LNFOD has trained 30 rural disabled people per year as development activists in a series of three 1-week workshops. Places on the training programme were shared equally between the member organisations, and 50 per cent of all trainees were women. In addition, the CBR programme was allocated places for disabled adults who were potential leaders in the programme.

The courses included an introduction to disability as a development issue, consciousness-raising on disability-rights issues, advice on how to set up and run local committees, and ideas on income generation. There was also some orientation on disabled children's issues, and visits were organised to both segregated and integrated schools. The organisation of these courses and the follow-up in the communities were the responsibility of the one salaried person within LNFOD and of its volunteer committee members. The main impact of the training has been in the raising of self-esteem and confidence of the individuals trained. The mutual support systems which have developed through the workshops and subsequent local meetings have fostered a greater sense of self-worth in the trainees and of control over their own lives:

> We used to feel isolated and suffered in silence. Now we meet and make our own decisions. (du Toit, 1995)

Similarly, the parents who have been trained have experienced a change in their attitude towards their disabled children and a greater appreciation of disability issues:

> Being involved with disabled people has taught me to handle my situation. My disabled child is now active in my family. (du Toit, 1995, p. 18)

Finally, disabled adults now feel committed to CBR-type activities, such as the challenging of negative attitudes, and the counselling of other disabled people and their families about education, employment and rehabilitation issues. They consider themselves responsible resource people in their communities and, in particular, they are concerned to support parents of disabled children:

> I now have the courage and understanding to approach parents to change their view of their children with disabilities, to seek education for them, and to organise for self-help. (du Toit, 1995, p. 17)

The development activists have formed support groups in which they plan their activities, such as holding community meetings and establishing self-help groups. Their awareness of CBR issues has given them the confidence to provide advice and information to families, and in this way they are performing part of the function of CBR workers. In fact, LNFOD has taken over the management of an NGO-run CBR programme in the south of Lesotho, and this provides them with the opportunity to integrate the two approaches.

The following section describes the reverse situation, where CBR workers are involved in setting up local disabled people's support groups, often with very little input from the national DPO.

THE ROLE OF CBR WHERE THERE IS NO DPO

CBR programmes invariably operate in communities where there is no DPO, and CBR workers are often instrumental in facilitating their development. In the following examples, the CBR workers provide a vital link between local groups and the national DPO and relevant government departments. They act as a channel of information and ideas, and are therefore in a position of power. The way in which this is handled is crucial to the long-term sustainability of the local group. Local DPOs are in danger of either becoming totally dependent on the CBR programme and, therefore, being ineffective, or of being left to develop so independently that they lack support and resources, and so flounder.

One of Africa's earliest rural CBR programmes, in Kibwezi, Kenya, began without the involvement of disabled people, but its staff have come to realise the drawbacks of this way of working. The Kibwezi programme targeted disabled children up to the age of 16, and neither provided services for adults nor considered helping them to set up a local support group. In 1990, the programme was evaluated, and this lack of involvement of disabled adults was highlighted as an issue of concern (Saunders and Zinkin, 1990). As a result of this, a local group began to meet as a separate entity from the CBR programme. The coordinator of the programme is now convinced of the importance of starting CBR programmes with the full involvement of disabled adults, if they are to be sustainable.

In Mozambique, the community-based support (CBS) team attached to the Ministry of Social Action in Mozambique provided a meeting room for a group of deaf school-leavers who had failed to make their voices heard in the national DPO. The group prioritised the development of a national sign language, and became involved with teaching small groups of deaf children as part of the national CBS programme. The group will soon form itself into an association and will apply for affiliate membership to the national DPO. The CBS team played a crucial role in reporting a neglected group of disabled people who, in turn, have made an invaluable contribution to community disability work by supporting the development of groups in many different provinces.

In South Africa, a working relationship between disabled people and occupational therapists has existed since the mid-1980s with the advent of an organisation known as Rural Action on Disability (RURACT), which is affiliated to the national DPO. Its responsibility is to promote CBR and develop networks throughout South Africa and the surrounding countries. RURACT has provided a useful forum for the development of thinking on CBR issues in the context of the disability-rights philosophy.

The Alexandra Health Centre's CBR programme in South Africa had, as one of its original aims, the establishment of a support group of, and for, disabled people. The process of facilitating the development of the Alexandra Disability Movement (ADM) has been documented from the point of view of the CBR implementer (Cornielje, 1993). The creation of a body of disabled people to whom rehabilitation workers would be accountable was one of the original objectives. Despite the difficulties of working in a politically divided society and the lack of quality leadership, ADM is increasingly playing a vital role in the development of rehabilitation services.

In Amawoti, disability was identified by the local civic committee as an issue to be addressed, and a committee was formed of concerned persons, which included disabled people and parents of disabled children. Subcommittees of interest groups have since been formed so disabled people meet separately as a subgroup, but they come together with the parents and civic committee members to form the Amawoti Disabled People's Association, as they do not wish to isolate themselves from the rest of the community. They consider it their role to raise awareness of the fact that disabled people are members of the wider group of disadvantaged and impoverished people in Amawoti, and they encourage others to be inclusive in their approach to development (SCF, 1994).

In Lesotho, the Scott CBR programme established contact with the national DPO, primarily to solicit help with the training of CBR workers and teachers. Close contact between the CBR programme and the DPO has been possible because Lesotho is a very small country and because of a good working relationship between the respective leaders. Parents' groups have been set up and, as membership is open to disabled people, the need for a separate DPO has not been identified.

In the above examples, the CBR programmes have provided the initial funding for the establishment of local DPOs and parents' groups, and it is unlikely that these groups would have been set up without this support. The local groups all have a role to play in the CBR programmes with which they are associated. In the case of Alexandra, this role was predetermined, and with the others it is being defined as the programmes develop. The Amawoti programme is somewhat different, as it does not use CBR terminology and it is a single organisation which is fulfilling both functions. Finally, membership of local DPOs is not always restricted to disabled people, and it is very common for disabled adults and parents to work together at a local level. The CBR programmes described are moving towards greater partnership with disabled people and parents. This is a dynamic process which necessitates the continual reappraisal of roles. One of the main purposes of SCF's regional meeting was to clarify the role of CBR workers in relation to DPOs, and it was agreed that this should be as follows (Miles, 1994):

- Mobilisation of parents and disabled people.
- Help with the formation of local parents' and disabled people's groups.
- Networking and dissemination of information between local and national DPOs.
- Empowerment and capacity-building of disabled people and their organisations.

The greatest and most urgent need was considered to be the capacity-building of DPOs. DPOs, especially at a local level, tend to lack funds and administrative and logistical support, and are generally less well-resourced than CBR programmes. More coordinated planning in the deployment of scarce resources would improve the situation, but the empowerment and capacity-building process will inevitably be slow—slower than most donors are likely to tolerate.

PARENTS AS ACTIVISTS

This final section addresses the issue of parents, their involvement in both CBR programmes and the disability rights movement, and the way in which they have come to realise that they face oppression in common with disabled adults. It is recognised that there are important differences between the experience of disabled people in Africa and that of disabled people in the U.K., for example, and that very real, often insurmountable, problems and conflicts exist between organisations of disabled people and those for them in industrialised countries. Similar tensions and conflicts have already arisen in southern Africa, and attempts have been made to understand and resolve them.

In southern Africa, the term 'parents' rather than 'families' tends to be used, as they have organised themselves into pressure groups, and are active in promoting and implementing CBR activities. In practice, they are primarily mothers' groups, as many women are abandoned by their husbands as a result of the birth of a disabled child, or upon diagnosis (Kisanji, 1995). Economic pressure to produce healthy children is very strong. Although mothers have been extremely effective in organising themselves into support groups, they have not achieved the same levels of recognition or success as the disability-rights movement, and what they have achieved is poorly documented. A major reason for the disparity between the two groups in southern Africa is undoubtedly gender-related, as DPOs tend to be led by men and parents' groups by women who are primarily the sole breadwinners for their families (Miles, 1994). SAFOD's progressive gender policy will, in time, redress this imbalance, but the fundamental inequalities between men and women in relation to childcare are likely to continue.

As parents have become more involved in the setting up of their own organisations and in CBR programmes, they have come into contact with broader disability issues. Parental involvement in the struggle for disability rights has effectively challenged the predominant attitude in SAFOD that parents neglected, overprotected or discriminated against their children. This attitude had been compounded by the lack of interest shown by DPOs in children's issues in general, but more specifically in those involving profound and multiple disabilities and in the consequences for their families. Not surprisingly, parents were unsure of their role and did not see disabled adults as their natural allies. A lack of concern for children's issues among DPOs is not peculiar to southern Africa, as the following quotation from the U.K. illustrates:

> I had been active in disability politics for more than ten years, but it was only when I became a parent that I realised that the moves forward that we have achieved for ourselves as adults with disabilities have not reached the lives of disabled children at all. (Rieser and Mason, 1992, cover note)

In Lesotho and South Africa, parents have argued that they are disabled by virtue of being the full-time carers of severely disabled children, and that together with their children they are affected by the stigma of disability. As a result, parents' organisations have been accepted as affiliate members of DPOs. This enables them to pursue their own agendas, which are quite distinct from those of disabled adults, while maximising the opportunity of being an ally of the disability-rights movement.

Parents also have a role to play in service provision. CBR implementers have trained mothers of disabled children as CBR workers in Lesotho and South Africa, and in many instances they have proved to be more effective and more dedicated than health workers, as McGlade and Aquino (1995) testify from their experience in the Philippines. Ideally, both parents and disabled adults should be employed as CBR workers, or as CBR team members. In this way, the needs of disabled children for role models and of parents for support are more likely to be met. Tensions inevitably exist between the two groups, especially where resources are scarce. However, through a process of constructive dialogue and a commitment to working in partnership, a mutually supportive relationship can be developed through which disabled adults and parents can teach each other a great deal.

CONCLUSION

The long-term goal of all CBR programmes should be to facilitate disabled people to take control of their own lives and to play a decisive role in any services that are created. In a recent survey of people living with acquired impairments in the U.K., services were seen as tending to remove choice and control because they were provided by others on their behalf (Todhunter, Pilgrim and Pearson, 1995). There is enormous potential in developing countries to leapfrog over the professional hurdles created by the rehabilitation industry in the west and to work directly with disabled people and parents to ensure that the services which are created are those that are most needed. The cultural bias in Africa towards collective, rather than individual, needs and responsibilities should be fully exploited by CBR.

Resource-driven service provision, based on the western model, is not sustainable and is of questionable value. Disabled people need access to mainstream services and to appropriate information in an accessible form. CBR has the potential to unlock and validate existing indigenous knowledge and information systems, while facilitating access to relevant information and ideas outside the community. I have argued that this should be done with the active participation of the consumers themselves, and with an understanding of disability as a development issue.

The danger inherent in CBR is that it may simply become a community version of IBR with the power still firmly in the hands of professionals, and with disabled people and their families in the role of passive recipients. It is important that programmes strive to develop services which have appropriately high standards while at the same time ensuring an equal partnership between consumer and professional. This will inevitably call into question some of the fundamental aspects of CBR, such as the practice of home visiting. The development of a mutually supportive relationship and an honest discussion of the different agendas of CBR workers, parents and DPOs have helped in redefining CBR as a consumer-focused strategy in southern Africa.

In summary, CBR workers have a key role to play in the development and capacity building of DPOs, especially at community level. They have access to information and resources which need to be shared. By feeding information about disability work at community level to the policy-makers at national level, they can provide an essential link between local and national issues. CBR teams should work together with DPOs to address poverty, and to tackle education and employment issues. At a political level, they can support the efforts of DPOs to run advocacy programmes and to develop policy and legislation on disability. It is crucial that CBR workers and donors recognise that the pace will inevitably be slow, and that it is in the long-term interests of disabled people to work with, rather than against, the disability-rights movement.

References

Barnes, C. 1993. (ed.) *Making Our Own Choices: Independent Living and Personal Assistant.* Derby: British Council of Organisations of Disabled People.

Charlton, J.I. 1993. 'Development and disability: voices from the periphery—Zimbabwe', in B.L. Mallory et al. (eds), *Traditional and Changing Views of Disability in Developing Societies: Causes, Consequences, Cautions.* Monograph 53. Durham: University of New Hampshire.

Cornielje, H. 1993. 'A local disability movement as part of a CBR programme', in H. Finkenflügel (ed.), *The Handicapped Community*. Amsterdam: Vrij Universiteit Press.

du Toit, M. 1995. *An Evaluation of the Lesotho National Federation of Organisations of Disabled Persons' Development Activists' Training Programme*. Maseru: Save the Children Fund.

Helander, E. 1993. *Prejudice and Dignity*. New York: United Nations Development Project.

Kisanji, J. 1995. 'Growing up disabled', in P. Zinken and H. Mcconachie (eds), *Disabled Children and Developing Countries*. Cambridge: MacKeith Press and Cambridge University Press.

Leaman, D. and Fricke, Y. 1991. *The Making of a Movement: SAFOD Evaluation*. Bulawayo: South African Federation of the Disabled.

Mbewe, M. and Lee, P. 1991. *SAFOD Development Activists' Handbook*. Bulawayo: South African Federation of the Disabled.

McGlade, B. and Aquino, R. 1995. 'Mothers of disabled children as CBR workers', in B. O'Toole and R. McConkey (eds), *Innovation in Developing Countries for People with Disabilities*. Chorley: Lisieux Hall Publications.

Miles, M. 1993. 'Different ways of community-based rehabilitation', *Tropical and Geographical Medicine*, 45: 238–41.

Miles, S. 1992. *The Relationship between SAFOD and SCF's Regional Disability Programme: A Discussion Paper*. London: Save the Children Fund.

———. 1994. *Partnership for Change: A Report of a Regional Disability Meeting*. London: Save the Children Fund.

Miles, S. and Medi, E. 1994. 'Community-based support for disabled children in post-war Mozambique', *Disasters*, 18: 284–91.

Momm, W. and Konig, A. 1989. *From Community-Based Rehabilitation to Community Integration Programmes: Experiences and Reflections on a New Concept of Service Provision for Disabled People*. Geneva: International Labour Organization.

O'Toole, B. 1994. 'Community-Based Rehabilitation', a paper presented at the World Conference on Special Needs Education: Access and Quality, Salamanca, Spain, 7–10 June 1994. Government of Spain in cooperation with UNESCO.

Philpott, S. 1995. *Amawoti: Responding to the Needs and Rights of People with Disabilities*. Durban: Centre for Social and Development Studies, University of Natal.

Rieser, R. and Mason, M. 1992. *Disability Rights in the Classroom: A Human-Rights Issue*. London: Disability Equality in Education.

Saunders, C. 1987. *Trip Report of a Visit to Southern Africa*. London: Save the Children Fund.

Saunders, C. and Zinkin, P. 1990. *An Evaluation of Kibwezi CBR Programme*. London: Save the Children Fund.

Save the Children Fund. 1994. *Children, Disability and Development: Achievement and Challenge*. London: Save the Children Fund.

Serpell, F., Mariga, L. and Harvey, K. 1993. 'Mental Retardation in African Countries: Conceptualisation, Services and Research', *International Review of Research in Mental Retardation*, 19: 1–39.

Todhunter, C., Pilgrim, D. and Pearson, M. 1995. *Living with Acquired Physical Impairment: Reality and Potential*, HACCRU Research Report 95110. Liverpool: Health and Community Care Research Unit, North-West Regional Health Authority and University of Liverpool.

UNESCO, ILO and WHO. 1994. *Community-Based Rehabilitation for and with People with Disabilities*. Joint position paper. Geneva/Paris: UNESCO, ILO and WHO.

Vanneste, G. 1995. *Daily Management of CBR Fieldworkers and Supervisors* (draft version). Dar es Salaam: ART/Comprehensive Community Based Rehabilitation Tanzania.

Werner, D. 1993. 'Preface', in H. Finkenflügel (ed.), *The Handicapped Community*. Amsterdam: Vrij Universiteit Press.

Werner, D. 1995. 'Strengthening the role of disabled people in CBR programmes', in B. O'Toole and R. McConkey (eds), *Innovations in Developing Countries for People with Disabilities*. Chorley: Lisieux Hall Publications.

PART 5

Political Life with a Disability: Disability Politics and Policy

Introduction

Osamu Nagase & Stuart Blume

Under a medical model of disability (see Part 1), politics tends to be 'reallocative'. Political engagement aims at securing more resources: for benefits, services, medical research and so on. It is typically professionals who engage in this kind of politics. A social model of disability leads to very different politics. Having defined the problems faced by people with disabilities as the results of discriminatory social practices, the political focus then moves to the transformation of those practices. The struggles of other marginalised groups (such as ethnic minorities) may be an inspiration here. The social model has stimulated political advocacy on behalf of people with disabilities: first in a few western countries, and then in Asia, Africa and Latin America. International and regional organisations of national advocacy groups, such as Disabled Peoples' International (DPI) and the African Union of the Blind, have played an important part in pressing for the rights of people with disabilities and in supporting the formation of advocacy groups.

For Part 5 we have chosen four articles that deal with political movements of disabled people, two from the west and two from Asia. As in other issues, while the politics of disability varies from one country to another, there are common elements as well. Social movements may cross national borders, and identity politics sometimes binds people across nations. Disability is one example of this.

Richard Scotch deals with the issue of disability as the basis for a social movement in the U.S.A. which started the independent-living movement in the 1970s. As Hayashi and Okuhira note, the U.S. movement has had an international impact. The political formation of the movement, Scotch argues, was not easy for disabled people because of the stigma of disability. People were reluctant to mobilise around the most stigmatised aspect of their identity. The redefinition of disability, therefore, from dependency to social exclusion, as being the result of constraints imposed by the environment, was needed for the establishment of the movement.

Scotch's paper, written before the passage and the implementation of the Americans with Disabilities Act (ADA) in 1990, which encouraged a great number of countries to adopt antidiscrimination legislation, does refer to some pre-ADA legislation banning disability discrimination. U.S. disability legislation, as well as international instruments such as the Standard Rules on the Equalisation of Opportunities for Persons with Disabilities, adopted by the UN in 1993, gave powerful momentum to the political participation of disabled people in different countries around the world. The beneficial cycle of mutual influences of the movement and the system is witnessed by developments in the U.S.A. in the 1980s and beyond.

Tom Shakespeare gives us another perspective on the disability movement, this time from Britain. Comparing British experiences with those of the U.S., he notes some of the things that led to a different emancipation politics—'the absence of a developed welfare state, the strong emphasis on individual rights, the fullest development of the free market and competitive values, and the virtual absence of collectivism'—in the U.S. Like Scotch, Shakespeare touches upon two dimensions of disability identity: as an oppressed group as well as a cultural minority, referring to the 'subversion of stigma: taking a negative appellation and converting it into a badge of pride'.

Self-organisation of disabled people in many parts of Africa and Asia took place after the International Year of Disabled Persons in 1981, declared by the UN, when Disabled Peoples' International (DPI) was established. The social model of disability, which was established by the disability movement and disability studies in Britain, was adopted by DPI, which was the first cross-disability international movement. A cross-disability movement was possible only when identification was not with a particular impairment (such as blindness or deafness) alone, but when the societal barriers against people with different impairments were acknowledged.

Shakespeare reminds us that even though 'all disabled people face a common exclusion, prejudice and discrimination, and the vast majority share a condition of poverty,' we must 'not … ignore differences between impairments.' (Though Shakespeare does not explicitly mention the cultural aspect in this context, different experiences of impairment do resemble those of different cultures. Think of deaf culture, as well as blind culture and autistic culture.) The experiences of impairments have gained more attention since the British movement faced difficulty in 'reaching beyond its core group' because of its 'tendency to downplay the role of impairments'. Rather than avoiding impairments, 'new ways of dealing with the issues of impairments' need to be worked out. Obviously, there is the concern that this brings us back to the traditional medical and individual models of disability, but this needs to be explored without bringing this medicalisation and individualisation back in.

Distribution of resources is another point raised by Shakespeare. While new social-movement theorists give less emphasis to these materialist aspects, Shakespeare argues that the British disability movement has been fighting 'for more resources to be channelled towards disabled people', and that it 'challenges the distributive logic of capitalism'.

This has also been one of the major aspects of the disability movement in Japan, though not explicitly mentioned by Reiko Hayashi and Masako Okuhiro, who present Japanese experiences. Modern political organisation of disabled people started in the 1970s with the Aoi Shiba group, which included people with cerebral palsy. Their well-known platform, announced in 1970, denied the 'able-bodied love and justice' that often killed disabled people, and it rejected 'able-bodied civilisation'. Aoi Shiba inspired later disability-studies scholars to question the current system of distribution of resources, just as (according to Shakespeare) happened in Britain. The development of the disability movement in Japan has two important elements, as discussed by Hayashi and Okuhiro, and includes (a) the unique national experiences demonstrated by Aoi Shiba, and (b) the U.S. independent-living movement. The formation of the international political disability movement of DPI in Singapore, with the participation of movements from Japan, U.K. and U.S.A. was in a sense inevitable. Different national experiences were coming together. The solidarity of the Japanese movement with those in other Asian countries, including South Korea and Thailand, could also be witnessed when the tragic tsunami hit Southeast Asia in December 2004, and joint relief and reconstruction efforts were set up. The experiences common to disability beyond national borders promotes regional and international solidarity.

The structural analysis of disability in the political sense also makes us look into development issues as well. The reader is invited to consider disability and development in the overall context of development, including the implementation of the Millennium Development Goals, to which the international community has committed itself.

The issue of development provides the major background to Anita Ghai's paper. Ghai argues that in 'a scenario marked by widespread poverty, disability is not even considered as a cause of vulnerability.' This helps explain why disabled people demanded that the census count disabled people, while in developed countries disabled people often protest *against* this, arguing that a census does not help them. The gender dimensions of disability are Ghai's major theme. She points out the exclusion of disabled women from both the disability agenda and the feminist agenda in the Indian context. Though the marginalisation of disabled women is not unique to India, the way it expresses itself there does reflect specific aspects of the Indian situation. Perhaps one of the most common factors affecting disabled women in developing countries is the role of the family. As Ghai puts it, in 'the absence of education, employment, infrastructure and a social-security system, autonomy is a formidable goal for women in India to attain, and more so for disabled women,' and 'the resolution of any issues concerning disability has to be done in the context of the family and community.' This also brings us to experiences in Japan (Hayashi and Okuhiro), where the murder of a disabled child by her mother in 1970 promoted the formation of the modern political disability movement Aoi Shiba.

Independent living, espoused mostly in developed countries, takes different forms in different socio-economic conditions. One solution for the family and the society, proposed by Ghai, is 'to tell the story of diverse women's experiences in as truthful a manner as possible.' Certainly, the creation of political space in which disabled women can share their lived experiences might lead to the formation of groups of disabled women in

India. In fact, that has been the case for disabled men.

The personal and lived experiences of disabled people, discussed in earlier Parts of this Reader, are essential to political life with a disability.

17

Disability as the Basis for a Social Movement: Advocacy and the Politics of Definition

Richard K. Scotch

Although 1 in 11 Americans of working age identify themselves as having a disability (McNeil, 1983), for most of them such self-identification does not translate into group consciousness or political action. Disabled individuals face many barriers to full participation in American society, but until recently there has not been a significant social movement of disabled people dedicated to removal of those barriers. Disabled individuals in non-institutional settings are geographically and socially dispersed, and this fact constitutes a barrier to collective political action.

Nevertheless, in the past quarter century, a small but growing number of disabled people have formed a community, both through informal interaction and the establishment of formal organisations. Following in the wake of the race, gender and other civil-rights movements of the 1960s, increasing numbers of disabled people embraced activism and political action, and demanded integration into the mainstream of American society. Groups first formed among individuals with similar disabling conditions, such as blind people and deaf people, and among disabled war veterans. By the 1970s, organisations had been formed that

---

Scotch, R. 1988. 'Disability as the basis for a social movement', *Journal of Social Issues*, 44 (1): 159–72.

crossed disability lines and encompassed individuals with a wide range of physical and mental impairments.

This paper discusses the barriers disabled people face in forming a social movement and how such barriers have been overcome. In addition, the relationship between the disability-rights movement and public policies of the past two decades is explored, together with the current status and prospects of the disability-rights movement.

This paper builds on research on the growth of the disability-rights movement since the 1960s, and the relationship between that developing movement and the passage and implementation of federal civil-rights legislation affecting people (Scotch, 1984). Drawing on archival materials and a series of interviews with advocates and public officials, this research traced organisational histories, and the development of linkages among movement organisations and between such groups and government agencies. While this previous work focused on a particular statute, Section 504 of the Rehabilitation Act, the current paper concerns the more general topic of the formation and mobilisation of the disability-rights movement.

BARRIERS TO ORGANISATION

As the study of social movements and collective behaviour indicates, exclusion and discriminatory treatment alone do not inherently generate collective identity or collective political action. For the estimated 36 million Americans with disabilities (Bowe, 1980), the creation of an effective social movement may be even more problematic than for other excluded groups. With the exception of a few organisations based in particular geographical locations or on particular physical impairments, people with disabilities do not constitute a group that acts politically 'for itself'. Non-disabled excluded groups such as racial and ethnic minorities may share geographical communities, workplaces, or religious and other voluntary associations. Many groups develop their own subcultures based on their collective history or social position. For the most part, this has not been true for disabled people.

The social and political isolation of the vast majority of the disabled population is reinforced by a number of factors. Disability is concentrated among the least powerful members of American society: those with low incomes, low education and low workforce participation (Asch, 1984a). Individuals with physical impairments may face major barriers to obtaining education and entering the workforce. Furthermore, there are many risk factors associated with working-class and lower-class life in the United States that may contribute to the onset of disability.

While those lacking economic and political resources are more likely to be disabled, disability is, nonetheless, spread across the various social classes and status groups in our society. If a disabled person's impairment does not result in institutionalisation, that person may spend nearly all of his or her time in the company of non-disabled individuals. Parents, neighbourhood friends, school classmates, fellow employees—most of the people with whom a disabled person associates are likely to be non-disabled. Even where circumstances lead to interaction with other individuals with disabilities, the physical or mental impairments involved may be so disparate as to discourage mutual recognition of a shared social status. Thus, disability is an individualised experience for most people.

Of course, there are exceptions. People with disabilities stemming from a single cause may already have a great deal in common, particularly if they already share occupational or other ties, as in the case of disabled war veterans or miners with black-lung disease. In cases such as these, perceptions of relatedness may lead to joint activities ranging from mutual support to political action. Even so, the medicalisation of these disabilities has often forced individuals to give up control over their lives and to experience undertones of moral stigma, which make political identification and action problematic (Zola, 1983).

Another exception is the shared subculture that may develop among disabled residents of institutions. Individuals being treated in long-term care facilities may construct a patient culture as a means of coping with common impairments or in response to the indignities of life in a total institution (Goffman, 1961a). However, only in rare instances have such bonds led to activism upon departure from institutional confines. One notable exception is the case of associations of ex-mental patients (Anspach, 1979).

In most circumstances, it may be more accurate to characterise people with disabilities as members of a social category rather than as an identifiable social or political group (Goffman, 1963). Disabled people not only lack the common demographic conditions to foster group awareness and activism, but the social status of being disabled can create serious disincentives for many to identify themselves as disabled and act collectively on that basis. To be perceived as disabled is typically to be seen as helpless and incompetent, and many individuals with physical impairments seek to disassociate themselves from disability, exercising what Goffman (1961b) calls 'role distance'. Such dissociation may or may not be successful, since disabling images are reinforced by the proliferation of architectural barriers, by providers of services to disabled individuals (Gartner, 1984), and by the very language used to characterise disability (Longmore, 1985). In either case, however, the unattractiveness of the role of disabled person can serve to discourage both self-identification as a member of an excluded group and the likelihood of political action flowing from that identification.

This lack of disability consciousness has been noted by Hahn, who wrote, 'Persons with disabilities are often understandably reluctant to focus on that aspect of their identity that is most negatively stigmatised by the rest of society, and to mobilise politically around it' (Hahn, 1985, p. 310). Boyte, in discussing research on blind men and women, noted:

> Escape out of the ghetto created by pervasive social expectations and assigned roles has almost always meant individual attempts to deny or render irrelevant one's disability—not to challenge the expectations themselves.... Thus the story of how a movement of self-assertion among the disabled emerged in the 1970s and continues today involves an exploration into changing self-perceptions as well as dominant social attitudes. (Boyte, 1984, p. 116)

Interaction among disabled people may reflect and even exaggerate the stigmatisation of disability practiced by the rest of society. In such instances, disabled individuals can deliberately distance themselves from each other or make invidious distinctions between good and bad impairments, rather than seek to develop social ties on the basis of common experiences and similar social positions.

The stigmatisation of disabled persons is reinforced and even created by the attitudes of providers of rehabilitation services (Krause, 1976). Limitations and dependency are attributed to disability, and the disabled person is encouraged to accept these as part of the rehabilitation process

(Anspach, 1979; Scott, 1969). By promoting the image of disabled people as dependent and in need of professional help, medical and rehabilitation professionals retain control over programme beneficiaries at the cost of severely constraining the disabled person (Zola, 1983). Those who seek to avoid such constraint may choose to present themselves and to conceive of themselves as non-disabled.

Even to accept one's disability while rejecting ascriptions of dependency is in itself no guarantee of participation in collective political activity. Those people who are most severely impaired, and thus perhaps most likely to identify themselves as disabled, may face the greatest handicaps to effective political action.

Perhaps more importantly, the rejection of prejudicial stereotypes can often be an act of individual self-assertion against personal troubles, rather than an attempt to correct public problems (Mills, 1959). In a society that celebrates the individual (Bellah et al., 1985), it is all too natural to seek solutions to our problems as individuals rather than as members of an excluded class. Those individuals best able to reject the disabled role may refuse to identify themselves as disabled, thus avoiding political involvement as a disabled person. On the other hand, those individuals who accept the role are at risk of accepting its handicapping connotations of dependency, and thus also avoiding political involvement.

Who, then, is left as potential organisers and participants in a social movement of disabled people? Those who accept an identity as disabled while denying the associations of incapacity that our society attempts to impose. In order to do this, it may be necessary to conceive of a world in which physical impairment need not be disabling, and in which prejudicial exclusion is proscribed.

However, 'disability' as a unifying concept that includes people with a wide range of physical and mental impairments is by no means an obvious category. Blind people, people with orthopaedic impairments, and people with epilepsy may not inherently see themselves, or be seen by others, as occupying common ground. Even greater divisions may exist between individuals with physical impairments and those with mental disabilities. Thus, another prerequisite for collective action may be the social construction and promulgation of an inclusive definition of disability.

Anspach has termed the efforts by disability-rights activists to redefine disability 'identity politics' an attempt to create a new public perception of disabled people as independent. In such politics, she writes, 'political goals and strategies often become a vehicle for the symbolic manipulation of persons and the public presentation of self' (Anspach, 1979, p. 766). Anspach describes identity politics as 'a sort of phenomenological warfare, a struggle over the social meanings attached to attributes' (Anspach, 1979, p. 773). However, while redefining disability may be an important prerequisite for the emergence of a social movement of disabled persons, redefinition has not been the only aim of that movement. Disability-rights activists have also sought a number of policy goals, from changes in admissions and hiring practices to the literally concrete changes involved in increased architectural accessibility. Nevertheless, in order for an active and broadly based social movement of disabled people to come about, a redefinition of disability was required—one that treated disability as a label for a group of people who had the potential for political action and who were unfairly excluded from mainstream social institutions on the basis of their physical or mental impairments. The next section of this paper briefly reviews the history of political organisations among disabled people, and discusses how disability-rights activists attempted to promote new definitions of disability through political action.

GROWTH OF THE SOCIAL MOVEMENT OF DISABLED PEOPLE

Some of the earliest formal associations of disabled people in the United States were organised between the two World Wars (Lenihan, 1976–77). These included the Disabled American Veterans (DAV) and the National Federation of the Blind (NFB). Each stressed the needs of its own constituency rather than more universal disability issues. While the DAV focused essentially on expanding government benefits for disabled veterans, the NFB challenged the paternalistic practices of rehabilitation agencies, and was often a militant supporter of equal rights for blind people. The NFB promoted some of the earliest civil-rights laws guaranteeing access regardless of disability: the white-cane and guide-dog laws. It is not surprising that blind people, because their disability allows a relatively high degree of participation in the mainstream of everyday life, were particularly active in claiming full social participation as their due.

Other organisations of disabled persons were established in the 20 years following the Second World War including the Paralysed Veterans of

America, the National Association of the Deaf, and the American Council of the Blind. These groups had varying degrees of political involvement, but none were oriented towards the general issue of civil rights for all disabled people (Asch, 1984c). For the most part, each sought to advance the position of its particular constituency group.

This situation changed dramatically in the late 1960s. At that time, important changes were affecting those who identified themselves as disabled. Medical technology was extending the lives of those with a variety of medical problems or injuries who previously would not have survived, and thus the number of active disabled adults increased. Medical and rehabilitative advances were giving those who in earlier times would have been totally incapacitated the potential to function in society, for instance, many who had contracted polio in the final epidemics of the 1950s. For growing numbers of disabled people, physical impairment was becoming less handicapping than the barriers of stereotyped attitudes and architectural constraints.

Another development was the increase in the number of people who remained socially active despite disabling injuries in childhood, adolescence and young adulthood. Most individuals who experienced disability as the result of polio, teenage automobile or diving accidents, or the Vietnam War, had clear memories of themselves as non-disabled, and many retained expectations of full economic and social participation. They had not incorporated a self-image of dependency, and sought to live as normal young adults, which was increasingly technologically possible.

Even for children whose disabilities came at birth and who grew up in the 1950s and 1960s, individual potential was stressed by the Spock-influenced middle-class parents of that affluent era, who promoted self-confidence and achievement in their children. This 'new generation' of disabled people was encouraged to think of themselves as capable of participation. As Asch has written:

> Many activists, then, are not people who were kept out of the mainstream as children; they had been in the mainstream and had never questioned their right to be there. So, when others questioned it, they were ready with armour and anger to fight to preserve their sense of themselves that the adult world was trying to shatter (Asch, 1984b, p. 551).

These aspirations of participation were promoted by the politics of the times. In the communities and colleges, there were many other groups seeking greater participation in social institutions, and more autonomy and control in their lives. Demands for full access by disabled people occurred in the wake of the widespread and highly visible social conflicts of the 1960s: the struggle for civil rights by black people and other racial minorities, the antiwar and student movements, and a revitalised feminist movement. A number of disabled people who had been active participants in these movements came to see their disability in the same political sense as blacks viewed their race or women their gender.

Along with this new consciousness came an appreciation of how change strategies used by other movements could be adopted: While models of change-oriented advocacy did not guarantee success, they did suggest a method for stirring up latent support among a constituency and among the general public, and for channelling that support toward influencing governmental and institutional decision-makers. The potential of integration into the societal mainstream motivated disabled people to form new organisations at the local and state levels, and to rebuild existing groups. A number of the newly formed organisations included individuals with a variety of disabilities: e.g., the Centres for Independent Living organised in Berkeley and a number of other communities, and Disabled in Action in several East Coast cities.

The growing potential for political activism, however, was not sufficient to ensure the growth of a broadly based and effective social movement. By the early 1970s, many grass-roots groups had been formed, but there had been little or no attempt made by these local organisations to join in influencing public policy. Contacts among the various organisations had begun, however, through the networking opportunities provided by the annual meetings of the President's Committee on the Employment of the Handicapped (PCEH). PCEH had been founded after the Second World War in order to promote the employment of disabled veterans. While PCEH was, for the most part, dominated by service providers and put traditional emphasis on education, rehabilitation and incrementalist approaches to change, it did sponsor annual meetings that attracted people concerned with disability issues from around the country. These meetings became a forum for communication among the younger, more militant disability-rights activists. Several remained in contact between meetings, and this evolving network helped organise demonstrations against President Nixon's vetoes of the Rehabilitation Act in 1972 and 1973. The demonstrations, in turn, helped strengthen personal and organisational ties among disabled activists.

This loose network evolved into a formal organisation at the 1974 PCEH meeting. Alternative workshop sessions were held in the conference hotel lobby, bringing together about 150 people to discuss discrimination issues not included in the formal programme. This group became the first national coalition of disability activists when it organised itself as the American Coalition of Citizens with Disabilities (ACCD), linking several local and single-disability organisations, while retaining the autonomy of each constituent organisation.

A steering committee was formed, and ACCD held its first formal meetings at the 1975 PCEH conference. By-laws were adopted, a board of directors chosen, offices opened in New York and Washington, and in 1976 a grant was obtained from the federal Rehabilitation Services Administration to permit the hiring of staff. ACCD was to become a major coordinating network of disability-rights groups through the 1970s, and a major advocate for incorporating civil-rights guarantees for disabled people into federal laws and regulations.

ACCD was not the only cross-disability organisation to develop in the mid-1970s. One of its major constituent groups, Disabled in Action, developed affiliates in a number of states, while in many localities and states coalitions of existing groups were organised. Several non-membership organisations that claimed national constituencies were formed as well, including the National Centre for Law and the Handicapped in South Bend, Indiana, and the Disability Rights Centre in Washington, D.C., one of the Ralph Nader advocacy centres. Some advocacy groups not exclusively oriented toward disability issues, such as the Children's Defence Fund, became heavily involved in disability-advocacy efforts. Furthermore, a number of established single-disability organisations built up their advocacy components, including the American Council of the Blind, the National Association of the Deaf, and the Paralysed Veterans of America.

Increasingly, the attention of the evolving disability-rights movement became focused on events in Washington, D.C., as the federal government considered and enacted policies prohibiting discrimination on the basis of disability in a number of institutional spheres. A community had grown up among the Washington-based advocates for disability rights who met regularly to compare notes, develop strategies, and divide up the various lobbying tasks. Positions on issues were debated and agreements were reached on public stances. Although, frequently, consensus was not obtained, a viable movement had been constructed. Changes in public policy by the federal government were critical elements in the growth of this movement.

THE ROLE OF THE STATE IN REDEFINING DISABILITY

The above discussion of barriers to political activism by disabled people suggests that a prerequisite to such activism was a redefinition of disabilities as impairments that are limiting only to the extent that constraints are imposed by the physical and social environment. The activists who created the various disability-rights organisations redefined disability in this way, and sought to have this redefinition institutionalised and accepted in public policy and by the general public.

However, the political and financial resources of most of the disability-rights organisations were extremely limited. A major proportion of their budgets in the late 1970s was provided by the federal government in the form of grants and contracts, and substantial amounts of this federal funding were used for newly initiated political activity. (Several organisations were major exceptions, such as the NFB.) The political impact of many disability-rights organisations in the late 1970s was extremely dependent on the support of agencies of the federal government.

The contribution of the federal government, however, extended far beyond financial support. The social movement of disabled people became better organised and more broadly based as the result of federal civil-rights activities. Contracts for training and technical assistance to local groups were received by a wide range of disability organisations. Disability-rights leaders were often sought out by federal policy-makers, thus making lobbying even easier to pursue. Activists were routinely asked to review draft policies and to testify at congressional hearings. These contacts served the further function of reinforcing the visibility of disability-rights activists and of legitimating their leadership role, both within the disability community and outside it.

The consultations and meetings organised by federal officials seeking policy input had another important impact on the disability-rights movement by fostering a network among locally based activists around the country. This network was also furthered by a number of federal agencies that created advisory committees on disability-rights issues, as well as by the annual PCEH conferences.

More important still, the government contributed to the redefinition of disability. Through such legislation as Section 504 of the Rehabilitation Act of 1973, and the Education for All Handicapped Children Act of 1975 (P.L. 94–142), federal policy-makers established disabled people as a class to be protected from discrimination by federal law, and made it illegal to exclude them from publicly supported programmes and activities. The programmatic effects of these statutes were far-reaching: They dramatically increased the accessibility of public education, employment, government services and public facilities to disabled people. Of equal or greater importance, however, were the definitions included in the new laws, which focused on a broad group of people in a way that aided the formation of a social movement.

There were two types of statutory definitions of disability, both extremely broad. The first, employed in P.L. 94–142, was categorical. Section 121a.5 of the law defined handicapped children as those evaluated as being mentally retarded, hard of hearing, deaf, speech impaired, visually handicapped, seriously emotionally disturbed, orthopaedically impaired, other health impaired, deaf-blind, multi-handicapped, or as having specific learning disabilities. P.L. 94–142 guaranteed these children a free and appropriate public education and related services in the least restrictive possible environment. Schools were mandated to provide individually appropriate services to children defined as handicapped, but, procedurally, all disabled children were accorded the same rights.

The second type of statutory definition was more functional in nature. Section 504, for example, defined a handicapped individual as any person who has a physical or mental impairment that substantially limits one or more major life activities, has a record of such an impairment, or is regarded as having such an impairment. Disabled people falling within this broad group were protected from discrimination in all federally supported programmes and activities. The centrality of government-sponsored definitions is emphasised by Hahn and Longmore, who state that 'the definition of disability is essentially determined by public policy. In other words, disability is whatever laws and implementing regulations say it is' (Hahn and Longmore, no date, p. 5). They point out that government definitions of disability have historically been influenced by rehabilitation and medical professionals. However, in the 1970s, federal definitions of disability were specified with the assistance of disability-rights advocates, and in several cases they were actually written by representatives of movement organisations (see Scotch, 1984).

Conventional interest-group explanations of policy changes characterise advocacy groups as shaping the development and implementation of public policies. In the case of disability-rights legislation in the 1970s, this process was largely reversed. Advocates for the disability-rights movement did not apply political pressure that resulted in the passage of these laws. Rather, the adoption and implementation of the laws contributed to the growth of national advocacy organisations representing disabled people, and reinforced their involvement with civil-rights issues. Civil-rights oriented statutes such as Section 504 and P.L. 94–142 became focal points for organising among disabled people, and provided a good opportunity for establishing policy-oriented coalitions of the new generation of grass-roots disability organisations.

The emphasis in this paper on the role of the state in providing resources and creating networks is consistent with the evolving literature on resource mobilisation in social movements (Freeman, 1982; McCarthy and Zald, 1977). The importance of network linkages and resource availability, however, has sometimes been stressed to the exclusion of any emphasis on the role of ideas and symbolic categories in framing issues—for example, in attempts to argue for structural over social-psychological modes of analysis. As Snow and others (1986) have recently pointed out, however, social-psychological and resource-mobilisation models are not mutually exclusive. The disability-rights movement is one in which the way an issue was framed had serious effects on both movement participation and the ability of the movement to influence public policies (as was also the case with the problem of drunk driving: Gusfield, 1981).

Ensuring access to public buildings or public services may be viewed as a social-welfare benefit or as a civil right. The former connotes dependency by the disabled person and largesse on the part of society. It suggests that we must approve of disabled people, their attitudes and behaviour, in order to help them, and that they must earn our approval by conforming to our expectations, however handicapping those expectations may be. Within this conception, helping disabled people is analogous to helping single mothers with dependent children—a qualified and rather grudging form of assistance. Further, providing access as a welfare benefit invites the rationing of accessibility, for welfare is typically given and withdrawn based on the limits of generosity of the giver rather than according to the needs of the recipient.

Alternatively, when access to societal institutions is defined as a right, it becomes virtually unconditional. Removing architectural barriers to public buildings becomes analogous to abolishing the poll tax, a necessary guarantee of equity in our society. Cost, inconvenience, or disapproval of the deprived group's behaviour becomes far less relevant to whether their lack of access should be remedied.

Of course, definitions and perceptions are not independent of social structure and political power; the efficacy of definitions typically depends on structural factors, not the least of which is the power held by their proponents. Nevertheless, as the tradition of scholarship dating back to Max Weber has demonstrated, ideas can influence social structures, just as social structures can generate ideas.

THE POLITICS OF DISABILITY IN THE 1980s

While disability has been less visible as a public issue in the 1980s, the growth of grass-roots organisations has continued around the country. The establishment of independent-living programmes, access to mass-transit systems, architectural accessibility, and other civil-rights oriented issues have been passed, along with attempts to maintain a number of benefit programmes in the face of federal cutbacks. One particularly visible issue has been public transportation, for the Reagan administration has substantially weakened federal requirements for accessibility, thus leading to many local debates over what services should be provided by financially besieged transit operators. While national organisations such as the Denver-based ADAPT have been active in this arena, much of the impetus for activism has been at the local level. However, conflict has continued between proponents of total access to transit systems and those supporting para-transit and other special services.

Nationally, organisations such as the Disability-Rights Education and Defence Fund and ACCD have continued to lobby Congress and federal agencies. However, many observers of the disability-rights movement have perceived a decline in its effectiveness and national influence. The Reagan administration has removed a number of advocacy-oriented individuals with ties to established movement organisations from administrative and advisory positions in federal agencies. Lowered expectations have dimmed the hopefulness of the late 1970s about promoting vigorous enforcement of civil-rights protections such as Section 504, and enacting new legislation prohibiting discrimination in private-sector employment. Optimism about further advances has been replaced by concerns about court decisions and administrative rulings that circumscribe the effectiveness of existing laws. A successful effort was made to prevent weakening 94–142, yet many local school districts have been accused of less than full compliance with the provisions of that statute. Clearly, the federal government has retreated from its activist role in promoting the rights of disabled persons and the growth of organisations seeking to support and extend those rights.

While during the 1970s disability advocates were often in a collaborative relationship with many federal officials, the relationship between disability-rights organisations and the federal government is now much more adversarial in nature. Similar tensions have been experienced by advocates involved with other issues, ranging from environmental protection to occupational safety to human services. Thus, the crucial change has been in the political environment rather than in the disability-rights movement itself.

On the positive side, although the disability-rights movement may have lost some of its political efficacy, its relationships with other 'progressive' movements may have been enhanced. Common opposition to Reagan administration policies may have helped to institutionalise the participation of disability-rights activists in the broad coalition of liberal-left advocacy groups in Washington. Similar partnerships have formed in a number of states and local communities, as social programme budgets have experienced severe fiscal constraints in the wake of federal reductions.

However, quite a different alliance has been formed around one important issue. Right-to-life advocates within and outside the Reagan administration have joined disability-rights organisations in seeking federal intervention in cases where medical treatment had been withheld from newborn infants with physical disabilities, i.e. the 'Baby Doe' cases. Section 504 has been cited as the legal basis for intervention in these cases, since it prohibits discrimination on the basis of disability in all federally supported programmes, including in hospitals. On the other side of these cases, feminist groups, civil libertarians, and health-care providers have opposed government intervention. The Supreme Court has ruled that the federal government may not intervene in such cases, but there is likely to be continuing public debate over the appropriateness of medical treatment for severely disabled newborns. Advances in medical technology are likely to generate other such debates involving the quality of life for disabled persons, the personal choice of parents and other family members, and the ability of health-care professionals to make informed decisions about sustaining life. The disability-rights movement will have a great deal to say on ethical and policy issues involving abortion, care for disabled newborns, the right to treatment, and the right to refuse treatment (see, for example, Asch, 1986). It remains unclear to what extent spokesmen for the disabled will be accepted as legitimate contributors in these debates by policy-makers, as experts rather than as unfortunate and axe-grinding victims. Having reconstructed their own definition of self, disability-rights activists must continue to influence the definitions of others, through reasoned debate and through political activity. The ability of movement leaders and grass-roots disabled advocates to be full participants will depend on both their organising ability and their acumen as issue entrepreneurs.

Equally unclear, due to its current political unpopularity, is the future of further extensions of government-guaranteed rights in the United States. Diminished funding for programmes that promote independence for disabled people, such as attendant care, independent-living centres, and facility modification to remove architectural barriers, may inhibit the political participation of many people with disabilities and thus limit their ability to mobilise politically. Political conservatism within government and the general public may mean that the catalytic role of public officials in promoting the growth of the disability-rights movement is over, at least for the present. Also unclear is the long-term impact of the policy gains of the 1970s. The large-scale entry of disabled Americans into schools, jobs and public life may have taken on a momentum of its own, or it may merely have reached a plateau of tokenism.

Progress should continue, even in the absence of government support, if disability-rights groups can raise the consciousness of the vast majority of disabled people who have not been involved politically and who may not share the political definition of disability promoted by the movement. However, redefinition of disability can no longer be expected to flow from court rulings and government policies. Community organising will be essential: to broaden participation in the movement, to build acceptance of a positive image of people with disabilities, and to sustain and expand the organisational infrastructure created by the movement in the 1970s. Organisation at the community level can create the resources necessary for the movement to be effective, and continue the extension of conceptions of disability that promote social and political participation.

Clearly, the emergence of a social movement of disabled people is no guarantee of major institutional changes. If the movement continues to grow at the local level, however, its power may be expected to accumulate. The more that people with disabilities become integrated into mainstream social institutions, the more their presence may lead to further institutional changes. And to the extent that more political definitions of disability become widespread, the disability-rights movement may be expected to continue to play an active role in American political and social life.

References

Anspach, R.R. 1979. 'From stigma to identity politics: Political activism among the physically disabled and former mental patients', *Social Science and Medicine*, 13A: 765–73.

Asch, A. 1984a. 'The experience of disability', *American Psychologist*, 39: 529–36.

———. 1984b. 'Personal reflections', *American Psychologist*, 39: 551–52.

———. 1984c. 'Understanding and working with disability-rights groups', in H. McCarthy (ed.), *Complete Guide to Employing Persons with Disabilities*. Albertson: National Centre on Employment of the Handicapped, Human Resource Centre, pp. 170–94.

———. 1986. 'Real moral dilemmas', *Christianity and Crisis*, 46: 237–40.

Bellah, R.N. et al. 1985. *Habits of the Heart*. Berkeley: University of California Press.

Bowe, F. 1980. *Rehabilitating America*. New York: Harper and Row.

Boyte, H.C. 1984. *Community is Possible: Repairing America's Roots*. New York: Harper and Row.

Elder, C.D. and Cobb, R.W. 1983. *The Political Uses of Symbols*. New York: Longman.

Freeman, J. 1982. (ed.) *Social Movements of the Sixties and Seventies*. New York: Longman.

Gartner, A. August 1984. 'Disabling images', *The Disability Rag*, pp. 3–4.

Goffman, E. 1961a. *Asylums*. Garden City: Anchor Books.

———. 1961b. *Encounters*. Indianapolis: Bobbs-Merrill.

———. 1963. *Stigma*. Englewood Cliffs: Prentice-Hall.

Gusfield, J.R. 1981. *The Culture of Public Problems: Drinking-driving and the Symbolic Order*. Chicago: University of Chicago Press.

Hahn, H. 1985. 'Introduction: Disability policy and the problem of discrimination', *American Behavioural Scientist*, 28: 293–318.

Hahn, H. and Longmore, P.K. (n. d.). 'The emergence of the study of disability and society at the University of Southern California'. Unpublished paper, University of Southern California.

Krause, E.A. 1976. 'The political sociology of rehabilitation', in G.L. Albrecht (ed.), *The Sociology of Physical Disability and Rehabilitation*. Pittsburgh: University of Pittsburgh Press, pp. 201–21.

Lenihan, J. 1976–77. 'Disabled Americans: A history', *Performance*, 27 (5–7): 1–72.

Longmore, P.K. 1985. 'A note on language and the social identity of disabled people', *American Behavioural Scientist*, 28: 419–23.

McCarthy, J.D. and Zald, M.N. 1977. 'Resource mobilisation and social movements: A partial theory', *American Journal of Sociology*, 82: 1212–41.

McNeil, J.M. 1983. *Labour Force and Other Characteristics of Persons with a Work Disability: 1982*. Series P-23, No. 127. Washington, D.C.: United States Bureau of the Census.

Mills, C.W. 1959. *The Sociological Imagination*. New York: Oxford University Press.

Scotch, R.K. 1984. *From Goodwill to Civil Rights*. Philadelphia: Temple University Press.

Scott, R.A. 1969. *The Making of Blind Men*. New York: Russell Sage Foundation.

Snow, D.A. et al. 1986. 'Frame alignment processes, micromobilisation, and movement participation', *American Sociological Review*, 51: 464–81.

Zola, I.K. 1983. 'Medicine as an institution of social control', in I.K. Zola (ed.), *Socio-medical Inquiries*. Philadelphia: Temple University Press, pp. 247–68.

18

Disabled People's Self-Organisation: A New Social Movement?

Tom Shakespeare

INTRODUCTION

Recent decades have seen disability become a hotly contested issue: in the political arena with the development of the disabled people's movement, and in academic debates. Political interventions have centred on issues of discrimination and segregation, moving beyond the traditional concerns about medical and welfare provision to focus on areas such as anti-discrimination legislation, the role of charity and cultural representation, segregation in transport and education, and innovations to increase autonomy (through centres for independent living). The academic debate has developed the concept of the social model, originally initiated within the Union of Physically Impaired Against Segregation (UPIAS), and has witnessed a conflict between the approaches of disabled and non-disabled researchers.

It is important to consider these developments as examples of praxis, the unity of theory and practice within struggle. However, because of the priority afforded to achieving change, there has been little space for considering the nature of the movement itself, historically and politically,

---

Shakespeare, Tom. 1993. 'Disabled people's self-organisation: A new social movement?', *Disability, Handicap and Society*, 8 (3): 249–64.

and the significance of new definitions of disability for the self-identity of disabled people. This article attempts to contribute towards this type of analytical self-awareness, using existing sociological theories about new social movements.

DISABILITY AND DIRECT ACTION

There are now several empirical histories of the disabled people's movement, both internationally and in Britain (Pagel, 1988; Driedger, 1989). These are useful beginnings, but are nevertheless rather brief descriptions, with little consideration of the causal factors involved in the expanding consciousness of disabled people. Rather than repeat existing material, I will point to parallels and differences between the disability movements in Britain and North America and other liberation campaigns before contextualising disability within new social-movement theory. There are significant differences between the disability movements in Britain and the U.S.A. Clearly, the U.S. has a different tradition of protest and social reform than Britain and much of Western Europe. The absence of a developed welfare state; the strong emphasis on individual rights, expressed in a written constitution; the fullest development of the free market and competitive values; the virtual absence of collectivism and an organised labour movement, are all important factors in explaining the different developments of disabled people's politics.

One of the main inspirations of the movement in the U.S. was the example of the civil-rights campaigns and women's movement of the late 1960s. Another was the widespread injury caused by the war in Vietnam, and the increase in the numbers of young disabled people. A large element of the movement in North America has stemmed from consumerism and self-help: for example, in the independent-living centres this emphasis plays a large part. This is a particularly U.S. tradition of self-reliance and of individual rights. Many writers focus on consumer involvement, whereas British approaches would stress political autonomy and democratic participation, not the market. U.S. disability campaigns focus on admitting disabled people to wider society, demanding the extension of existing social rights to them as a group. In Britain, although this citizenship stress is an important (and developing) emphasis, there has been a radical rejection of social normality, and a structural stress on changing the system that produces disability.

In Britain, as in North America, direct action is a very important part of the disabled people's movement: for example, the Campaign for Accessible Transport (CAT) and the Campaign Against Patronage (CAP). Both groups have organised highly visible and controversial actions: for example, a demonstration in London's Oxford Street, which involved wheelchair users chaining themselves to buses; and regular blockades of television fund-raising spectaculars such as Telethon and Children in Need. Such mobilisations are reminiscent of the tactics of women suffragists in the years before the First World War, but also of the struggles of the 1960s: there is an unsubstantiated story that New York wheelchair users enlisted the support of the Weather Underground to dynamite undropped kerbs in the early years.

The civil-rights movement was influential for subsequent liberation struggles, not just because of the content of demands, but also through the techniques and manner of struggle:

> When traditional legal channels have been exhausted, disabled persons have learned to employ other techniques of social protest, such as demonstrations and sit-ins. (DeJong, 1983, p. 12)

This development is important not just instrumentally, in the securing of specific changes and reforms, but because direct action challenges popular perceptions of disabled people, and empowers and inspires participants. Aldon Morris's history of the early U.S. civil-rights movement suggests that its importance for black people was two-fold:

> One, it was the first time that large masses of blacks directly confronted and effectively disrupted the normal functioning of groups and institutions thought to be responsible for their oppression. The hallmark of the modern civil-rights movement is that these mass confrontations were widespread, and sustained over a long period of time in the face of heavy repression. Two, it was the first time in American history that blacks adopted non-violent tactics as a mass technique for bringing about social change. (Morris, 1984, p. xi)

This comment could be applied, for example, to Stop Telethon demonstrations, and to actions against inaccessible transport. The latter is a form of segregation not so divorced from the segregated buses which were one of the first targets of the civil-rights movement:

> Buses became the first target of the movement because members of the black community had begun to see bus discrimination not as a private misery but as a public issue and a common enemy. (Morris, 1984, p. 48)

Morris sees the direct-action orientation as emphasising the 'here and now'. This immediacy seems obvious in the urgency of contemporary disabled people's struggles, and through the impact of direct action on the streets, as non-disabled people are forced to confront their stereotypical attitudes. Jenny Morris has written of the feelings of power that collective action engenders:

> The obvious challenge that we were mounting to people's assumptions was also a source of my sense of power. Indeed, each time I had to explain to a non-disabled friend why I was going on such a demonstration, I was very conscious of the way that this issue challenges the root of our oppression, and that even to explain my motivations very briefly brings people up short against the core of their own prejudice. (Morris, 1991, p. 191)

Direct action has a number of important elements. It is a way of focusing attention on the institutions and environments that create disability: the inaccessible transport, the demeaning television charity spectaculars. It is an overtly political act, showing that disability is a matter of social relations, not medical conditions. It is a chance for disabled people to 'do it for themselves', without the help or participation of non-disabled people, thus prefiguring the claims of the disability movement to autonomy, independence and power. It is an empowering process for participants, creating a sense of solidarity, purpose and collective strength which enhances and develops the movement.

When CAT blockaded Oxford Street, and during other demonstrations, the police force has found it difficult to deal with wheelchair users and other mobility-impaired people. Proceedings against arrested protesters at Horseferry Road Magistrates Court had to be terminated, as the building was inaccessible to disabled people. These ramifications of direct-action protest illustrate the way style and method can reinforce the message and content of the campaign.

Popular opinion cannot come to terms with disabled radicalism, preferring to think disabled people are happy with their situation. In an editorial coinciding with the Oxford Street demonstrations, the *Times'* leader (29 September 1990) suggested that, while everyone was sympathetic to disabled people (after all, anyone could become disabled, and it was no one's fault), the militants must be careful not to alienate public opinion:

> Militancy, unlawful demonstrations, and the disruption of city life may relieve the feelings of the disabled. But such tactics will eventually alienate the public support on which the disabled have to rely.

Of course, this fairly common opinion indicates that many people have still not understood that the basic claim of the disability movement is that disability results from social relations, not impairment, and therefore society does not merely face responsibilities towards 'the disabled' but is culpable in creating disability in the first place.

In the recent Institute of Public Policy Research (IPPR) report, *Equal Rights for Disabled People: The Case for a New Law*, Oliver and Barnes summarise recent developments as follows:

> The move towards self-organisation has prompted increasing numbers of disabled people to adopt a shared political identity, which in turn has helped to build a new mood of confidence. Disabled people no longer ask for change but demand it. They are prepared to use a whole range of tactics in pursuit of their demands, including direct action and civil disobedience. (Bynoe, Oliver and Barnes, 1991, p. 12)

These features of the disability movement—a shared political identity, the use of direct action—indicate the importance of developing parallels with other social movements. In 1976, Safilios-Rothschild suggested:

> The time may be ripe for the disabled to generate a social movement patterned after the at-least partially successful examples of the Black Movement and the Women's Movement. (Safilios-Rothschild, 1976, p. 45)

Each liberation struggle was the work of the subject peoples themselves, be they black, gay or women:

> Perhaps the most striking thing about feminism is the extent to which it has been a movement of women and not just for women. (Banks, 1986, p. 106)

Political change did not rely on the lobbying of professionals, or the use of electoral methods. Each of these constituencies has historically been disempowered: black people and women being disenfranchised totally, others being electorally invisible. Disabled people, too, have been disenfranchised: several writers have shown the obstacles to registration and voting, let alone effective political participation. Oliver (1990) argues that conventional party politics has failed disabled people, who have become a marginalised underclass. The solution has been grass-roots campaigning activity, self-organisation, direct democracy and direct action, inspiring struggles that rely on passion as much as logical persuasion, as Olive Banks argues for first-wave feminism:

> During this period, women and men were stirred not only by the intellectual arguments put forward but even more, perhaps, by the emotional impact of the struggle itself. (Banks, 1986, p. 140)

Thus, there were the civil-rights marches, the Stonewall Riot, the Miss World demonstration, and, more recently, Greenham Common, Telethon and Outrage. All these campaigns have implicitly worked through a wider conception of politics, classically encapsulated in the feminist slogan 'The personal is political'.

IDENTITY AND GROUP CONSCIOUSNESS

Above, I have made reference to disability identity in connection with the empowering role of direct action. Much academic work has discussed disabled people's identity, but the majority has focused more on 'identifying' disabled people, through empirical or clinical investigation, taking disability to refer to medically assessable impairment and functional limitation. I am concerned with identity in a political sense: with identifying as part of an oppressed group, with part of a cultural minority.

This process of identification seems the reverse of what William Ryan called 'blaming the victim', because it is about converting private woes into public wrongs. It is about 'the victim' refusing that label, and instead focusing attention on the structural causes of victimisation. It is about the subversion of stigma: taking a negative appellation and converting it into a badge of pride.

Recent Anglo-American homosexual politics shows a similar process, as gay men and women take on the word 'queer', a traditional insult, and make of it a strengthening identifier, referring to the new tendency of direct action, pride and political struggle. Similarly, many disabled activists and performers use the word 'cripple', or 'crip', in a way which they would find offensive if non-disabled people adopted it. In both these cases, the words refer to a wider development, which is the assertion of group identity in the face of oppression, constructed through a political and cultural struggle focused on pride. And this pride is about the assertion of a positive identity, personally and collectively, in the face of prejudice and discrimination.

The key to this development is that people are 'doing it for themselves'. The British Council of Organisations of Disabled People (BCODP) and similar disabled people's organisations came into being against existing charities and pressure groups which worked *for* disabled people, on their behalf. BCODP said that this must be the action of disabled people themselves, mass action rather than elite action. This dichotomy is familiar from previous struggles. For example, the National Association for the Advancement of Coloured People, based in the U.S., was a white-dominated organisation for much of its early history. By contrast, the Southern Christian Leadership Conference was formed and controlled by black people, and it subsequently took over the leadership of the struggle, and was itself later superseded, to an extent, by more radical black-consciousness groups. In contemporary British gay politics, there is the conflict between the political strategies of the Stonewall Group and Outrage. The former is an elite group who lobby for change at the top: for example, having tea with John Major, the British prime minister at the time. The latter is a radical, participatory, direct-action group trying to change popular consciousness, not just laws.

I conclude, firstly, that liberation struggles have to be led and controlled by the colonised group itself, and, secondly, that liberation must involve the most widespread possible action and mobilisation, rather than mere changes in elites or legislation; the latter would parallel a *coup d'état*, rather than the intended revolution. Ethel Klein makes a distinction between the feminist sympathy of men (an 'abstract, ideological commitment to equality') and the feminist consciousness of women (an 'internalised political perspective derived from personal experience'):

> ... feminist support based on abstract commitments to social justice and equality is diffuse, and has a relatively weak and short-term impact on people's political choices. In contrast, support based on personal experience and solidarity with the experiences of other women, on feminist consciousness, fosters a vigilant commitment to the pursuit of sex equality. (Klein, 1984, p. 7)

So, identifying as a member of an oppressed group and organising to effect social change are critical.

In Britain, the explicitly political character of the struggle, and the extent to which it is an 'indigenous' struggle, has been recognised from the start, in the UPIAS/Disability Alliance split. In the U.S., this issue was also being recognised, though perhaps more cautiously. DeJong concludes, rather tentatively:

> One of the most vexing issues in the future will be the role of able-bodied persons in the movement. In some quarters, it is strongly felt that only disabled consumers should hold significant leadership positions. The issue finds a parallel in the civil-rights movement, at the stage when whites were asked to relinquish their leadership roles in black-advocacy organisations. (DeJong, 1983, p. 26)

Irving Zola makes the claim more strongly:

> I do not claim that no one else can help or understand us; rather, I would argue that, as with women and blacks, we have reached that point in history where having been there is essential in determining where to go. (Zola, 1983, p. 57)

The latest British developments in this 'indigenous' tendency came at the 1992 Researching Disability conference, when disabled people told non-disabled researchers that they had no right to be researching the disability experience, showing that even the academic study of disability has felt the politicising effects of the movement.

Is this development valid? Can only disabled people speak for other disabled people? Disability is less of a unitary concept than race and gender: the experiences of people with visual impairment, restricted growth or spinal injury will differ markedly, and factors such as the onset of the condition will also influence the experience, as well as the obvious dimensions of race, class and gender. It is important not to ignore differences between impairments, despite the tendency of writers to gloss over difference in favour of the totalising and unifying role of oppression. Clearly, all disabled people face a common exclusion, prejudice and discrimination, and the vast majority share a condition of poverty. But beyond this, there are variations. Can I, as a person with restricted growth, effectively speak for or write about someone with cerebral palsy or visual impairment? I can identify with the basic social experience, but the details can be no clearer to me than they would be to anyone else, disabled or not. If a non-disabled person cannot describe or represent my experience, then can I describe or represent the experience of someone with a different impairment? Does this undermine either the claim for disabled unity or the denial of a role to non-disabled people? I think not, on the basis that the social oppression is the most immanent aspect of the experience; however, the issue of advocacy and identity is rather more confused than has so far been suggested.

The crucial issue regarding identity is the process whereby individual people with impairment come to recognise themselves as disabled, focusing on the social oppression which is basic to that condition. People are socialised into particular ways of viewing disability which are based on individualised and medicalised attitudes. Disability is widely seen as individual medical tragedy, by disabled people as much as by non-disabled people.

This problem parallels the experience of other subaltern groups. For example, there is a wide Marxist literature on 'false consciousness', whereby proletarians fail to recognise the true nature of the social relations which render them powerless and alienated, and seek individual explanations, or have recourse in religion, or perhaps nationalism and other divisionary ideologies. Feminist writers have used psychoanalytical concepts in the discussion of 'internalised oppression', whereby women absorb the patriarchal world view, and hold discriminatory attitudes to themselves and other women.

Here, I wish to focus on identity formation as a part of the growth of group consciousness which leads to social movements: collective political action by subaltern groups. Ethel Klein highlights the issue when she argues:

> Having a hard life and being a member of an exploited group does not, in itself, lead to political unrest. People often blame themselves for their difficulties. Only when they see that their problems are shared by other people like them, the group, can they attribute the source of their concerns to social conditions, such as discrimination, and look to political solutions. (Klein, 1984, p. 2)

She isolates a three-stage process of political consciousness from her study of the women's movement: first, affiliation, through a process of group membership and sharing of interests; second, a rejection of traditional definitions for that group's status in society; and finally:

> Personal problems become political demands only when the inability to survive, or to attain a decent life, is seen as a consequence of social institutions or social inequality rather than of personal failure, and the system is blamed. (Klein, 1984, p. 3)

Clearly, these three steps are demonstrated in the development of the disabled people's movement. However, it may be more difficult for people with impairment to identify as disabled, as socially oppressed, than it is for women, blacks or gays. The oppression is couched in terms of paternalistic support and charity. The dominance of professionals is well-nigh total. The very real element of physical impairment restricts activity and reinforces 'natural' explanations of disability. The possibilities of people with various impairments coming together in a political struggle are reduced by the tendency of medicine and welfare to arbitrarily divide up the constituency: separation of the old from the young, or segregation of people with different physical conditions who nevertheless share similar social experiences.

And the downside of the disability movement, made more understandable by factors such as those just enumerated, is that it does not reach out to the total constituency of disabled people. It has proved less successful in developing positive identity and group consciousness beyond the relatively active, relatively young, middle-class elements. It is rare for this to be specifically acknowledged; because critics are always eager to undermine the movement, it has become difficult to make such criticisms from within it. In the U.S., there has been more openness:

> Notably absent from the movement's constituency are older persons with severe physical impairments resulting from strokes or other degenerative conditions. While the movement's philosophy may have direct relevance to older disabled persons, the movement has focused its concern elsewhere. (DeJong, 1983, p. 6)

While the movement in Britain is far more representative, there are some similar tendencies. Age-wise, it has tended to be skewed towards younger people, whereas the distribution of impairment in the population is overwhelmingly towards older people, especially women. Only recently have women's voices been explicitly recognised within the movement, or those of black and Asian disabled people.

Part of the reason for the difficulties the British movement has had in reaching beyond its core group has been the tendency to downplay the role of impairment, of the physical condition. Given that the majority of unpoliticised disabled people identify first and foremost via their particular physical impairment, it is an obstacle to their development if this is ignored by the theoreticians of the struggle. Recent work has begun to rectify this gap (Morris, 1991; Crow, 1992; French, 1993). In order to reach out and foster collective identity, the disabled people's movement will have to work out new ways of dealing with the issue of impairment, and of developing conscienticisation among the wide majority of disabled people. Central to this will be cultural and artistic representations by disabled people themselves, because only through challenging images, and depicting the contradictions, will progressive conceptions emerge.

NEW SOCIAL MOVEMENTS

Alan Scott's study of this phenomenon, the most recent fixation of sociologists, defines the term as follows:

> A social movement is a collective actor constituted by individuals who understand themselves to have common interests and, for at least some significant part of their social existence, a common identity. Social movements are distinguished from other collective actors, such as political

> parties and pressure groups, in that they have mass mobilisation, or the threat of mobilisation, as their prime source of social sanction, and hence of power. They are further distinguished from other collectivities, such as voluntary associations or clubs, in being chiefly concerned to defend or change society, or the relative position of the group in society. (Scott, 1990, p. 6)

He goes on to discuss race, gender, sexuality, peace and environment groups, but not disability. In fact, none of the major theorists mention disability. However, Michael Oliver (1990) has argued that the disabled people's movement is a new social movement in that it has the following features: marginalisation from traditional politics, the link of the personal with the political, a critical evaluation of society, and post-materialism.

To a certain extent, the important qualifier in the equation is 'new'; these movements are very much seen in distinction to previous political forces, chiefly the working-class and socialist movements. There is a tendency to downplay all elements of continuity, and to stress instead the rupture existing between traditional forms of protest and 'new' developments. All these 'new social movements' (including the disability movement) do share some basic features. They have arisen since the Second World War, mainly since the 1960s; however, this fact must not be allowed to obscure earlier forerunners, such as the suffragists of the early twentieth century (or the National League of the Blind and Disabled). They are outside conventional party politics or trade union/corporate activity. Partly as a result of this second factor, they have recourse to 'unconventional' tactics and forms of political mobilisation: popular protest taking new forms such as marches, demonstrations, blockades, boycotts, sit-ins, etc. But these techniques are perhaps not so very new; mass action has been a feature of popular uprisings for centuries. Moreover, in the absence of strike action as a potential weapon, these techniques are the obvious alternatives. Perhaps an important aspect is the self-consciousness and preparation involved in mounting such activities: rarely spontaneous, often carefully planned to influence opinion-formers, the media, etc.

However, while all these groups look superficially similar in terms of tactics, many of which are adopted from each other to suit the particular instance (in this context, note the Scottish nationalist movement's borrowing of tactics pioneered by the 'Outrage' gay and lesbian campaign in the 1990s), there are significant reasons to question the catch-all description of 'new social movement'. It is my contention that this term obscures important differences between two types of contemporary popular struggle: the 'post-materialist' tendency, on the one hand, and the 'liberation' movements, on the other. While they may share tactics and overlapping constituencies of support, there are fundamental distinctions between the two approaches.

Take the idea, reiterated by Oliver, that new social movements, including the disabled people's movement, are characterised by a shift in values to post-materialism. This originates with authors such as Inglehart, who have contrasted the historical trend of social movements, for example the workers' movement, with new developments. A simple opposition is drawn between the traditional claim for more resources, the materialist position, and the modern post-materialist value consensus:

> The presence of materialist or post-materialist values proves to be the most important single influence on whether a given individual will support new social movements. (Inglehart, 1990, p. 64)

The survey evidence for this 'value switch' is simplistically designed, the results weak, and the case is certainly overstated.

Most of the struggles mentioned above are about resource allocation: women, black people and disabled people are crucially concerned with their economic exploitation and poverty. Within feminism there is a central concern with equal pay, with gender inequality in the marketplace, with discriminatory benefit systems, etc. The whole thrust of the British disability movement is for more resources to be channelled towards disabled people, and it challenges the distributive logic of capitalism. It would be more accurate to suggest that new social movements are often concerned with the interrelations of the market and the welfare state. Perhaps there is relevance in Offe's (1987) stress on those groups which occupy a marginal labour-market role, such as women domestic workers, older people, migrant workers, disabled people, and the 'decommodified or peripheral groups'.

A second criticism of new social-movement theory is the tendency, for example in the work of Melucci (1989), to suggest that these struggles are not concerned with politics or the political process, but are centred on civil society and the control of information, not production. The latter point was refuted above. The former suggestion neglects the struggle to establish citizenship rights: political rights to vote; legal rights (for example, the age of consent, custody of children); and, above all, social rights. The most relevant of these is the growing campaign in Britain for anti-discrimination legislation. Claus Offe seems to highlight the crucial issue:

> The opposition is primarily not between old and new values but between conflicting views of the extent to which different elements of modern values are satisfied. (Offe, 1987, p. 88)

The movements of women, black people and disabled people have shown that these constituencies have not benefited from post-war developments in both living standards and social rights, and they have demonstrated the continuing inequalities in access to both political and economic power. So Brand, quoting Klandermans, is fundamentally incorrect to argue that:

> ... new social movements are not concerned with questions of distribution, economic power or political power. (Brand, 1990, p. 25)

Part of the important challenge of the liberation movements has been to widen the concept of the political by suggesting that personal, domestic and social relations are as political as voting and democratic representation. This is clearly not the same as a lack of concern with politics. Moreover, as such constituencies are marginalised from the political process, unrepresented either by political parties or corporate interests, there is often little choice but to operate in this way.

Another supposed difference between old and new social movements relates to the question of interests. Connected with the lack of concern for resource allocation has been the argument that new movements are protesting at their own economic situation not out of personal grievances but as a result of their value orientation. Dalton, Kuechler and Burklin, (1990) have argued:

> Activists in new social movements often hold intense feelings about their cause, but these sentiments fall short of the primordial frustration-aggression emotions that spawned food riots and tax revolts in the eighteenth century and the revolutionary movements of the nineteenth. Moreover, student protesters and environmental activists are not primarily drawn from the ranks of the socially deprived. (Dalton, Kuechler and Burklin, 1990, p. 7)

This may or may not be accurate in terms of the 'post-materialist' wing of the new social movements: the anti-nuclear, green and peace campaigns. But it seems less relevant with regard to liberation struggles. Women, black people, gays and disabled people are very clearly mobilising in defence of their objective interests: social being and social consciousness have the potential to come together in a manner directly paralleling the Marxist conception of the proletariat. Dalton et al. are wrong to suggest that the distinguishing feature of new social movements is that

> ... they lack the narrow special-interest appeal to any one social grouping. New social movements are not drawn from the socio-economically disadvantaged or from repressed minorities. (Dalton, Kuechler and Burklin, 1990, p. 12)

The term 'interest group' has an ambiguity which might usefully focus the distinction here: on the one hand, those who are 'interested in' a cause—who have a value commitment; and, on the other, those who 'have interests' in the sense of a real stake in the outcome. Everyone has interests in world peace, global environmental survival, and so forth. However, there is a significant difference between these comprehensive benefits and the more localised and personally specific benefits arising from progressive social relations in terms of gender, race, etc. Thus, there is a real distinction to be drawn between interests as subjective preference, and interests as an objective social category.

Alan Cawson distinguishes welfare pressure groups from traditional interest groups such as trade unions and employers' organisations. The latter owe their existence to their common position in relation to capital, their role in the division of labour. As a result of this, they have economic power and influence. As well as a dual economy between competitive and monopoly capital, there is a dual politics between such corporate interests and the pluralistic world of competing interest groups:

> The competitive group is formed by voluntary interaction: the corporate group consists of individuals having a common location in the socio-economic structure of society. (Cawson, 1982, p. 38)

Thus, social pressure groups such as Shelter and Child Poverty Action Group (CPAG), representing the interests of welfare-state clients, do not have the power of corporate interests:

> They do not possess socio-economic leverage—they have no clout—because the clients they represent are not among the economically productive whose cooperation is a prerequisite of successful policy. (Cawson, 1982, p. 43)

My suggestion is that this dichotomy needs to be enlarged to include the distinction I have made above between the two forms of competitive-interest groups; within the field of disability, Disability Income Group (DIG) or Disability Alliance (DA) would be distinguished from BCODP. Both are competitive-interest groups, but the former are not indigenous or representative. However, they do gain considerable funding and have a measure of consultative input into government policy:

> ... many of these organisations, which for many years have acted as both charities and disability pressure groups, have built up close working relationships with official policy-makers, which gives them a degree of credibility but relatively little power. (Barnes, 1991, p. 218)

In contrast to this role, the excluded, but representative, pressure groups who are interest groups in the true sense, straddle the corporate and competitive sectors and have resorted to new social-movement tactics in order to achieve political and social change. Frank Wilson distinguishes corporatist and pluralist forms of politics, in a distinction similar to that between DIG/DA/RADAR and BCODP above:

> The established groups seek to perpetuate their monopolies by co-opting or vigorously opposing new groups claiming to represent the same interests. ... The government often subsidises the privileged groups and denies such funding to unofficial bodies. (Wilson, 1990, p. 69)

Oliver has pointed out that organisations for disabled people outnumber organisations of disabled people by about 100 to 1, and receive far higher levels of funding. Moreover, Wilson goes on to discuss the role that 'official' groups have in formulating and administering government policy, which echoes the role of DIG in administering the independent-living fund. By contrast, those groups outside the process are left in a situation of 'residual pluralism':

> Frustrated by their inability to gain a hearing for their concerns from the policy-makers, outside groups resort to unconventional methods, such as demonstrations, boycotts, political strikes, sit-ins and even violence, to

> draw the attention of the public or the policy-makers to their concerns. (Wilson, 1990, p. 71)

Now I wish to move from criticising new social-movement theory to discussing those elements that have clear relevance to the disabled people's movement. Alan Scott has suggested that a key feature of new social movements is the stress on autonomy at the level of the personal (the focus on consciousness, personal power, etc); in the challenge of restrictions on freedom; and in what he calls the 'autonomy of struggle':

> ... the insistence that the movement and those it represents be allowed to fight their own corner without interference from other movements, and without subordinating their demands to other external priorities. (Scott, 1990, p. 20)

In focusing on autonomy, there is a parallel with the recent work of David Held (1987), who suggests that this concept has the potential to bring together new left and new right positions in a new, radical democracy. Carl Boggs makes similar claims:

> What emerge from the experience of local movements are the broad outlines of a radical democracy that rests upon a deeper conception of political involvement. (Boggs, 1986, p. 49)

Certainly, the disabled people's movement exemplifies the notion of autonomy that Scott has described. Colin Barnes echoes both Scott and perhaps Held:

> ... throughout the 1980s, BCODP and its member organisations produced a wealth of policy initiatives which, when implemented, will benefit not only them but the disabled population generally. Furthermore, these strategies owe as much to the political ideologies of the right as they do to those of the left. These include enabling disabled people to free themselves from unnecessary and costly bureaucratic regulation; to earn a living rather than live off the state; to achieve a degree of personal autonomy comparable to that of their non-disabled peers; and to expand their role as consumers. (Barnes, 1991, p. 224)

The central values of the disabled people's movement are autonomy, integration and independence. Features such as the U.S. consumer perspective, the independent-living movement, and the indigenous disability culture have a libertarian and grass-roots emphasis that reflects, to an extent, this comment by the new social-movement theorist, Brand:

> New social movements insist not only on the expansion of direct democratic forms of political participation but also on the widening of opportunities for social self-organisation. The cultural pluralism of the movements and their emphasis on autonomy also suggest a more reflexive way of political integration which is more responsive to different cultural norms and varying lifestyles. (Brand, 1990, p. 27)

In this struggle, the forms taken by the organisation and the campaign have significance:

> The organisational forms of the movement are not just 'instrumental' for their goals; they are a goal in themselves. Since collective action is focused on cultural codes, the form of the movement is itself a message, a symbolic challenge to the dominant codes. (Melucci, 1989, p. 60)

While not overstressing the semiotic component, it is clear that disabled people's self-organisation challenges the myth of passivity and the objectification of disabled people. Disabled people, like children, are meant to be seen and not heard; they are meant to be grateful, not angry; they are meant to be humble, not proud. In challenging all these preconceptions and discriminatory ideologies, the movement is making progress everyday, even before attaining the central political objectives. To quote Melucci again:

> The actors mobilise to regain control of their own action. They try to reclaim the right to define themselves against the criteria of identification determined by an anonymous power and systems of regulation that penetrate the area of 'internal nature'. (Melucci, 1989, p. 61)

The British focus on terminology and the social model parallels this claim by Melucci: the rejection of medical identifications of disability in favour of the new structural analysis.

A third feature of the disability movement which echoes Melucci's analysis is the exposure of underlying oppressive ideologies and social relations; what had seemed to be altruistic benevolence is shown to be paternalistic domination. Charities are identified as being promoters of oppressive ideologies; health and welfare professionals are exposed as being insensitive, overbearing and patronising. Penetrating the mask of concern and care, the real power struggles have been revealed:

> The function of contemporary conflicts is to render visible the power that hides behind the rationality of administrative or organisational procedures, or the 'show business' aspects of politics. (Melucci, 1989, p. 76)

In this way, it is not only the central structures and institutions that are being challenged, but also the 'molecular' level of daily life and relationships.

Returning to the prefigurative nature of much new social-movement politics—Melucci quotes McLuhan's 'the medium is the message'—a parallel might be drawn with Lenin's concept of consciousness. People's understanding of their social being increased and developed as they participated in mass action and mobilisation. As in Maoism, the revolution is an educative process.

CONCLUSION

The mobilisation around disability as a social movement is important for disabled people themselves, and also for the conceptualisation of disability. Self-organisation and direct action challenge prevailing stereotypes of powerlessness and objectification. This is important in the formation of disabled people's own identity, just as it is in breaking down patterns of prejudice and discrimination. In making 'personal troubles' 'public issues', disabled people are affirming the validity and importance of their own identity, rejecting both the victimising tendencies of society at large and their own socialisation. In short, the issue is the development of individualisation through the solidarity that a mass movement brings. New social-movement theory, in combining divergent political phenomena and overstressing the novelty of these developments, fails to theorise this process usefully.

References

Banks, O. 1986. *Becoming a Feminist.* Brighton: Wheatsheaf.

Barnes, C. 1991. *Disabled People in Britain and Discrimination.* London: Hurst and Co.

Boggs, C. 1986. *Social Movements and Political Power*. Philadelphia: Temple University Press.

Brand, K.W. 1990. 'Cyclical aspects of new social movements', in R.J. Dalton and M. Kuechler (eds), *Challenging the Political Order*. Cambridge: Polity Press.

Bynoe, I., Oliver, M. and Barnes, C. 1991. *Equal Rights for Disabled People*. London: IPPR.

Cawson, A. 1982. *Corporatism and Welfare*. London: Heinemann.

Crewe, N.M. et al. 1983. *Independent Living for Physically Disabled People*. San Francisco: Jossey-Bass.

Crow, Liz. 1992. 'Including all our lives: Renewing the social model of disability', in J. Morris (ed.), *Encounters with Strangers: Feminism and Disability*. London: Women's Press, pp. 5–9.

Dalton, R.J., Kuechler, M. and Burklin, W. 1990. 'The challenge of new movements', in R.J. Dalton and M. Kuechler (eds), *Challenging the Political Order*. Cambridge: Polity Press.

DeJong, G. 1983. 'Defining and implementing the independent living concept', in N.M. Crewe et al. (eds), *Independent Living for Physically Disabled People*. San Francisco: Jossey-Bass.

Driedger, D. 1989. *The Last Civil-Rights Movement: Disabled Peoples' International*. London: Hurst and Co.

French, Sally. 1993. 'Disability, impairment or something in between?', in J. Barton et al. (eds), *Disabling Barriers, Enabling Environments*. London: Sage.

Held, D. 1987. *Models of Democracy*. Cambridge: Polity Press.

Inglehart, R. 1990. 'Values, ideology and cognitive mobilisations in new social movements', in R.J. Dalton and M. Kuechler (eds), *Challenging the Political Order*. Cambridge: Polity Press.

Klein, E. 1984. *Gender Politics*. Cambridge: Harvard University Press.

Melucci, A., Keane, J. and Mier, P. 1989. *Nomads of the Present: Social Movements and Individuals Needs in Contemporary Society*. Philadelphia: Temple University Press.

Morris, A.D. 1984. *The Origins of the Civil-Rights Movement*. New York: Free Press.

Morris, J. 1991. *Pride against Prejudice*. London: Women's Press.

Offe, C. 1987. 'Challenging the boundaries of institutional politics', in C.S. Maier (ed.), *Changing Boundaries of the Political*. Cambridge: Cambridge University Press.

Oliver, M. 1990. *The Politics of Disablement*. London: Macmillan.

Pagel, M. 1988. *On Our Own Behalf: An Introduction to the Self-organisation of Disabled People*. Manchester: Greater Manchester Council of Disabled People Publications.

Safilios-Rothschild, C. 1976. 'Disabled persons' self-definitions and their implications for rehabilitation', in G.L. Albrecht (ed.), *The Sociology of Physical Disability and Rehabilitation*. Pittsburgh: University of Pittsburgh Press.

Scott, A. 1990. *Ideology and New Social Movements*. London: Unwin Hyman.

Wilson, F.L. 1990. 'Neo-corporatism and the rise of new social movements', in R.J. Dalton and M. Kuechler (eds), *Challenging the Political Order*. Cambridge: Polity Press.

Zola, I.K. 1983. 'Developing new self-images and interdependence', in N.M. Crewe et al., *Independent Living for Physically Disabled People*. San Francisco: Jossey-Bass.

19

The Disability-Rights Movement in Japan: Past, Present and Future

Reiko Hayashi & Masako Okuhiro

Only two decades ago, Japanese society did not perceive the confining of disabled persons in institutions for life as a human-rights violation. Today, the disability-rights movement in Japan boasts 90 centres for independent living throughout the country that provide community-based services and also do advocacy work. It also supports the independent-living movements of disabled people in other Asian countries. Its goal is the realisation of nationwide consumer-directed personal-attendant programmes that enable persons with any disabilities, regardless of their severity, to live independently in their communities. This paper introduces the history of the disability-rights movement in Japan, which has been the driving force both for change in social norms and policies and for improving the lives of disabled persons and their families.

After examining pre-movement conditions, this paper describes a radical movement of people with cerebral palsy, active from the 1960s through the 1980s, within the cultural milieu of Japanese society. Furthermore, it recounts the emergence of the independent-living movement in the 1980s and discusses the current disability-rights movement, including

Hayashi, R. and Okuhiro, M. 2001. 'The disability-rights movement in Japan: Past, present and future', *Disability and Society*, 9: 855–69.

the successes of independent-living centres and the challenges they face as providers of community-based care.

This paper is based on a review of documents, as well as interviews of personnel working for centres for independent living and disability-rights advocates in the spring of 2000. The interviewees were asked about their personal history: their childhood experiences; their experiences in school, if they attended one, and in institutions; their first contact with, and their involvement in, the disability-rights movement; and their current activities and future directions. The personal history of these interviewees embodies the disability-rights movement that freed people from confinement in parents' homes or institutions to living independently and actively in society.

JAPAN'S TRADITIONAL APPROACH TO WELFARE

A centralised government was established in Japan in 1874, and the Social Relief Regulation was enacted to provide rice to the extremely poor and the indigent—elderly, young, sick or disabled. Blood relatives and neighbours, however, were expected to support the underprivileged; consequently, governmental relief was severely limited. As the nation waded through the First World War and the depression that followed, the labour movement intensified. Laws were introduced to expand governmental obligations to the poor, together with medical insurance and a pension programme for employed workers. Disabled citizens, however, were still assumed to be dependents of their parents and siblings, and no public policies existed to support them (Ministry of Health and Welfare, 2000).

After the Second World War, three welfare laws were enacted: the Public Assistance Law, the Child Welfare Law, and the Law for the Welfare of People with Physical Disabilities. The Law for the Welfare of People with Physical Disabilities, enacted in 1949, was the first national policy in support of disabled persons. It was, however, enacted to provide rehabilitation services to disabled veterans to restore their vocational capabilities. Under this law, occupational rehabilitation facilities were established in some cities. Disabled persons other than veterans were still left to depend on their blood relatives or receive public assistance for their survival. A small minority were sent to live in only a few publicly funded alms houses (Tateiwa, 1990; Ministry of Health and Welfare, 2000). In 1961, the National Pension was inaugurated. This system was initially developed only for employed workers. Later it was expanded to cover the self-employed and farmers, and eventually it became a universal national pension. Employers and workers paid into it, and workers received the benefits when they reached retirement age. A supplementary and provisional system with non-contributory pensions (welfare pensions) was also adopted out of consideration for fatherless households, people with disabilities, and those who had already reached a certain age and did not have sufficient time to contribute (Ministry of Health and Welfare, 2000). For disabled persons, the National Pension included the Welfare Pension for People with Disabilities. The amount of the pension, however, depended on the income of family members as well as the severity of the impairments. Even though the disabled persons were adults, their parents and other family members were expected to support some of them. Therefore, many disabled persons could not receive the pension, and were kept dependent on blood relatives or had to enter residential institutions, which had been rapidly established in the 1960s (Wakabayashi, 1986; Tateiwa, 1990).

FROM HOME CONFINEMENT TO INSTITUTIONAL SEGREGATION

The 1960s saw the parents of disabled persons organise themselves to demand residential institutions for their disabled children. Social norms and government policies demanded they care for their children even through adulthood. The parents said that institutions would be needed when they were no longer able to care for their children. As the post-Second World War economic recovery gained momentum, Japanese society began to respond to these 'welfare' demands. Residential institutions for disabled persons were built, and the institutions for occupational rehabilitation initially established for disabled veterans were turned into residential facilities for other disabled persons (Tateiwa, 1990; H. Kondo, interview, 26 May 2000). These institutions became places for disabled persons to live permanently, segregated from the wider society. At the same time, many disabled persons still remained hidden in their parents' homes. It became common for disabled children to be separated from their families at an early age and sent to residential facilities. Many of those children lived there until they reached 18 years of age, and were then moved to residential facilities for adults to live there the rest of their lives (Irube, 1990).

These residential institutions implemented strict rules to control all aspects of the residents' lives. It was a life of segregation and obedience, without privacy. The living conditions were often harsh and the human rights of the residents were customarily violated.

A woman who stayed in an institution for disabled children for 10 years witnessed the maltreatment of children. Some who became sick were left without proper medical treatment and died. She recalled children with severe impairments who were left in unsanitary conditions and never bathed. They smelled badly, and flies gathered over them and laid eggs in their bed sores (Kim, 1996).

Surgeries were often performed on disabled children. Parents of those children gave consent for the surgeries in the hope of a cure or at least an improvement. In reality, the opposite was common. In many cases, their physical functions weakened because of the surgeries. For example, a child who was able to walk lost this ability as a result of four surgical operations while he was institutionalised (K. Onoue, interview, 17 May 2000). Disabled persons who experienced surgery as children or who witnessed the deterioration of their fellow residents following surgical procedures now suspect that they were used as guinea-pigs for the professional advancement of their doctors (Irube, 1990; Kim, 1996).

A standard practice in these institutions was to perform hysterectomies on women who menstruated, in order to make the staff's work easier. Disabled women were simply not regarded as women. Whenever they menstruated, staff would complain and urge them to get a hysterectomy. Sometimes the staff would ignore a resident's wishes and get permission for the surgery from her parents. A woman had to be extremely assertive to avoid this surgery (K. Irube, interview, 17 May 2000). Sexual abuse towards female residents was also common. Onaka (1990) reports incidents of a male staff member fondling female residents' breasts each time he bathed them. Verbal abuses by staff were also prevalent, such as 'you are a burden to society' and 'your parents should have killed you.' Male and female residents were often bathed together by male staff. Toilet facilities for residents had no doors. Protest against such abuses was not an option. Residents needed daily assistance, and were thus forced to accept humiliation by the staff and their inferior position in society. They cried quietly in their beds while tolerating these daily abuses.

Beyond these obvious violations of human rights, living conditions in these institutions were very harsh. The daily schedules of the residents were often determined or modified for the convenience of the institution, rather than that of the residents. For example, in a residential institution for children, the time for getting up was 6:30 a.m. To be ready by that time, children were awakened as early as 4 a.m. to dress, assisted by a limited number of staff. In winter, there was no heating. Trembling from the cold and without assistance, some children took hours to change their clothes (Kim, 1996). In an institution for adults, staff were scheduled to prepare futons for sleeping at 4 p.m., and they often came as early as 1 p.m. to prepare the room for the residents to sleep. All window shades were closed in the early afternoon. Residents who had the courage to complain were blacklisted. They were scolded, not only by staff but also by other residents, who argued they had no right to complain since they could not do anything by themselves (Suzuki, 1995).

In institutions for children, residents were ranked by the severity of their impairments. Children with less severe impairments were favoured by teachers and staff. They then adopted an 'elite' attitude, and considered themselves superior to residents with more severe impairments. The mission of these institutions was to train the residents to overcome their impairments and become as much like able-bodied persons as possible. Children whose impairments made it impossible for them to walk were pressured to try. Children with severe physical impairments were often neglected and left on their beds. Their beds became their whole world (K. Onoue, interview, 17 May 2000; Kim, 1996; Irube, 1990).

Having visitors and going out with family members were special events for institutionalised children. It was, however, strictly limited by institutional rules. In many cases, they were allowed to visit their families only once or twice a year (typically New Year's Day), and to have visitors as seldom as once or twice a month (Irube, 1990; Higuchi, 1998). Children who were abandoned in front of the institution or whose parents disappeared after they entered the institution had no one to visit during the holidays, nor did anyone come to visit them. With no knowledge of the outside world, they remained confined in the institution until they reached 18 years of age, when they were moved into an institution for adults. Residents who had visitors tended to be treated better by staff than those who had no visitors. Families would sneak in snacks (against institutional rules) for their hungry children, who were forced to endure a restricted diet (Kim, 1996; Higuchi, 1998).

In institutions for adults, the residents were treated as if they were children. Staff were patronising towards the residents. A handbook published by a coalition of residential institutions for their staff focused on the functional limitations of disabled persons, and depicted them as people of weak character who needed constant supervision. The handbook stated that the staff should be teachers foremost, and scold residents to make them behave (Onaka, 1990). Residents had to ask permission to do anything. Yokoyama (1998) recalls that, in the institution where he lived, no resident was given permission to go out during the winter. The official reason for the denial was to protect the residents from getting cold outside. Newspapers for the residents were censored. Advertisements for housing were cut out so the residents would not dream of leaving the institution. Onaka (1990) describes an incident that can be perceived as intentional institutional neglect: a doctor instructed an institution to allow a disabled resident to try an electric wheelchair so that he could move around without the assistance of volunteers. It took 2 years and 6 months for the institution to allow him the trial. Then, after the trial, in which the resident proved that he could control the electric wheelchair, it took a further 8 years for the resident to receive one.

THE EMERGENCE OF THE DISABILITY-RIGHTS MOVEMENT

The disability-rights movement in Japan was born alongside the other social movements of the 1960s and 1970s, among them the anti-Vietnam war, student, environmental and feminist movements, and the Buraku liberation movement. (The Buraku people are Japanese citizens whose ancestors belonged to the lowest caste during the Samurai Era, 150 years ago. They are still discriminated against today.) Disabled people began to raise their voices in protest against discriminatory treatment. One incident that happened in the Fuchu Ryoiku Centre is described below. This section also introduces the Aoi Shiba, a group of people with cerebral palsy that had a great influence on the disability-rights movement in Japan in the 1970s and 1980s. They criticised the 'able-bodied culture', and changed the perception of disabilities among disabled people and among the wider population as well.

The Fuchu Ryoiku Centre Battle

The Fuchu Ryoiku Centre was a residential institution of the type described in the previous section. Opened in 1968, it was considered a model institution under the welfare policies of the left-leaning Tokyo governor, Taturo Minobe. In reality, it was not an exception regarding the maltreatment of its residents. For disabled persons to be accepted into the Centre, their parents had to sign a waiver eliminating the requirement of their consent for any surgical procedures performed on their adult children. This enabled the doctors of the Centre to perform any surgery, including lobotomy and autopsy, without parent notification. As a result, residents were used as guinea-pigs by the doctors for medical research (Kyukyoku, 1998). During the induction, disabled persons were stripped naked and photographed. Residents wore pyjamas 24 hours a day and lived in bedrooms shared by many. There was a notice in the building stating, 'Do not feed except the meals provided by the Centre'. The residents were not allowed to make any contact with persons outside the institution, except for once-a-month visitations. They were allowed to go out only once every 3 months, when their parents submitted a request in writing. Verbal abuses by staff were common, especially when the residents received toilet assistance. 'One who can't wipe his own ass has no right to be concerned about his hairstyle. Cut your damn hair!' (Wakabayashi, 1986)

After having their requests for better treatment repeatedly ignored, some Fuchu Ryoiku residents began a hunger strike in 1970 to protest their chronic maltreatment at the Centre. Although the hunger strike did receive some media attention, the Centre made no policy changes. In 1972, triggered by lay-offs of sympathetic staff, the residents' union called for sit-ins in front of the Tokyo municipal building. This time they gained strong support from labour and student activists, who helped them to set up and sustain the sit-ins. The sit-ins lasted for more than a year. It forced the government to look into the living conditions in residential institutions. The incident also led the disabled participants to think about life alternatives. They had been given only two options in their lives: they had to live with their parents or in an institution. They began to consider the possibility of living independently in the community (Wakabayashi, 1986; Kyukyoku, 1998).

Aoi Shiba

The origin of Aoi Shiba goes back to a school established in 1932 and a friendship group started in 1957 by its graduates. In 1932, the first school for the physically disabled, Komyo Gakko, was opened in Tokyo by the efforts of a few motivated educators who were influenced by the democracy movement of the early twentieth century. This became the only school where children with cerebral palsy could get an education in Japan. The school accepted children from affluent families. These students received an education in literature, art and music. Graduates of the school reached adulthood around the end of the Second World War, and in 1947 they started a literature club known as Sinonome. They printed a journal to publish their essays, poems and haikus. While the majority of people with cerebral palsy in Japan remained hidden from view, confined to their parents' homes, these fortunate elite braved curious gazes to enter occupational rehabilitation institutions. Some even entered colleges. However, once they completed their training or education, they learned the stark reality that there was no place for them in society. Even organisations for disabled persons did not welcome persons with cerebral palsy (Wakabayashi, 1986).

In 1957, some of these educated elite established a group called Aoi Shiba for people with cerebral palsy. At first, the activities of the group were limited to recreation and socialisation, activities which other organisations of disabled persons had been providing to their respective members. However, the group began to develop a deeper awareness of social issues involving those with cerebral palsy. In 1961, they held their first meeting with the Japanese government's Ministry of Health and Welfare. They requested twelve policy changes, including an increase in the Welfare Pension for People with Disabilities. Their demands included items that current disability-rights advocates would strongly oppose, such as the establishment of permanent residential facilities (Wakabayashi,

1986). Although some of their demands are viewed with contempt from our current perspective, it should be noted that this meeting held with the government of Japan by a group of people with cerebral palsy—a group discriminated against even by people with other disabilities—was a historically important achievement.

As Aoi Shiba grew, it was joined by two other groups of persons with cerebral palsy. One, a small residential institution called Kurume-en, was created by a progressive welfare worker who encouraged the residents to express their opinions and exercise their freedom for the first time in their lives. Another, the Maharaba Colony for persons with cerebral palsy, was a commune lead by a left-leaning Buddhist monk who helped the residents realise that they had to free themselves from the social norms of an ableist society (Wakabayashi, 1986). These two groups presented stronger social awareness than Aoi Shiba's founding elite, who wanted less conflict with mainstream society.

Aoi Shiba's leadership changed hands as it absorbed these new groups, and so did its direction, as marked by its response to a child-killing incident in Kanagawa prefecture. In 1970, a mother killed her 2-year-old disabled child. This led to a petition drive by an association of parents of disabled children to halt the criminal prosecution of the mother. Such petitions were not new. Usually, the petitions blamed the limited number of institutions for the disabled, and citizens felt great sympathy for the parents. Influenced by this public outcry, the District Attorney's office was reconsidering prosecution. However, this time Aoi Shiba publicly criticised the parents' movement. They accused the parents of being representatives of an ableist society which nurtured a eugenic ideology that labelled disability as a fate worse than death. They successfully counter-petitioned the court to judge the mother according to the law, and she was prosecuted (Wakabayashi, 1986; Tateiwa, 1990; Nagase, 1995).

Disabled persons had been taught to be childlike, lovable, always smiling, appreciative and apologetic towards able-bodied persons. They had been taught self-pity and dependence at home, in institutions and in society. Aoi Shiba's new leadership helped them realise that ableist society judged them as 'an existence which should not exist'. It encouraged them to aggressively represent themselves for self-protection (Nagase, 1995). They also implored people with disabilities to refuse ableist society's 'love and justice', which they recognised as pity and oppression. Finally, they stated that they would not solve problems. They understood from their personal experiences that easy solutions to problems would lead to dangerous compromises. They believed that exposing problems was their mission (Okahara, 1990; Tateiwa, 1990). Aoi Shiba sent organisers to establish branches in many areas in Japan. They continued to raise their voices in protest against ableism. They, among others, participated in sit-ins to stop inaccessible buses, worked against the compulsory segregation of disabled children in separate schools, and organised protests against the Eugenics Protection Law, which legalised abortion when the foetus had disabilities (Wakabayashi, 1986; Yamamoto, 1995; Yokoyama, 1998). Aoi Shiba was the leading force to establish a coalition of disability-rights organisations, Zenshoren, in 1976. Zenshoren, a progressive coalition of people with diverse disabilities, also organised various protests against ableist policies (Wakabayashi, 1986).

Challenges in the Disability-Rights Movement

As with other political organisations, Aoi Shiba faced internal conflicts. One of these was related to the involvement of non-disabled persons in the movement. Toyota (1988) recalls that some of those able-bodied supporters were left-wing radicals who had goals beyond the liberation of disabled people. They wanted to exploit the energy of this oppressed group to help their political factions fight against the social system. They tried to take control over the activities of disabled persons and their organisations. To establish a 'disability authority', some disabled persons declared that non-disabled persons should be just 'hands and legs', meaning the non-disabled should attend to the needs of disabled persons but not express their opinions. They felt that the non-disabled should acknowledge the parts they played in ableist society and should work as 'hands and legs' for free as redemption for their role as oppressors (Toyota, 1988). Having been eliminated from society and never considered employable, some disabled persons found it difficult to comprehend that their able-bodied supporters had to earn a living. Some labelled working for money as 'impure'. The idea of paying for personal attendants did not cross the minds of early activists in the movement. In some extreme cases, volunteer attendants who were a few minutes late for their appointments received strong verbal rebukes and were condemned as oppressors. Those who wanted to quit their volunteer positions for personal reasons were also berated. This desire to establish disability authority, born of their experiences of being abused by ableist society, caused angry outbursts towards non-disabled persons around them. Many non-disabled supporters refused to accept subjugation and the expectation that they should provide free labour but have no voice in the movement (Kyukyoku, 1998).

Another problem they encountered was in assigning 'ranks' to oppressions. This was during a time when many oppressed groups raised their voices to be heard by the wider Japanese society. Some of these included Koreans and the Buraku people. There came to be a ranking of oppressions in which sexism was labelled lightest. There was a sense that ableism and Buraku-discrimination were critically important, while sexism was not. When a mother killed her disabled child, the disability movement saw *mothers* as enemies. 'Mothers, do not kill!' was their slogan, not 'Parents, do not kill!' The disability-rights movement failed to acknowledge the intersection of sexism and ableism in such incidents. When women could validate their social status only as mothers who bore 'healthy' children for their husbands' families, those who bore disabled children were condemned to live in shame with the children. While the murder of a child should doubtless be denounced, so should sexism (Yonezu, 1998). By ignoring other oppressions in society, the movement became an uncomfortable place for many.

Aoi Shiba experienced inner organisational conflicts because of differences in opinion on many issues. Many left the organisation with heavy hearts. Yet, with all of its weaknesses, Aoi Shiba should be remembered as a radiant star in Japan's modern disability-rights movement. Those who stayed, those who left for various reasons, and those disabled persons who did not join the organisation but learned disability pride because of its existence: all acknowledge that Aoi Shiba helped change their lives forever. Many of the leaders of the current disability-rights movement had their consciousness raised by the Aoi Shiba movement and have continued to be active as a result.

LIVING IN THE COMMUNITY

As consciousness was raised in the 1970s within the disability-rights movement, some disabled activists left the confinement of their institutions or their parents' homes and started new lives in the community, supported by volunteer attendants. They were determined not to go back to their former situations even though their lives were at risk (K. Onoue, interview, 17 May 2000). Managing their own lives 24 hours a day with volunteer attendants presented enormous challenges, including recruiting volunteers, keeping them and arranging their time schedules. Many found themselves constantly on the phone trying to get attendants. Soon they were competing for the same volunteers with other disabled persons (Yokoyama, 1998). Their personal needs for daily living in the community led them into negotiations with their local governments in many regions. They demanded that the government create or expand programmes, such as home-helper services, and provide funds to allow disabled citizens to directly hire personal attendants (Kyukyoku, 1998).

In the 1980s, disability-rights organisations put more energy into negotiating with regional governments to improve the daily lives of disabled persons, rather than leading protests in response to discriminatory incidents. During the 1970s, their negotiations with governments tended to be protest-oriented. At that time, getting patronising and insincere government personnel merely to listen to what disabled persons were saying was as important as the content of their demands. By the 1980s, government agencies were getting used to the presence of disabled people at the negotiation table and disability-rights organisations began making requests based on research findings. Their requests expanded beyond the immediate personal needs of activists to include benefits for 'ordinary' disabled persons (K. Onoue, interview, 17 May 2000).

The 1980s was a time when people started to consider independent living within the community as an alternative to institutional living when their parents became old or their care-giving siblings fell ill. For example, in 1980, the Osaka Aoi Shiba chapter surveyed disabled persons about their living conditions. The survey consisted of 100 questions about daily life, employment, education and medical necessities. The purpose was to study the situation of those disabled persons living with their parents or living in institutions. The data they gathered on about 200 respondents revealed some situations of serious concern. For example, it was typical that a disabled person did nothing but sit in front of the TV all day alone, except when going out with a volunteer once a month. It was also common that a disabled person bathed only once a month because the parents were getting too old to give bathing assistance. Having presented their findings to the Osaka City government, Osaka Aoi Shiba then negotiated with the City for several years to establish a personal-attendant programme which would satisfy the needs of disabled persons. They recommended same sex 'home helpers' who could not only do housekeeping tasks, but also personal-care assistance such as bathing and toilet support. They demanded the right to select their helpers, as well as the right to dismiss them. In 1986, the Personal Attendants Programme for Physically Disabled Persons was started in Osaka City. At first the programme provided assistance for a maximum of only 12 hours a month per person, and the hourly wage for the helper was 650 yen. However, the programme progressed, and by 1999 the city was providing 153 hours of assistance a month per person at an hourly wage of 1,400 yen (Onoue, 2000).

In some areas, disability-rights organisations started their own personal-attendant programmes. The members of these organisations had faced difficulties obtaining high-quality attendants as well as in getting an adequate supply of attendants. Helpers from municipal governments tended to be inflexible regarding what they would do. Also, disabled persons had to wait for the helper to arrive at their home. They could not change their schedule and go out when they wanted. Some helpers were patronising and domineering. These pioneers of independent living learned from experience how to educate and handle their helpers. The personal-attendant programmes hired and educated attendants and coordinated them with their clients for a fee. By becoming service providers, the disability-rights organisations helped expand the opportunities of independent living to disabled persons who wanted to leave their institutions or parents' homes but did not know how. They faced strong criticism from some of their peers from the 1970s, who still believed that assistance should be 'pure', without monetary compensation. However, in spite of some dissension, the programmes developed in response to the demand within communities. Disabled people continued their negotiations with local governments to increase funding for personal attendants (Kyukyoku, 1998; Yokoyama, 1998).

Besides the issue of personal attendants, disability-rights organisations were active on many fronts in the 1980s. For example, in the Osaka area they started some 'workshops for the disabled', supported by grants from local governments. These grants were established originally by parents' movements in the 1960s. These new workshops included a soap shop, bakeries and print shops (Irube, 1990). The major difference between these workshops and traditional ones was that these were founded and managed by disabled persons. The workshops were located in the community, and disabled workers participated in planning, production, sales and management. By contrast, traditional workshops were usually established and controlled by the non-disabled, often the parents of the disabled workers. In those 'sheltered work shops', disabled persons were assigned to menial tasks, and had little or no voice in organisational decision-making (K. Onoue, interview, 17 May 2000).

Disability-rights organisations expanded the definition of 'workshops' as well. Some groups received a workshop grant to establish offices where people could receive information, do networking, plan for negotiations, and participate in other activities. Shared homes with personal attendants were opened and supported by such grants, as well as 'experimental' facilities for independent living, where disabled persons could try living independently in the community, assisted by 'total strangers', for the first time in their lives (M. Kawakami, interview, 16 May 2000).

Beyond their community activism, some disabled women fell in love with their male attendants, got married, became mothers, and raised families (Irube, 1990; M. Saito, interview, 19 May 2000). These women would have once been forced to get hysterectomies while living without any measure of independence in institutions. When disability-rights advocates decided they needed their voices heard in a city assembly, a mother who required 24-hour attendant care ran for the position and won in 1990. When she first appeared at the City Hall, city employees talked to her attendant even though she was the city assembly person. She is now serving her third term, and city employees talk directly to her. (K. Irube, interview, 17 May 2000).

ADVOCATES FROM THE UNITED STATES

The 1981 International Year of Disabled Persons prompted visits by advocates from the United States, including the pioneers of the U.S. disability-rights and independent-living movements, Ed Roberts and Judy Heumann. Roberts, a quadriplegic and respirator-user, entered the University of California, Berkeley, in 1962, notwithstanding the reluctance of university officials and a complete lack of accommodations. Encouraged by his action a few more students with severe disabilities enrolled at this university in the next few years. They formed a group known as the Rolling Quads, and worked to make the campus and surrounding community accessible. Roberts also founded the first centre for independent living in 1972 (Pelka, 1997, pp. 266–67; Shapiro, 1993, pp. 41–73). Heumann, who won a disability-based discrimination lawsuit in New York, became the first wheelchair-using teacher in New York City's public school system in 1970. She founded Disabled in Action, a political action group, and organised demonstrations and sit-ins protesting President Richard Nixon's veto of the Rehabilitation Act of 1972. She joined Roberts at the Centre for Independent Living in Berkeley in 1973. In 1977, disability-rights activists occupied the federal building in San Francisco for 25 days, demanding that the Carter administration implement Section 504 of the Rehabilitation Act of 1973. The action nurtured a sense of pride and solidarity in the disability community (Pelka, 1997, pp. 152–54; Shapiro, 1993, pp. 55–73). As the U.S. movement broadened its purview, disability-rights activists challenged institutionalised oppression, segregation, and the lack of basic rights such as physical accessibility, equal employment, housing and transportation.

By the time of the visits to Japan in 1981, the U.S. disability-rights movement had established several centres for independent living in American cities. The centres, administered by disabled people, provided advocacy work as well as social services to support disabled people living in the community (Lifchez, 1979; Levy, 1988; DeJong, Batavia and Mcknew, 1992). At that time, Ed Roberts was the director of the California State Department of Vocational Rehabilitation, and Judy Heumann was the deputy director of the Centre for Independent Living in Berkeley. They and other U.S. advocates attended conferences in many Japanese cities, and impressed participants with disabilities tremendously with their descriptions of the centres for independent living, as well as with their credentials as important officials in government and community agencies.

Among the Japanese in attendance were those who had kept their distance from the disability-rights movement of the 1970s. Some had felt uncomfortable with the aggressive strategies Aoi Shiba took then. Others were still children then, living in institutions. They grew up listening to teachers who warned that Aoi Shiba was a dangerous and extremist organisation and forbade them from approaching the group. Motivated by the stories of these U.S. advocates, some Japanese participants took advantage of a scholarship programme offered by a foundation that enabled them to go to the United States and study at the centres for independent living there (Higuchi, 1998). Thus, a new breed of advocates was trained in the United States in 1980s.

ESTABLISHING CENTRES FOR INDEPENDENT LIVING IN JAPAN

In 1986, the first centre for independent living modelled on those in the U.S. was opened in a suburb of Tokyo, staffed mainly by those trained in the United States. Different from the protest-oriented organisations of the 1970s, the new centre for independent living established a business office and offered the following fee-based services: an independent-living programme, peer counselling, and a personal-attendant programme. The independent-living programme equipped its participants with the social skills, behaviours and attitudes they would need to live within the community, and it offered classes to raise their self-confidence, motivation for life and self-esteem. Although established segregated schools for the disabled offered physical-rehabilitation training to their students, they ignored their crucial need for the social skills and self-confidence required to live in the community. Thus, the independent-living programme was essential for disabled persons who were inspired to live independently. Peer-counselling sessions were developed by combining information from co-counselling, peer-counselling and therapy methods and practices in other countries with knowledge about uniquely Japanese situations. The personal-attendant programme hired and trained attendants, and coordinated them with clients. Members of the centre also provided the support to found more centres for independent living in other areas of Japan (Nakanishi, 1996; Higuchi, 1998; Tsutsumi, 1998; H. Kondo, interview, May 26, 2000; S. Nakanishi, interview, June 1, 2000).

In 1991, the Japan Council on Independent-Living Centres (JIL), an association of centres for independent living, was established to coordinate the independent-living movement. To join JIL, organisations have to fulfil certain requirements. First, both the president and the director of the organisation, as well as a majority of its board of directors, must be disabled persons. Second, the organisation must provide a 'packaged service' consisting of at least two out of the following four programmes: peer counselling, a personal-attendant programme, a housing service and an independent-living programme. Finally, they must admit all disabled clients, regardless of the type or severity of their disabilities (JIL, 2000a). Advocacy organisations from the 1970s that had already been providing various services to the community, as well as the more recently founded centres for independent living, joined JIL. Activists trained in the protest movements of the 1970s, along with new advocates educated in the U.S., joined forces to establish nationwide consumer-directed personal-attendant programmes. The membership started with 10 centres in 1991. By the spring of 2000, there were 90 centres for independent living in Japan associated with JIL. JIL provides assistance for the creation of new centres, promotes cooperation among existing centres, and strives to gain public recognition for the centres' work in order to receive government contracts and private foundation grants to help maintain and advance their activities. It also educates the general public about human-rights violations of disabled persons and advocates the eradication of all such violations.

While providing services, the centres for independent living have, both jointly and separately, continued negotiations with governmental agencies to increase official support for attendant services. As a result, one quarter of all Japanese citizens now live in regions where disabled persons can receive more than 8 hours of attendant services daily, provided by government agencies. In Matsuyama City, Takamatsu City, and 17 regions in Tokyo, disabled persons can receive round-the-clock attendant services covered by government agencies (SSK, 2000).

THE DISABILITY-RIGHTS MOVEMENT: INTO THE FUTURE

In Japan's traditional welfare society, disabled people were assumed to be taken care of physically and financially by their parents and siblings, even after reaching adulthood. Life choices for the majority of persons with severe impairments were limited to either living with parents or living in institutions for their entire lives. In the 1970s, the modern disability-rights movement was born as disabled persons protested against human-rights violations in residential institutions, segregated schools and

Japanese society. Eventually, some of these pioneers left their institutions or their parents' homes to live in the community, determined never to return. They had to recruit volunteer attendants themselves, and when that failed they faced starvation, sitting in their own excrement, and other terrible hardships. Those courageous people who overcame these challenges became even more motivated and determined activists. Their continuous negotiations with local governments made it possible for disabled persons to receive funds and attendant services, enabling them to survive in the community. By the 1990s, people with disabilities no longer had to be activists to live independently (K. Onoue, interview, 17 May 2000).

Advocates from the United States introduced the philosophy and practices of their centres for independent living, inspiring disabled persons from Japan to train in U.S. centres and return to open Japan's first centre for independent living. More centres were created, and in 1991 the Japan Council of Independent-Living Centres was established to coordinate the independent-living movement.

Both national and regional governments have gradually come to accept the idea of consumer-directed, community-based programmes. In 1996, the Ministry of Health and Welfare established the City-Town-Village Living Support Programme for Disabled Persons, and contracted out its services to three centres for independent living in the Tokyo area. In 2000, Machida City also contracted out its Home Helper Programme for Disabled Persons to a centre for independent living in the city (H. Kondo, interview, 26 May 2000). Furthermore, the Japanese government plans to implement the National Attendant Insurance Programme for Disabled Persons in 2005, which will contract out its services to community-based agencies. This presents the centres for independent living in Japan with an opportunity to show their competence as providers of community-based services and to become a national network of services contractors. Such an accomplishment would establish the concept of consumer-controlled services in every aspect of the service-delivery system. In the new millennium, besides establishing the public standing of the centres for independent living as major providers of community services, the disability-rights movement in Japan must continue its advocacy work on many fronts. Issues of importance include:

- creating accessible communities, including accessible transportation systems (H. Kondo, interview, 26 May 2000; JIL, 2000b);
- outreach to disabled persons living in institutions (Kishida, 2000; S. Nakanishi, interview, 1 June 2000);
- greater involvement in the Ombudsperson system, now dominated by able-bodied professionals, to protect the human rights of institutionalised persons (JIL, 2000b);
- expanding independent-living services to persons with psychiatric or intellectual disabilities (Nakanishi, 1996);
- providing their knowledge and expertise to movements outside of Japan.

The disability-rights movement in Japan has begun supporting independent-living movements in other Asian countries. Japanese advocates visit Asian countries to introduce their citizens to the philosophy and practices of the centres for independent living. Disabled persons from those countries are now being trained in Japan's centres for independent living. Japanese advocates hope that other Asian countries will be able to avoid the creation of segregated institutions which, once created, will be hard to abolish (S. Nakanishi, interview, 1 June 2000). The disability-rights movement in Japan has come a long way, and there remains much to accomplish.

References

DeJong, G., Batavia, A.I. and McKnew, L.B. 1992. 'The independent-living model of personal assistance in long-term care policy', *Generations*, 16: 89–95.

Higuchi, K. 1998. *Enjoy Jiritu Seikatu* (Enjoy Independent Living) (in Japanese). Tokyo: Gendai Shokan.

Irube, M. 1990. *Harikiri Oyabunnoo Kurumaisu Hanjyouki* (The Activities of an Energetic Boss in a Wheelchair) (in Japanese). Toyonaka: Aznokai.

Japan Council on Independent-Living Centres (JIL). 2000a. *Japan Council on Independent-Living Centres*. Online: http://www.dl.dion.ne.jp/~jil.

———. 2000b. *Shogaisyato Kenri Yogo* (Disabled Persons and the Protection of their Rights) (in Japanese). Tokyo: Japan Council on Independent-Living Centres.

Kim, M. 1996. *Ikirukotono Hajimari* (Starting to Live) (in Japanese). Tokyo: Chikuma Shobo.

Kyukyoko, O. 1998. 'Kaijosya towa nanika' (What are attendants?) (in Japanese), *Gendai Sisou* (Modern Thinking), 26 (2): 176–83.

Levy, C.W. 1988. *A People's History of the Independent-Living Movement*. Lawrence: University of Kansas.

Lifchez, R. 1979. *Design for Independent Living*. California: University of California Press.

Ministry of Health and Welfare 2000. *Social Security Policies in Japan*. Japanese Ministry of Health and Welfare. Online: http://www.mhw.go.jp/english/ssp_inj/services.

Nakanishi, M. 1996. *Jiritu Seikatu Centre No Tanjo* (The Birth of the Centre for Independent Living) (in Japanese). Tokyo: Human Care.

Nagase, O. 1995. *Difference, Equality and Disabled People: Disability Rights and Disability Culture*. Master's thesis. The Hague: Institute of Social Studies.

Okahara, M. 1990. 'Seidotositeno aijou' (Love as a social structure) (in Japanese), in J. Asaka et al. (eds), *Sei no Giho*. Tokyo: Fujiwara Shoten.

Onaka, F. 1990. 'Sisetuno sotode ikiru' (Living outside of institutions) (in Japanese), in J. Asaka et al. (eds), *Sei no Giho*. Tokyo: Fujiwara Shoten.

Onoue, K. 2000. 'Osaka-si zensin syogaisya kaigonin haken jigyo hassokuno keika' (The process of establishing the home-atendants programme for disabled persons in Osaka City) (in Japanese), *SSK KHJ*, 1517: 48–49.

Pelka, F. 1997. *The Disability-Rights Movement*. California: ABC-CLIO.

Shapiro, J.P. 1993. *No Pity: People with Disabilities Forging a New Civil-Rights Movement*. New York: Times Books.

SSK. 2000. *Zenkoku Kakuchino Jyudo Zensinsei Syogaisyano Sensinkaigoseido Siryo* (Resource Manual of Personal-Attendant Programmes for Physically Disabled Persons in Japan) (in Japanese). Tokyo: Japan Association of Personal-Attendants Programmes.

Suzuki, T. 1995. 'Are you ready?', in M. Kishida and M. Kim (eds), *Watashiwa Onna* (I Am a Woman). Kobe: Choseisya.

Tateiwa, S. 1990. 'Hayaku yukkuri: jiritsu seikatsu undo no seisei to tenkai' (Fast and slow: the establishment and activities of the independent-living movement) (in Japanese), in J. Asaka et al. (eds), *Sei no Giho*. Tokyo: Fujiwara Shoten.

Toyota, M. 1998. 'Tojisya gensoron' (Illusion of the primary party) (in Japanese), *Gendai Sisou* (Modern Thinking), 26 (2): 100–13.

Tsutsumi, A. 1998. 'Peer counselling', *Gendai Sisou* (Modern Thinking), 26 (2): 92–99.

Wakabayashi, K. 1986. *Kiseki: Aoi Shiba no Kai* (The Way: Aoi Shiba Association) (in Japanese). Tokyo: Self publication.

Yamamoto, K. 1995. 'Nakuso yuseihogoho dataizai kaeyo boshihoken' (Abolish the eugenics law that penalises abortions; reform the welfare of mothers and children law) (in Japanese), *Fukushi Rodo* (Social Work), 66: 123–29.

Yokoyama, T. 1998. 'Kaijo wo dou ichizukerunoka' (How do we define personal assistance?) (in Japanese), *Gendai Sisou* (Modern Thinking), 26 (2): 84–90.

Yonezu, T. (1998). 'Omosa kurabeya atomawashi karawa nanimo umarenai' (Nothing emerges from comparing the severity of oppressions and labelling one as less severe) (in Japanese), *Gendai Sisou* (Modern Thinking), 26 (2): 224–42.

20

Disabled Women: An Excluded Agenda of Indian Feminism

Anita Ghai

My purpose in this essay is to locate disabled women within the women's movement as well as the disability movement in India. While foregrounding the existential realities for disabled women in the Indian scene, I underscore the reasons for their absence from the agenda of Indian feminism. I conclude by reflecting on the possibilities of inclusion within Indian feminist thought.

INTRODUCTION

I must submit at the beginning that my understanding of the issues and related questions has been predominantly influenced by my own experiences as a disabled Indian woman advocating for the other disabled people in India. My initial engagement with the issue of oppression began as I negotiated my socio-cultural and political positioning as a woman in a traditionally patriarchal society. A closer acquaintance with the developing intellectual discourse on feminism, especially in my own country, indicated how the movement that originated essentially as a response to oppression experienced by women excluded disabled women.

Ghai, A. 2002. 'Disabled women: An excluded agenda of Indian feminism', *Hypatia*, 17 (3): 49–66.

It was painful and disillusioning to realise that disabled women occupy a multifarious and marginalised position in Indian society, based on their disability and also on socio-cultural identities that separate them into categories constructed according to such properties as caste, class and residential position. Disabled women thus can have plural identity markers that make their daily experience perplexing and difficult. The recognition of such forces in my own existence, especially those that affect me because I am a disabled woman (Ghai, 1998, p. 35), shifted my focus per se to the disability movement.

The disability movement in India has aimed its protest at the segregation and discrimination experienced by the disabled. My personal experience of the disability movement, however, indicated to me that the gender-based bias women must contend with everyday in a patriarchal society also permeates the disability movement. It is not as if disabled women have not resisted such marginalisation. However, the task of locating the 'self' under such conditions has been daunting.

To gain an insight into the issues confronting disabled women in India, I begin by looking at the general disability scene in India and the dynamics of the feminist movement as well. I am aware that a western audience may experience a sense of *déjà vu* with regard to many of the following arguments. All the same, arguments are significant for an understanding of the specifics of Indian reality. Without getting into a debate about the areas of communality between disabled woman in Washington, D.C., Toronto and London, I restrict myself to a candid analysis of the experiences of disabled women in India.

THE INDIAN CONTEXT AND THE DISABILITY MOVEMENT

India, often described as an emerging superpower, has a population of one billion, out of which approximately seventy million are characterised as disabled. Public consciousness of the issues and concerns that affect the lives of those with disabilities is a fairly recent phenomenon. It was only in the forty-ninth year of India's independence that the first legislation advocating equal rights for disabled people came into effect. Though notified five years ago, the act still awaits proper implementation.

Notwithstanding the legislation, the state continues to be largely apathetic. Owing to a complete lack of public planning, responsiveness to any specific condition such as disability is missing. Consequently, the physical environment is largely inaccessible and inconvenient. Dissemination of information in formats accessible to people with sensory impairments is very restricted. For instance, there is a single televised sign-language news bulletin per week for people with hearing impairments. The range of accessible reading materials for people with vision impairments is also extremely limited. The non-availability of other assistive technology devices such as electrically powered wheelchairs at affordable prices adds to the miseries experienced by disabled people.

An example of indifference is the nationwide protests that people with disabilities had to undertake in order to be counted as a category in the forthcoming census. Notwithstanding some small steps toward inclusion, the lives of disabled people remain mired in inhumane patterns of helpless cynicism, political inertia, and resistance to social innovation. In this climate, long-term solutions are neither sought nor found.

The state continues to rely on the voluntary sector for the provision of basic services for disabled people, although this sector, stretched beyond its resources, is unable to serve even a miniscule proportion of those in need. Needless to say, the disabled are relegated to the margins in every avenue of opportunity, be it education, employment, transportation, or any other significant area of life. While disability advocates in the developed world have progressed from issues of service delivery and rehabilitation to an engagement with the multiple nuances and meanings of disabled existence, the developing world continues to agonise over securing the very basic elements that disabled people need to survive.

Thus, the meaning of disability in India is embedded in this basic struggle for survival. The predominantly elite, educated (and therefore privileged) group of disabled activists within the disability movement does not inquire into the subtle conceptual and cultural nuances that influence the nature of this survival. Most of the time, an agenda borrowed from western counterparts lacks the reflexivity to analyse the Indian context, in which disability is not a singular marker. In a scenario marked by widespread poverty, disability is not even perceived as a cause of vulnerability and total helplessness. As I argue elsewhere (Ghai, 2001, p. 29), for poor families living a hand-to-mouth existence the birth of a disabled child or the onset of a significant impairment in childhood is a fate worse than death. It is truly the proverbial last straw on the camel's back, jeopardising the entire family's existence.

The situation is worse because, in addition to hopeless life conditions, disabled people often have to contend with cultural constructions marked by negativity and stigmatisation. Within the Indian cultural context, disability implies a 'lack' or 'flaw' leading to a significantly diminished capability; images of the disabled also are associated with deceit, mischief and devilry. Disabled people sometimes are depicted as suffering the wrath of God, and being punished for misdeeds that either they or their families have committed—a kind of penance or retribution for past misdeeds. Yet another strand of this cultural construction conceives of disability as eternal childhood, where survival is contingent upon constant care and protection. Here, the emphasis is on images of dependency, thereby reinforcing the charity/pity model. Consequently, charity and philanthropy have remained the predominant response to the predicament of disability. Even today, many institutions regularly receive food, old clothes and money from wider society, which makes these charitable gestures not out of a sense of commitment to the issue of disability but as a response to a cultural expectation to do one's *dharmik* (religious) duty toward the needy, in the same spirit as alms are given to beggars.

This 'altruistic' paradigm is reflected in governmental policies, which until very recently looked at disability as a welfare issue. Even now, most government efforts are targeted at strengthening non-governmental organisations, without making any direct interventions. Western disability studies often fail to comprehend the reality of disability in India, which is marked by a complex amalgam of class, gender and caste issues. Feminism, with its emphasis on multiple oppressions, is the key to guiding disability studies and research toward an understanding of the pluralities that characterise the experience of disability in India.

This list, though not exhaustive, illustrates the underpinnings of the negative cultural identity given to those with disabilities. Historically, alternative narratives have indicated instances where disabled people have been considered children of a 'lesser god', a status that provides spaces, in spheres of religious or metaphysical discourse, where the ability to transcend the body stands as a distinct possibility (Ghai, forthcoming). By not acknowledging the centrality of the physical body, these alternatives did provide the possibility for a dignified negotiation of difference. Even though assigning such a status to disabled people implied renunciation of their material bodies (in service to the god), such narratives did offer a metaphysic that was more humane than the oppressive lives that characterised disability. However, this option was largely available to disabled men only. That only few women could avail themselves of such alternatives was reflective of a patriarchal society which viewed disability as an additional stigma beyond the stigma of being a woman. However, a position that provided such a space historically may not have the same implications in present-day India. A recurrent change in the meaning of the body raises significant questions regarding the whole notion of transcendence of the body and its location in the patriarchal discourse.

However, contemporary constructions (Miles, 1999, p. 233) of disability in India do not draw systematically on historical and cultural research. They largely portray disabled people as possessing a medical identity, perceived from a predominantly health and welfare perspective. This western medical model, which focuses on the clinical dimensions of impairment, dominates policy. For instance, the latest Indian human development report states that 'physical disabilities are genetic, biological and even birth defects, and future research must focus on the causes of such disabilities' (Shariff, 1999, p. 148). Such a policy stance makes medical intervention, without any regard for cultural analysis, the sole instrument for addressing disability. The Indian milieu offers very little understanding of the social model of disability, which argues that it is society that disables people with impairments, and therefore that any meaningful solution must be directed at societal change rather than at the individual. Rather than locating the disability in the body, the social model conceives of disabled people as an oppressed group in society.

In its attempt to highlight the centrality of disability as an organising principle of life, and therefore to move it from the margins of social consideration, the disability movement has promoted sweeping generalisations about disability and handicap without regard for differences in kind and degree of impairment, or different adaptations to impairment. Consequently, the disability movement advances a few select agendas —mostly those that address the concerns of middle-class men. As I have argued elsewhere:

> The problem, however, arises when their fight for 'disability rights' subsumes agendas that are visible and significant only for the very privileged of the

> disabled. Concessions in air travel, hotels, and special parking facilities, though undeniably necessary, are meaningful only to a select population of the disabled. The truth is that these issues do not resonate in the lives of the majority of disabled, who are further marginalised by virtue of their class, caste, rural (rather than urban) residence and, most strikingly, gender. What is and should be more significant for them are the issues of education, employment, residence, technological aids and accessibility, to name a few. The reality, however, is that the majority of disabled are still fighting to secure the 'bare minimum'. (Ghai, 2001).

That there might be a gender dimension to disability has only recently been realised. Das and Agnihotri (1999) indicate that the incidence of disability is intersected (or influenced) by gender. In an extrapolation of the available statistics, they have indicated that disabled women are marginalised much more than disabled men. Disability legislation also adopts a gendered approach, with the result that out of twenty-eight chapters outlining various issues, not a single one addresses the problems of disabled women. This approach reflects the general attitude toward disabled women in India. In Hindi, the phrase *Ek to ladki, upar se apahij* translates as 'First a girl, and then disabled.' That is, both congenital and acquired disabilities for a girl child are seen as additional rather than initial liabilities. Opportunities to improve the quality of life of a disabled girl are virtually nonexistent. Already living a life of subordination without education and employment, women could do without the burden of disability. A mother lamented: 'Wasn't it enough that we have a hand-to-mouth existence? Why did God have to punish us further by giving us a *langri* (lame girl)' (Ghai, 2001, p. 31).

In a culture where being a daughter is considered a curse, being a disabled daughter is a fate worse than death. She has to contend with both her role as daughter, when what was desired was a son, and with her disability. The desire for sons has to be understood in the context of the ritual value of sons as well as the social and economic burden of bringing up daughters (Johri, 1998, p. 78). The construction 'daughter as burden' is rooted in the culture, which looks at daughters as *parai* (outsider), that is, one who will go to another home. Johri elaborates: 'One of the religious duties of a father is *kanyadan*, the unreciprocated gifting of a virgin to the husband and his family. Giving dowry becomes a part of this ritual.' However, the implicit understanding in this practice is that whatever you give must be perfect. A disabled bride must be compensated for. If compensation is not possible, then compromises, such as marriage to a widower, have to be made.

Disability in a son, on the other hand, though traumatic, is more acceptable, as he does not have to be given away. While many authors have used traditional versions of *Manusmrti*,[1] for the present purpose I follow the interpretation of Wendy Doniger and Brian K. Smith (1991, Chapter 9). Law 72 states: 'Even if a man has accepted a girl in accordance with the rules, he may reject her if she is despised, ill or corrupted, or if she was given with something concealed.' This is followed by Law 73: 'If anyone gives away a daughter with a flaw and does not mention it, that gift from the evil hearted daughter-giver may be annulled' (Doniger and Smith, 1991, pp. 205–6). Consequently, a culture in which arranged marriages are the rule inherently puts disabled women in a difficult position. However difficult it may be, the possibility exists for 'normal' women to resist this cultural arrangement. Some disabled girls of the upper or middle class might be able to negotiate the difficulties inherent in arranged marriages, albeit with a great deal of compromise. Disabled sons retain the possibility of marriage, as they are not gifts but the receivers of gifts. Disabled men, as with non-disabled men, seek 'normal' women as wives, and therefore participate in the devaluing of people because of disability.

The preference for a son in the wider Hindu society of India, in keeping with its religious philosophy, has now been coupled with modern technology that provides a way to determine the sex of an unborn foetus. The most recent census counts 927 females to every 1,000 males in the Indian population. That is lower than the ratio recorded in 1981, which was 934 females to 1,000 males. The census of 2001 is expected to show a further decline in the ratio, a reflection of the practice of

[1] *Manusmrti* consists of 2,685 verses encompassing representations of life in the world–how it is and how it should be. *Manusmrti* is a fundamental text of the dominant form of Hinduism as it emerged historically. It provides the most influential construction of the Hindu religion and Indian society as a whole. A study of Hindu family life, concepts of body, sex, attitudes to money and material possessions, politics, caste and social practices, among many others, requires a knowledge of *Manusmrti*.

aborting female foetuses (Krishnaji, 2000, p. 1161). In a society where there is widespread female infanticide, aborting imperfect children will not cause any stir or rancour. This becomes clear in respect to the feminist campaign against amniocentesis as a sex-determination test. While there is an ongoing discussion of the ethical contradictions that prenatal sex testing poses for feminists, prenatal testing to identify and abort children at risk of disabilities does not get addressed (Menon, 1996).

For disabled women themselves, these issues become secondary, because cultural stereotyping denies them the role of motherhood. As elaborated by Sudhir Kakar, a psychoanalyst (1978, p. 56), whether a woman's family is poor or wealthy, whatever her caste, class or religion, whether she is a fresh young bride or exhausted by many pregnancies and infants, an Indian woman knows that motherhood confers upon her a purpose and identity that nothing else in her culture can. Each infant borne and nurtured by her safely into childhood, especially if the child is a son, is both a certification and redemption of her ability, role and status as a woman. Disabled women are, however, denied this fulfilment, as both marriage and consequent motherhood are difficult achievements in a socially restrictive environment. (It is worth mentioning that single motherhood in the Indian culture is the privilege of only very elite women. In general, having a child out of wedlock evokes stigmatisation.) The denial of a woman's 'traditional roles' to disabled women creates what Michele Fine and Adrienne Asch (1988) term 'rolelessness', a social invisibility and cancellation of femininity that can impel disabled women to pursue, however hopelessly, the female identity valorised by their given culture but denied to them because of their disability.

A great deal of thoughtful work by Indian feminists analyses the impact of the evaluative male gaze. However, the essential difference between being sexual objects and objects of 'the stare' has not been understood. If the male gaze makes normal women feel like passive objects, staring turns a disabled object into a grotesque sight. Disabled women contend not only with how men look at women, but also with how an entire society stares at disabled people, stripping them of any semblance of resistance. Neither Indian feminism nor the Indian disability movement acknowledges that disabled women are doubly pinned by the dominant male gaze and the gaze of a culture that constructs them as objects to be stared at.

In a culture where any deviation from a normally accepted archetype is seen as a marked deviation, the impaired body becomes a symbol of imperfection. The myth of the beautiful body defines the impaired female body as unfeminine and unacceptable. Disability is thus constituted as being profoundly 'Other' in our society. The roots of such thinking are found in Indian mythology. Lakshmana, brother of Lord Rama, cuts off the nose of Shurpanakha, sister of King Ravana, who shows interest in him. That Lakshmana can only respond to what he considers unacceptable behaviour by disabling the 'ugly female' indicates how disability and de-sexing are equated in the Indian psyche.

This kind of reasoning is echoed the culture of Punjab in north India, where, although girls are allowed to interact with their male cousins, they are not allowed to sleep in the same room with them. Disabled girls, on the other hand, are under no such prohibitions. This reflects what Harlan Hahn (Thomson, 1997, p. 25) calls 'asexual objectification', and also evidences disregard for the danger of sexual violation to which disabled girls are exposed. The assumption that sexuality and disability are mutually exclusive also denies that people with deviant bodies experience sexual desires, and refuses them recognition as sexually typical despite their differences.

Indian feminist scholarship has looked at embodiment along the axes of caste, class, and historical phases such as the impact of colonisation; however, the impaired body has not been considered as having analytical consequence. Seemanthini Niranjana points out: 'Focus on the body has been a symbolic one, where the body is perceived as sign or code, important to the extent that it is speaking about a social reality other than itself. Suggestive as it may be to speak of the body as representing encoded social meanings, as an image of society or even a metaphor for society, the question remains whether these perspectives can acknowledge the materiality of bodies, not merely as they are formed/represented in a culture, but how they constitute the lived reality of persons' (Niranjana, 1997, p. 106). Though this analysis takes up the issues of cultural spaces and the male body, there is no mention of the disabled body.

This omission reflects a historical practice that continues to render the disabled invisible in a manner very similar to the invisibility experienced by blacks in a white racist society. As Robert Young (1999) argues, 'In such a society it is necessary for the African-American subject to be rendered invisible in order to enable the Euro-American subject (whiteness) to preserve the illusion of autonomy, rationality and control' (cited in Erevelles, 2000, p. 35). Erevelles's application of this analysis to disability pursues a similar argument. She says that a (non-disabled) subject, upon encountering its Other (the disabled subject), finds it necessary to suppress the memory of this deviant image to support the illusion of normalcy and wholeness. That these claims to wholeness are themselves illusions becomes vividly apparent when one examines how constructions of a normative self are in fact predicated on the existence of a disabled Other.

It is ironic that feminists engaged with the issue of difference, united in their attempts to empower the powerless, and resolved to transform social inequalities, have not picked up on the issues concerning the meaning of impairment for disabled women. While the disability movement's failure to acknowledge disabled women can be fathomed as reflecting the patriarchal character of a society it accepts and aims to be included in, at least within India, its disregard by the feminist movement, which claims objectivity through its theoretical deconstruction of oppressive social suppositions, is less understandable.

What is especially anguishing is that Indian feminist thought fails to recognise that the problematisation of women's issues applies equally to disabled women's issues. In principle, some disabled women might have benefited from the activities of some women's groups, but no documentation exists of specific instances. On the other hand, ample evidence abounds that disabled women are victims of domestic violence and sexual violation. However, when the national Indian media gave widespread coverage to a story about a woman with cerebral palsy who had been abused by her father, women's groups gave no more than a perfunctory response. Further, Indian feminist scholars have not attempted to develop theoretical responses appropriate to the situation of disabled women.

Only after major newspapers reported nineteen days later that fourteen mentally challenged girls were forced to undergo hysterectomies at Sassoon General Hospital in Pune (a city in the state of Maharashtra) did Indian women's groups intervene. Situated in a large rural community, developmentally disabled girls received care in an institution in which they were prevented from wearing pyjamas with drawstrings or sanitary napkins with belts, because it was claimed that the girls might use these to commit suicide. While the girls were deprived of the means to manage their menstrual periods, the boys were issued pyjamas complete with drawstrings that could equally be used as a noose. Apparently, the officials did not have the same concern about boys committing suicide. To deal with the problem of menstrual hygiene, the hospital decided to perform hysterectomies. The protest by women's groups was invaluable, because the operations stopped after the first fourteen girls. However, this incident was not translated into a broader effort to open a dialogue about the enforced sterilisation of developmentally disabled women, which indicates that Indian feminists still do not see women with disabilities as an important and enduring constituency.

While there is a strong emphasis on mainstreaming women's concerns for self-development in the national policy document (Ministry of Women and Child Welfare, 2000) on the empowerment of women, the paradox of a hierarchy within a hierarchy is evident because discussions about certain groups of women considered lower class or caste, or of a tribal or other minority, continue to be couched in 'welfare' terms. Unlike western countries, race is not a significant distinguishing factor in India. Disabled women are not even mentioned in this document, which highlights a vision for the Ministry of Women and Child Welfare.

It is not as if no other issues have been neglected within the Indian feminist discourse. For instance, as Bhargavi Davar (1999) points out, mental health has not been a topic to which feminist discourse has paid a lot of attention. Even Davar, however, fails to look at the issue of disability when addressing mental health. Research on national mental health omits discussion of women with disabilities, which reflects a presumption that their mental health issues will 'obviously be different' (IFSHA: A Report on Women, Violence and Mental Health, 1999). This reflects the skewed attitude of mainstream feminists who, while sensitively exploring distress as a major component of a woman's life experience, conveniently leave disabled women out of their focus.

It could be argued that by emphasising this exclusion by feminists and women's groups I am ignoring the possibilities of resistance, which, in the face of non-recognition, can only be attributed to a sheer will to survive. Taking this into consideration, I could argue that women with disabilities have formed support groups and are in the process of challenging dominant constructions of disabilities. However, owing to the absence of discussion among disabled people in general about differences in disabilities and impairments, no group exists to collectively pursue the concerns of disabled women, and thus to influence both the disability movement and the women's movement. Right now, the voices of disabled women are restricted to academic settings, where a double-oppression hypothesis is expounded. This hypothesis takes the standpoint that disabled women experience a double disadvantage, as they fare worse than either disabled men or non-disabled women, socio-economically, psychologically and politically. Disability compounds their already marginal status as women.

Many feminist thinkers in the field of disability have objected to this 'double disadvantage' approach, since the literature does not empower disabled women. Jenny Morris says:

> I always feel uncomfortable reading about our lives and concerns when they are presented in these terms. When Susan Lonsdale writes, 'For women the status of "disabled" compounds their status of being female to create a unique kind of oppression' (Lonsdale, 1990, p. 82), I feel burdened by the disadvantage. When Margaret Lloyd states that the issue for disabled women is 'the dilemma of identity for an individual experiencing multiple disadvantage and oppression' (Lloyd, 1992, p. 82), I feel a victim. ... Such writings do not empower me. We have to find a way of making our experiences visible, sharing them with each other, and with non-disabled people, in a way that—while drawing attention to the difficulties in our lives—does not undermine our wish to assert our self-worth. (Morris, 1996, p. 2)

While Morris is absolutely right in her stance, the problem is that even the double-disadvantage hypothesis fails to produce concrete action as the outcome of the feminist discourse, and practice does not move beyond tokenism and rhetoric. A feminism which is cognisant of differences between women is very similar to the struggle in India, which is engaged as a political movement. Both have had to fight continuously for mainstream feminism to acknowledge the dangers inherent in adopting a universal category of 'woman', and by default excluding those living on the periphery and margins. Says Elizabeth Weed: 'For those outside mainstream feminism, women's experience has never ceased to be problematic. The common ground of sisterhood long held as white feminism's ideal was always a more utopian than representative slogan. Worse, it was coercive in its unacknowledged universalism, its unrecognised exclusions' (Weed, 1989, p. 24).

Indian disabled women experienced this exclusion when feminist theory and practice in India continued to ignore their experiential realities of discrimination, ignorance and neglect. The feminists reinforced the construction of disabled women as being outside the hegemony of normalcy. Consequently, the much-needed political action has not been forthcoming. The resistance offered by disabled women has only led to a superficial acknowledgment of differences, an implicit assumption that the core issue is gender. The perceived need is therefore to raise the gender issues adequately enough to address all women's lives, regardless of their backgrounds and differences. At least, this recognition is responsible for the emergence of a discourse about difference; but I cannot ignore the reality that this discourse has not been able to achieve much, if any, change—either in increasing acceptance of disabled women's concerns in social policy or in enhancing the quality of their lives. What could be the reasons for the failure of Indian feminists to acknowledge and empathise with the existential realities of disabled women? Although it is difficult to posit a clear answer to this query, my interviews with active leaders in the field offer insights into the reasons for this exclusion. In the following section, my aim is to share some of the concerns expressed by feminists and women's activists. However, before doing so, it is appropriate to briefly consider the situation of the Indian women's movement.

REASONS FOR EXCLUSION

The women's movement in India, according to Nandini Gandhi and Nandini Shah, has no beginning or origin: 'It has always existed as an emotion, as an anger deep within us, and has flowed like music in and out of our lives and consciousness and actions' (Gandhi and Shah, 1992, p. 15), Within the movement today, diverse streams are based on ideology, class, community, and rural or urban locations all over India. The movement evinces deep concern for what are conceived as basic societal issues. These include poverty, class and caste inequalities, labour-related injustice, wages and employment, population technologies, sati (self-immolation by widows), dowry, and female foeticide. With time, many other issues, such as domestic violence, childhood sexual abuse, and sexuality have become dominant concerns of both feminist theoreticians in academia and activists in the women's movement. The emphasis of Indian feminism has been not on individual issues but rather on collective issues with significant political ramifications. Nonetheless, the feminist agenda in India, as in other countries, has focused on a reconfiguration of gender constructions in society by questioning patriarchal norms. This has focused action on programmes aimed at recasting traditional gender roles.

The common thread in this attempt to reinvent gender identities has been the experience of oppression shared by all women. Ironically, the movement's exhaustive list does not include disability oppression, despite the fact that disability cuts across all categories and may be associated with the experience of many of the other oppressions against which the women's movement is fighting. One reason highlighted by theorists and activists alike has been that disabled women have not participated in the movement's meetings and actions. Consequently, accounts neither of their lives nor of their challenges to feminist theory have immediacy.

While this explanation may have some merit, it also underlines the inability of the feminist movement to consider what may prevent women with disabilities from actively participating in the movement's work. In a country where it is not unusual to develop structural amnesia with regard to a particular category of persons, there are few opportunities for disabled women to create an immediate presence and speak for themselves. Yet, the feminist agenda and the women's movement have not remarked on these conditions. Possibly, the experience of disability is imagined to be opaque, intransitive and idiosyncratic. In the case of a sustained discourse about disability in Indian feminist theory, the mistaken belief that biological impairment prevents people from evolving as full social, psychological, political, aesthetic and cultural beings continues to prevail. Another feature that emerged from many interviews was the recurrent use of disability as an analogue for other kinds of limitations. For example, one respondent stressed that 'being a woman is the biggest form of disability' (Bhasin, 2000). Another observed: 'Disability is like belonging to the lowest possible' (Bhattacharya, 2000). There are several ways of understanding these analogies.

One option is to look at the socio-cultural meanings ascribed to female bodies and those assigned to disabled bodies. Both are excluded from full participation in public and economic spheres; both are conceived in opposition to a norm that is assumed to possess natural superiority. Such comparisons can be both emancipatory and oppressive.

If the objective of invoking such comparisons is to understand the lived experience of different people and to grasp their authenticity, the potential is immense. However, if the categories operate only at a metaphorical level, such comparisons can lead to a total erasure of the category that is being invoked. It is true that analogy is a rhetorical device that is meant to enable the move from more familiar to relatively unknown terrain in order to understand how a set of relations evident in one sphere might illuminate the other. However, if a comparison or parallel pits one set of relations against the other, as is the case of women against disability, the strategic advantage of the analogy gets lost.

Without devaluing such metaphorical moves, I wish to focus on what gets 'valorised' and what gets 'suppressed' in the process. My argument is that such analogising results in a suppression of the harsh reality of the lives of disabled women, limited by conditions much more difficult than usual to transcend. A shift from theoretical/metaphorical to the material is essential to render visible the 'cultural constructions' that have supported the currently flawed conceptualisations of disability and womanhood.

According to Nivedita Menon (2000), another, more fundamental, reason for the total absence of disability as an issue in the Indian women's movement, and the comparative lateness of its emergence in western women's movements, could be that feminists all over the world have usually assumed 'women' to be a category that is self-evident. That is, there is an unsupported assumption that all women, regardless of their differences from one another, have shared concerns. This abstraction of 'women' emerged from a feminist positing of 'difference' as a challenge to the abstract category of 'citizenship', which assumed masculinity as the norm. Up to the late 1970s, 'sisterhood is global' seemed an unquestionable feminist truth. Challenges from women of colour and other stigmatised and marginalised groups of women showed the category of 'women' to be another abstraction, which in turn assumed white, middle-class, heterosexual women (without disability) to be the norm. In India, this kind of challenge has come from feminists of minority communities. The charge is that the women's movement has assumed the Hindu upper-caste woman to be the norm, and this critique has emerged most clearly in the debates over the Uniform Civil Code (UCC). The debates were about the demand for a common set of personal laws that would apply to religious communities in India. The opposition came from the belief that the emerging uniformity would essentially represent the voices of the majority (which in this case was Hindu women), thereby marginalising women from minority groups.

Menon, a vociferous activist in the women's movement and a political scientist by profession, feels that the invisibility of disability within feminism occurs because of mechanisms similar to those that have made women in general invisible in the larger society. But as a feminist who felt disturbed by the neglect of disability issues, she thinks that the movement has the potential to grow and change. Another reason for the failure to represent women with disabilities is that within the Indian women's movement there are far too many issues and far too few resources. Consequently, action has been oriented to the dramatic patterns that resonate in the lives of the majority of women who are able and normal, rather than the minority who fail to exercise voice or agency. Notwithstanding these reasons, it is important to articulate the expectations that Indian feminism has aroused in disabled women. In the next section, I examine the possibilities evoked by these expectations.

EXPECTATIONS FROM FEMINISM

Notwithstanding the current reality of the exclusion of disabled women within the Indian women's movement, I would argue that simply deciding to include them is insufficient. The problem cannot be resolved so easily by merely adding disabled women as another category to the list of matters or kinds of issues requiring attention. Offering a feminist account of disabled women is problematic because it requires including them in the discourse. However, writing a subject such as disabled women into the ongoing discourse necessitates a certain exercise of power to construct that subject in some form, to give her shape, and to breathe life into her. This cannot be accomplished without knowing how she might construct herself.

This process thus requires some reflexivity. To explore the possibilities authentically and adequately requires that the process have a dialogical character. It is vital that both feminist discourse and practice engage in a concerted dialogue with disabled women and with the disability movement, so that a more inclusive theory as well as practice can emerge. To quote Mairian Corker:

> It is often argued that theories are too complex for *ex-post facto* explanation rather than for use by disabled people; they may lead to confusion and the paralysis of analysis. This is always a danger, if complexity of life is overemphasised, and if the need to understand fully is placed ahead of the need to act more effectively, because disabled people can be turned into interested spectators, rather than proactive participants of a strong social movement.... Theories which reduce or simplify disabled people's experience, particularly those which fail to conceptualise a dialogic relationship between disability and impairment, can have the same effect. (Corker, 1999, p. 639)

According to Corker, the resolution of these problems might come by following the example of Leonard (1997) in creating a paradigm of communication rooted in discursive strategies rather than structure. Failure to create these spaces even unintentionally does not alleviate the asymmetry of power relations. Feminist discourse has developed without disabled women taking a hand in shaping it. What now can be done about feminists' inattention to disabled girls and women, and how would feminist discursive attention look and read if, initially, they had been involved in its development?

Do we need a different kind of feminist theory to account for disabled women? As Rosemarie Garland Thomson observes (1997, p. 24), feminist theory can challenge the persistent assumption that disability is a self-evident condition of physical inadequacy and private misfortune whose politics concern only a minority of women. Feminist disability praxis would uphold women's right to define their physical differences and their femininity for themselves, rather than conforming to the social interpretation of their bodies. Such praxis could address some of the specific issues currently addressed by feminists, ones that do not look different when seen through the lens of a disability perspective.

One matter that, though within the ambit of feminist thought, seems different from a disability perspective is the issue of caring for the mothers of disabled children in India. As I elaborate, 'Although the stress of impairment impacts upon both the parents, it is usually the mother who bears the brunt of the child's disability' (Ghai, 2000). Instances abound where women have been divorced, abandoned or tortured because they have given birth to a disabled child. Given the preference for sons, blame on the mother is severe in the instance of a disabled girl child. The fantasy of maternal omnipotence holds mothers responsible for providing care. Home care is usually the only option; there often is no question of choice. Indian feminists who have debated over the ethics of caring, and who are now in the process of initiating a debate over equality in caring (Davar, 1999, p. 207), have not taken note of the conditions in which disabled people, and especially women, are placed. Within the traditional Indian system, the mother has been a source of succour for the children, especially for girls with disabilities (Ghai, 2001, p. 21). In the absence of social and community support, disabled women have relied largely on the care provided by their mothers, who undoubtedly have carried the extra burden. While it is perfectly justified to engage with their experiences of oppression in caring, the attempt to destabilise traditional notions in the absence of adequate alternative provisions might end up working against disabled women. In such a context, it is worthwhile to engage with the cautionary note given by Anita Silvers: 'Far from vanquishing the patriarchal system, substituting the ethics of caring for ethics of equality threatens an even more oppressive paternalism' (Silvers, 1995, p. 52).

Another significant area where feminist questioning would be invaluable concerns the idea of independent living as espoused by disability theorists in the west. In the absence of education, employment, infrastructure and a social-security system, autonomy is a formidable goal for women in India to attain, and more so for disabled women. The resolution of any issues concerning disability has to be in the context of the family and community. Indian feminists, with their grasp of the Indian reality, are equipped to devise options that can merge with the specific Indian context of the familial and the social.

One possible solution would be to apply Susan Bordo's view that the concrete experiences of exclusion have neither to be grounded in theory nor given a theoretical response. Rather, as new narratives begin to emerge, the major task is to tell the story of diverse women's experiences in as truthful a manner as possible. The only requirement is to listen, to become aware of one's own biases, prejudices and ignorance, so that a process of stretching the borders of what Minnie Bruce Pratt (in Bordo, 1990, p. 138) calls the 'narrow circle of self' can begin.

As Bordo explains, 'No matter how attentive the scholar is to the axes that constitute social identity, some of the axes will be ignored and some selected' (Bordo, 1990, p. 140). An inescapable fact of human embodiment, as Friedrich Nietzsche pointed out, is that '... an eye turned in no particular direction, in which the active and interpreting forces, through which alone seeing becomes seeing *something*, are supposed to be lacking; these always demand of the eye an absurdity and a nonsense. There is *only* a perspectival seeing, *only* a perspectival knowing' (Nietzsche, 1887; see English edition of 1969, p. 119; emphasis in original).

Perspectival knowing is never really pure. It is always influenced by our political, social and personal interests. Even in acting on the desire to embrace our differences, we are unavoidably centric. Mere recognition of difference does not assure that we will construct an adequate representation of difference. Further, constant attention to difference might create and construct Others who are unheard of and therefore unfamiliar. As Michel Foucault reminds us, 'Everything is dangerous, and every new context demands that we reassess the main danger' (Foucault, 1983, p. 232).

Thus, what is needed is not merely a strong commitment to create spaces where different voices can share their realities and be heard, but also an active integration of differences among and within women. However, for this possibility to become a reality, feminist discourse will need to go beyond a mere recognition of binaries. What is required is a consideration of the multiple constraints that inhibit the articulation of difference. This task is an arduous and a complex one, especially when heterogeneity serves as a mere tool to hide homogeneous understanding.

References

Bhasin, Kamla. 2000. Conversation with the author, New Delhi, 25 November.
Bhattacharya, Jaya. 2000. Conversation with the author, New Delhi, 5 November.

Bordo, Susan. 1990. 'Feminism, postmodernism and gender scepticism', in Linda Nicholson (ed.), *Feminism/Postmodernism*. New York and London: Routledge.

Corker, Mairian. 1999. 'Differences, conflations and foundations: The limits to "accurate" theoretical representation of disabled people's experience?', *Disability and Society*, 14 (5): 627–42.

Das, D. and Agnihotri, S.B. 1999. 'Physical disability: Is there a gender dimension?', *Economic and Political Weekly*, 33 (52): 3333–35.

Davar, V. Bhargavi. 1999. *Mental Health of Indian Women: A Feminist Agenda*. New Delhi: Sage.

Doniger, W. and Smith, B.K. 1991. *The Laws of Manu*. New Delhi: Penguin.

Erevelles, Nirmala. 2000. 'Educating unruly bodies: Critical pedagogy, disability studies, and the politics of schooling', *Educational Theory*, 50 (1): 25–47.

Fine, Michele and Asch, Adrienne. 1988. (eds) *Women with Disabilities: Essays in Psychology, Culture and Politics*. Philadelphia: Temple University Press.

Foucault, Michel. 1983. 'On the genealogy of ethics', in Hubert Dreyfus and Paul Rabinow (eds), *Beyond Structuralism and Hermeneutics*. Chicago: University of Chicago Press.

Gandhi, Nandini and Shah, Nandita. 1992. *The Issues at Stake: Theory and Practice in the Contemporary Movement in India*. New Delhi: Kali for Women.

Ghai, Anita. 1998. 'Living in the shadow of my disability', *The Journal*, 2 (1): 32–36.

———. 2000. 'Mothering a child of disability', *The Journal*, 2 (1): 20–22.

———. 2001. 'Marginalisation and disability: Experiences from the third world', in M. Priestley (ed.), *Disability and the Life Course: Global Perspectives*. Cambridge: Cambridge University Press.

Intervention for Support, Healing and Awareness (IFSHA). A conference on women and sexual abuse. C52, Second Floor, South Extension, Part II, New Delhi, India.

Johri, Rachana. 1998. 'Cultural constructions of maternal attachment: The case of a girl child', Ph.D. dissertation, University of Delhi, India.

Kakar, Sudhir. 1978. *The Inner World: A Psychoanalytic Study of Childhood and Society in India*. Delhi: Oxford University Press.

Krishnaji, N. 2000. 'Trends in sex ratio', *Economic and Political Weekly*, April: 1161–66.

Leonard, P. 1997. *Postmodern Welfare*. London: Sage.

Lloyd, M. 1992. 'Does she boil eggs? Towards a feminist model of disability', *Disability, Handicap and Society*, 7 (3): 207–21.

Lonsdale, Susan. 1990. *Women and Disability*. London: Macmillan.

Menon, Nivedita. 1996. 'The impossibility of "justice": Female foeticide and feminist discourse on abortion', in Patricia Uberoi (ed.), *Social Reform, Sexuality and the State*. New Delhi: Sage.

———. 2000. Conversation with the author. New Delhi, 5 December.

Miles, M. 1999. 'Can formal disability services be developed with South Asian historical and conceptual foundations?', in Emma Stone (ed.), *Disability and Development*. Leeds: The Disability Press.

Ministry of Women and Child Welfare. 2000. *Policy Document on Empowerment of Women.* Government of India.

Morris, Jenny. 1996. (ed.) *Encounters with Strangers: Feminism and Disability.* London: The Women's Press.

Nietzsche, Friedrich. 1887. (English edition 1969) *On the Genealogy of Morality.* New York: Vintage.

Niranjana, Seemanthini. 1997. 'Femininity, space and the female body: An anthropological perspective', in M. Thapan (ed.), *Embodiment: Essays on Gender and Identity.* New Delhi: Oxford University Press.

Shariff, Abusaleh. 1999. *India—Human Development Report: A Profile of Indian States in the 1990s.* London: Oxford University Press.

Silvers, Anita. 1995. 'Reconciling equality to difference: Caring for justice for people with disabilities', *Hypatia,* 10 (1): 30–35.

Thomson, Rosemarie Garland. 1997. *Extraordinary Bodies.* New York: Columbia University Press.

Young, Robert. 1999. 'Invisibility and blue eyes: Towards a theory of African-American subjectivity', *Revista Canaria de Estudios Ingleses,* 39: 169–90.

Weed, Elizabeth. 1989. *Introduction, Terms of Reference, Coming to Terms.* New York and London: Routledge.

Further Reading

Albrecht, G.L., Seelman, K.D. and Bury, M. 2001. *Handbook of Disability Studies*. London: Sage.

Albrecht, Gary and Devlieger, Patrick. 1999. 'The disability paradox: high quality of life against all odds', *Social Science and Medicine*, 48: 977–88.

Bickenbach, J.E. 1993. *Physical Disability and Social Policy*. Toronto: University of Toronto Press.

Bickenbach, J.E., Chatterji, S., Badley, E.M. and Üstün, T.B. 1999. 'Models of disablement, universalism and the ICIDH', *Social Science and Medicine*, 48: 1173–87.

Devlieger, P., Rusch, F. and Pfeiffer, D. 2003. (eds) *Rethinking Disability: Emergent Definitions, Concepts and Communities*. Antwerp: Garant.

Edgerton, R. 1993. *The Cloak of Competence*: Berkeley: University of California Press.

Frank, G. 2001. *Venus on Wheels*. Berkeley: University of California Press.

Goffman, E. 1959. *The Presentation of Self in Everyday Life*. Garden City: Double Day/Anchor Books.

———. 1963. *Stigma: Notes on the Management of Spoiled Identity*. Englewood Cliffs: Prentice-Hall.

Grandin, T. 1995. *Thinking in Pictures and Other Reports from My Life with Autism*. New York: Vintage.

Gritzer, G. and Arluke, A. 1985. *The Making of Rehabilitation: A Political Economy of Medical Specialisation, 1890–1980*. Berkeley and Los Angeles: University of California Press.

Guyatt, M. 2001. 'Better legs: Artificial legs for British veterans of the First World War', *Journal of Design History*, 14: 307–25.

Hahn, H. 1985. 'Towards a politics of disability: definitions, disciplines and policies', *Social Science Journal*, 22: 87–105.
Ingstad, B. and Reynolds Whyte, S. 1995. *Disability and Culture*. Berkeley: University of California Press.
Leder, D. 1990. *The Absent Body*. Chicago: University of Chicago Press.
Oliver, M. 1990. *The Politics of Disablement*. London: Macmillan.
Oliver, M. and Barnes, C. 1998. *Disabled People and Social Policy: From Exclusion to Inclusion*. London and New York: Longman.
Pfeiffer, D. 2000. 'The devils are in the details: The ICIDH2 and the disability movement', *Disability and Society*, 15 (7): 1079–82.
Scheer, Jessica and Groce, Nora. 1988. 'Impairment as a human constant: Cross-cultural variation and historical perspectives on variation', *Journal of Social Issues*, 44 (1): 23–37.
Stiker, H-J. 1999. *A History of Disability*. Ann Arbor: University of Michigan Press.
Stone, D. 1984. *The Disabled State*. Philadelphia: Temple University Press.

Index

A

D

E

F

G

H

N

O

P

Q

R

V

W

Z